Current Concepts in Head & Neck Pathology

Guest Editor

MARY S. RICHARDSON, MD

SURGICAL PATHOLOGY CLINICS

surgpath.theclinics.com

Consulting Editor
JOHN R. GOLDBLUM, MD

December 2011 • Volume 4 • Number 4

SAUNDERS an imprint of ELSEVIER, Inc.

W.B. SAUNDERS COMPANY
A Division of Elsevier Inc.

1600 John F. Kennedy Boulevard ● Suite 1800 ● Philadelphia, Pennsylvania 19103-2899

http://www.surgpath.theclinics.com

SURGICAL PATHOLOGY CLINICS Volume 4, Number 4
December 2011 ISSN 1875-9181, ISBN-13: 978-1-4557-1157-4

Editor: Joanne Husovski

Surgical Pathology Clinics (ISSN 1875-9181) is published quarterly by Elsevier Inc., 360 Park Avenue South, New York, NY 10010. Months of issue are March, June, September, and December. Business and Editorial Office: Elsevier Inc., 1600 John F. Kennedy Blvd., Ste. 1800, Philadelphia, PA 19103-2899. Accounting and Circulation Offices: Elsevier Inc., 3251 Riverport Lane, Maryland Heights, MO 63043. Periodicals postage paid at New York, NY and at additional mailing offices. Subscription prices are $184.00 per year (US individuals), $212.00 per year (US institutions), $91.00 per year (US students/residents), $230.00 per year (Canadian individuals), $240.00 per year (Canadian Institutions), $230.00 per year (foreign individuals), $240.00 per year (foreign institutions), and $112.00 per year (international & Canadian students/residents). Foreign air speed delivery is included in all *Clinics'* subscription prices. All prices are subject to change without notice. **POSTMASTER:** Send address changes to *Surgical Pathology Clinics*, Elsevier, 3251 Riverport Lane, Maryland Heights, MO 63043. Customer Service: 1-800-654-2452 (US). From outside the United States, call 1-314-447-8871. Fax: 1-314-447-8029. E-mail: JournalsCustomerServiceusa@elsevier.com (for print support) and JournalsOnlineSupport-usa@elsevier.com (for online support).

Reprints. For copies of 100 or more, of articles in this publication, please contact the Commercial Reprints Department, Elsevier Inc., 360 Park Avenue South, New York, NY 10010-1710. Tel. (212) 633-3812; Fax: (212) 462-1935; E-mail: reprints@elsevier.com.

Printed in the United States of America.

Contributors

CONSULTING EDITOR

JOHN R. GOLDBLUM, MD
Chairman, Department of Anatomic Pathology;
Professor of Pathology, Cleveland Clinics,
Lerner College of Medicine, Cleveland Clinic,
Cleveland, Ohio

GUEST EDITOR

MARY S. RICHARDSON, MD
Professor of Pathology and Laboratory
Medicine and Director of Surgical Pathology,
Medical University of South Carolina,
Charleston, South Carolina

AUTHORS

E. LEON BARNES, MD
Professor of Pathology and Otolaryngology,
Department of Pathology, University of
Pittsburgh Medical Center, Pittsburgh,
Pennsylvania

JUSTIN A. BISHOP, MD
Assistant Professor, Johns Hopkins Medical
Institutions, Baltimore, Maryland

REBECCA D. CHERNOCK, MD
Department of Pathology and Immunology,
Washington University School of Medicine,
St Louis, Missouri

ANGELA C. CHI, DMD
Associate Professor, Division of Oral
Pathology, Department of Stomatology,
College of Dental Medicine, Medical
University of South Carolina, Charleston,
South Carolina

SAMIR K. EL-MOFTY, DMD, PhD
Department of Pathology and Immunology,
Washington University School of Medicine,
St Louis, Missouri

JOAQUÍN J. GARCÍA, MD
Assistant Professor of Laboratory Medicine
and Pathology, Mayo Clinic College of
Medicine, Rochester, Minnesota

JAMES S. LEWIS Jr, MD
Department of Pathology and Immunology,
Washington University School of Medicine,
St Louis, Missouri

SUSAN MÜLLER, DMD, MS
Professor, Department of Pathology and
Laboratory Medicine, Emory University
Hospital; Department of Otolaryngology–Head
and Neck Surgery, Emory University School of
Medicine, Atlanta, Georgia

BRAD W. NEVILLE, DDS
Distinguished University Professor, Division of
Oral Pathology, Department of Stomatology,
College of Dental Medicine, Medical University
of South Carolina, Charleston, South Carolina

MARY S. RICHARDSON, MD
Professor of Pathology and Laboratory
Medicine and Director of Surgical Pathology,
Medical University of South Carolina,
Charleston, South Carolina

JAMES J. SCIUBBA, DMD, PhD
Consulting Staff, Milton J. Dance, Jr. Head and
Neck Center, Greater Baltimore Medical
Center, Baltimore, Maryland

RAJA R. SEETHALA, MD
Assistant Professor of Pathology and
Otolaryngology, Department of Pathology,
University of Pittsburgh Medical Center,
Pittsburgh, Pennsylvania

BRUCE M. WENIG, MD
Department of Diagnostic Pathology and
Laboratory Medicine, Beth Israel Medical
Center, St. Luke's-Roosevelt Hospitals,
New York, New York

WILLIAM H. WESTRA, MD
Professor of Pathology, Oncology, and
Otolaryngology–Head and Neck Surgery,
Johns Hopkins Medical Institutions, Baltimore,
Maryland

Contents

Lichenoid changes in the oral mucosa can be encountered in a wide range of lesions and can have varied etiologies. Immune-mediated disorders, including lichen planus, mucous membrane pemphigoid, discoid lupus erythematosus, and graft-versus-host disease, can have clinical and histologic overlaps. Lichenoid reactions to dental materials, such as amalgam, or to many systemic drugs are also well documented. Dysplasia of the oral cavity at times can also express a lichenoid histology, which may mask the potentially cancerous component. Proliferative verrucous leukoplakia, an unusual clinical disease, mimics oral lichen planus clinically and requires careful correlation of the clinical and pathologic features.

This article presents various odontogenic cysts and tumors, including periapical cysts, dentigerous cysts, odontogenic keratocysts, orthokeratinized odontogenic cysts, lateral periodontal cysts, glandular odontogenic cysts, ameloblastomas, clear cell odontogenic carcinomas, adenomatoid odontogenic tumors, calcifying epithelial odontogenic tumors, squamous odontogenic tumors, ameloblastic fibromas, ameloblastic fibro-odontomas, odontomas, calcifying cystic odontogenic tumors, and odontogenic myxomas. The authors provide an overview of these cysts and tumors, with microsopic features, gross features, differential diagnosis, prognosis, and potential diagnostic pitfalls.

The sinonasal tract (SNT) includes the nasal cavity and paranasal sinuses (maxillary, ethmoid, frontal, and sphenoid) and may give rise to a variety of nonneoplastic and neoplastic proliferations, including benign and malignant neoplasms. The benign neoplasms of the SNT include epithelial neoplasms of surface epithelial origin, minor salivary gland origin, and mesenchymal origin. The spectrum of malignant neoplasms of the SNT includes epithelial malignancies, sinonasal undifferentiated carcinoma, malignant salivary gland neoplasms, neuroectodermal neoplasms, neuroendocrine neoplasms, melanocytic neoplasm, and sarcomas. This article concentrates on some of the more common types of benign and malignant neoplasms.

The most common malignancy to involve the oral cavity and oropharynx is squamous cell carcinoma (SCC). Because these oral cancers share an origin from the squamous epithelium, the pathology of oral SCC might be expected to be uniform and its diagnosis repetitive. In reality, the morphologic diversity in SCC, along with the propensity for reactive processes of the oral cavity to mimic SCC histologically, renders its diagnosis one of the more challenging in surgical pathology. This article discusses variants of oral and oropharyngeal SCC and highlights those features that help distinguish human papillomavirus–related from human papillomavirus–unrelated SCC.

Benign and malignant lesions of the larynx and hypopharynx present an interesting and diverse spectrum of diagnostic entities, which may be infrequently encountered in routine surgical pathology practice. This article places emphasis on illustrating the classical pathologic characteristics, differential diagnosis, clinical significance, and presentation of common lesions unique to these sites. The initial diagnosis of these lesions is via small endoscopic biopsy. Many of the entities have overlapping histologic features which necessitate optimizing the information available in a small sample. The focus of this article is to provide useful criteria to enable separating the more common types of lesions encountered in these sites.

Malignant salivary gland epithelial tumors are histologically diverse with at least 24 recognized distinct entities. In general, malignant tumors account for 15% to 30% of parotid tumors, 40% to 45% of submandibular tumors, 70% to 90% of sublingual tumors, and 50% of minor salivary tumors. Common malignancies include mucoepidermoid carcinoma, adenoid cystic carcinoma, acinic cell carcinoma, salivary duct carcinoma, carcinoma ex pleomorphic adenoma, polymorphous lowgrade adenocarcinoma, and myoepithelial carcinoma. Each tumor type has its own unique histologic variants and prognostic pathologic features, and only mucoepidermoid carcinomas have a formalized grading system. The molecular pathogenesis of certain tumors, such as mucoepidermoid carcinoma and adenoid cystic carcinoma, has recently begun to be elucidated.

Although at least 24 distinct histologic salivary gland carcinomas exist, many of them are rare, comprising only 1% to 2% of all salivary gland tumors. These include epithelial-myoepithelial carcinoma, (hyalinizing) clear cell carcinoma, basal cell adenocarcinoma, cystadenocarcinoma, low-grade salivary duct carcinoma (low-grade cribriform cystadenocarcinoma), oncocytic carcinoma, and adenocarcinoma not otherwise specified. Few tumors (clear cell carcinoma and basal cell adenocarcinoma) have unique molecular correlates. Benign tumors, although histologically less diverse, are far more common, with pleomorphic adenoma and Warthin tumor the most common salivary gland tumors. Many benign tumors have malignant counterparts for which histologic distinction can pose diagnostic challenge.

Bone Lesions of the Head and Neck   1273

Samir K. El-Mofty, James S. Lewis Jr, and Rebecca D. Chernock

This article describes the clinical, radiographic, and pathologic features of tumors and tumorlike lesions affecting the bones of the head and neck region. Emphasis is placed on common bone lesions affecting the craniofacial skeleton, particularly those that occur with more frequency or those that are unique to this part of the skeleton. Several of these lesions pose a diagnostic challenge to the pathologist. To ensure that a correct diagnosis is rendered, it is of utmost importance that accurate and detailed clinical and radiographic information is available.

Surgical Pathology Clinics

RELATED INTEREST

Otolaryngologic Clinics of North America, February 2011 (Vol. 44, No. 1)
Oral Medicine
Vincent D. Eusterman, MD, DDS and Arlen Meyers, MD, MBA, *Guest Editors*

THE CLINICS ARE NOW AVAILABLE ONLINE!

Access your subscription at:
www.theclinics.com

Are There Challenges in the Interpretation of Head and Neck Specimens?

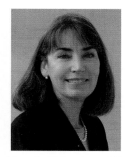

Mary S. Richardson, MD
Guest Editor

The spectrum of possible diagnoses posed by the mingling of diverse tissue types present in the region of the head and neck can be challenging for all involved in the daily practice of surgical pathology. The purpose of this issue is not to cover every aspect of head and neck pathology but rather to have well recognized experts provide a foundation for diagnosis of critical entities in this region. Articles in this issue focus on aspects of interpretation that can be especially vexing in the head and neck, including salivary gland lesions, craniofacial bone lesions, odontogenic lesions, lichenoid lesions of oral mucosa, sinonasal tract, oral cavity and oropharynx, and larynx and hypopharynx. The articles are designed to offer a practical reference for the everyday interpretation of biopsies and excision specimens.

Additionally, this issue includes state of the art review, key reference articles, and suggestions of ancillary testing. In each article there are high quality photomicrographs to complement the text. The diagnostic boxes and appropriate caveats may be used to further clarify relevant points in difficult areas where the diagnosis significantly alters the therapeutic intervention.

It is hoped that this text will provide a succinct reference for evaluation of the morphologic details of a wide variety of head and neck lesions as well as the manner in which to approach the evaluations of biopsies. This goal will be achieved if the articles presented in this issue of *Surgical Pathology Clinics* are useful to the daily practice of the general surgical pathologist.

I wish to acknowledge Dr Jean Lewis for her suggestions on the larynx and hypopharynx article. Also I would like to thank our editor Joanne Husovski for her suggestions, patience and encouragement. Lastly, this project would not have been possible without the unwavering support of my family, David, Conor, and Colin.

Mary S. Richardson, MD
Medical University of South Carolina
171 Ashley Avenue, MSC 908
Charleston, SC 29425, USA

E-mail address:
richardm@musc.edu

surgpath.theclinics.com

THE LICHENOID TISSUE REACTIONS OF THE ORAL MUCOSA: ORAL LICHEN PLANUS AND OTHER LICHENOID LESIONS

Susan Müller, DMD, MS[a,b,*]

KEYWORDS

- Lichen planus • Lichenoid reactions • Graft versus host disease • Oral dysplasia
- Proliferative verrucous leukoplakia

ABSTRACT

Lichenoid changes in the oral mucosa can be encountered in a wide range of lesions and can have varied etiologies. Immune-mediated disorders, including lichen planus, mucous membrane pemphigoid, discoid lupus erythematosus, and graft-versus-host disease, can have clinical and histologic overlaps. Lichenoid reactions to dental materials, such as amalgam, or to many systemic drugs are also well documented. Dysplasia of the oral cavity at times can also express a lichenoid histology, which may mask the potentially cancerous component. Proliferative verrucous leukoplakia, an unusual clinical disease, mimics oral lichen planus clinically and requires careful correlation of the clinical and pathologic features.

OVERVIEW

Oral lichen planus is a chronic inflammatory disease of unknown etiology.[1–5] The disease can wax and wane over a long period of time and disease severity varies greatly. There are several clinical as well as microscopic mimics of oral lichen planus (**Table 1**). Oral lichenoid lesions from systemic drug exposure or local allergic contact hypersensitivity are well documented.[1] Other immune-mediated diseases, including graft-versus-host

Key Features
ORAL LICHEN PLANUS

1. Can present clinically as asymptomatic reticular lesions or as erosive lesions; however, should be bilateral

2. Basal cell degeneration a hallmark of the disease and should be present for diagnosis

3. Presence of a well-defined band-like lymphocytic infiltrate subjacent to the basal cells

4. Direct immunofluorescence nonspecific or nondiagnostic

[a] Department of Pathology and Laboratory Medicine, Emory University Hospital, Emory University School of Medicine, 1364 Clifton Road, NE, Atlanta, GA 30322, USA
[b] Department of Otolaryngology–Head and Neck Surgery, Emory University School of Medicine, 1365 Clifton Road, NE, Atlanta, GA 30322, USA
* Department of Pathology and Laboratory Medicine, Emory University Hospital, 1364 Clifton Road, NE, Atlanta, GA 30322.
E-mail address: susan.muller@emory.org

Surgical Pathology 4 (2011) 1005–1026
doi:10.1016/j.path.2011.07.001
1875-9181/11/$ – see front matter © 2011 Elsevier Inc. All rights reserved.

Table 1
Causes of oral lichenoid reactions

Oral Lichenoid Drug Reactions	Oral Lichenoid Contact Reactions
Antibiotics	Dental metals
• Tetracyclines	• Nickel
Antifungals	• Palladium
• Ketoconazole	• Silver
• Amphotericin B	• Gold
NSAIDS	• Bismuth
• Naproxen	• Metallic mercury
• Ibuprofen	• 1% Ammoniated
• Diclofenac	mercury
• Indomethacin	• 0.1% Mercury
• Aspirin	chloride
Antimalarials	• Tin
• Choroquine	• Chromium
• Quinidine	• Cobalt
Antihypertensives	• Copper
• Propranolol	• Beryllium
• Enalapril	Other dental materials
• Hydroclorothiazide	• Glass ionomer
Antidiabetics	• Porcelain
• Glipizide	• Composite
• Insulin	• Acrylate compounds
Miscellaneous	Flavoring agents
• Gold	• Eugenol
• Penicillamine	• Cinnamon (cinnamic
• Allopurinol	aldehyde)
• Zidovuine	• Mint (mentha
• Antimycobacterials	piperita)
• Benzodiazepines	• Balsam of Peru
• Lithium	• Tartar control
	toothpaste
	• Menthol

Abbreviation: NSAID, nonsteroidal anti-inflammatory drug.

disease (GVHD), mucous membrane pemphigoid (MMP), and lupus erythematosus, can share common clinical and histologic features with oral lichen planus.[2] The variable presentation of oral lichenoid lesions requires that both the clinician and pathologist have broad knowledge of the differential diagnoses. There have been documented cases of malignant transformation of oral lichen planus although the exact incidence is unknown.[3] What is more common and of importance to pathologists is oral epithelial dysplasia with a lichenoid pattern. A prominent band-like, chronic inflammatory cell infiltrate can be present subjacent to the basal cells similar to lichen planus; however, on close examination, the features of epithelial dysplasia, including an abnormal maturation, mitoses, and/or dyskeratosis, can be appreciated. Finally, proliferative verrucous leukoplakia needs to be considered when a patient with multiple oral lichenoid lesions shows histologically varying degrees of dysplasia, verrucous carcinoma, or conventional squamous cell carcinoma.

ORAL LICHEN PLANUS
Overview

Lichen planus is a relatively common immune-mediated disease that affects the skin, nails, and mucous membranes.[6] Lichen planus is a chronic disease that undergoes periods of exacerbations and remissions. The pathogenesis of lichen planus is unknown but is thought to be a T-cell–mediated immune response. Next to cutaneous lichen planus, the oral lesions are the most common presentation. Oral lichen planus is the only disease manifestation in up to 35% of patients. Oral lichen planus is nearly always bilateral or multifocal.[1] In the oral cavity there are 3 major presentations: reticular, erythematous, and erosive.

In the reticular form, which is most common, the lesions present as white papules, plaques, or lace-like reticulations, also known as Wickham striae (**Fig. 1**).[7] The reticular form is often seen on the buccal mucosa although the dorsal and lateral tongue can also be affected. When lichen planus presents on the dorsal tongue, it often appears as thickened hyperkeratotic plaques (**Fig. 2**).

Erythematous and erosive lichen planus often have more typical reticular areas on the periphery of the lesions. Oral lichen planus is unusual on the palate and not seen in the floor of the mouth. Gingival involvement of lichen planus clinically presents as desquamative gingivitis and clinically can be difficult to distinguish from MMP (**Fig. 3**). In some patients, the only presentation of oral lichen planus is erythematous and erosive lesions of the attached gingiva. This form of the disease may involve focal areas or affect all the gingiva. The facial gingiva is most commonly affected, although in severe cases the palatal/lingual gingiva may be involved. A gingival/genital variant can also occur.

Biopsies of lichen planus ideally include intact epithelium rather than just the ulcerative component. Because the diagnosis of lichen planus requires evaluation of the basement membrane zone, biopsies from ulcerative areas lacking any epithelium are nondiagnostic. When a clinician is familiar with both the clinical and histologic features of lichen planus and relays the information to a pathologist, the diagnosis can be more definitive.

Microscopic Features

Lichen planus can exhibit a variety of histologic features depending on whether the biopsy was from a hypertrophic, atrophic, or erosive lesion.

Fig. 1. Typical clinical appearance of oral lichen planus from the buccal mucosa characterized by white papules and lace-like reticulations. These lesions are generally bilateral and affect other sites in the oral cavity.

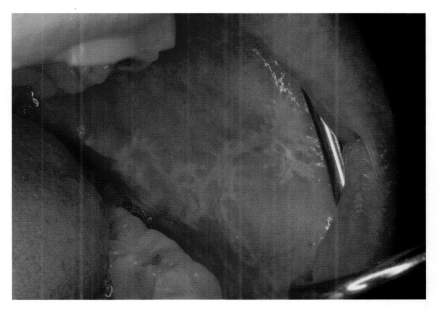

Both orthokeratosis and parakeratosis may be present. The hallmark of lichen planus is interface dermatitis with liquefaction (hydropic degeneration) of the basal cells (**Fig. 4**). The epithelium can be atrophic or acanthotic and the rete ridges may exhibit a sawtooth pattern (**Fig. 5**A). Dyskeratotic keratinocytes, known as Civatte (colloid, hyaline, or cytoid) bodies, can be seen at the lamina propria–epithelium interface and appear as eosinophilic globules (see **Fig. 5**B).[8] Subjacent to the basal cells at the basement membrane zone is a band-like inflammatory cell infiltrate composed predominately of T lymphocytes. Rarely, a few plasma cells may be present, but neutrophils and eosinophils are not seen. The inflammation is superficial rather than deep and a perivascular infiltrate is not generally seen. If the biopsy is from an ulcerated lesion (erosive lichen planus), many of the typical histologic hallmarks of lichen planus are lost. Reportedly, in up to 50% of oral lichen planus, cases lack clinico-pathologic correlation.[9] Epithelial atypia should not be seen in oral lichen planus. Dysplasia in what otherwise appears to be a lichenoid lesion should be diagnosed as epithelial dysplasia rather than lichen planus. One exception is when there is a superimposed candidal infection, which can cause reactive atypia.

Immunopathology

Direct immunofluorescence of oral lichen planus is nonspecific.[6] Fibrin deposited in a granular or linear pattern along the basement membrane zone is present (**Fig. 6**). Although this finding is not diagnostic for oral lichen planus, it can eliminate other vesiculobullous diseases, which mimic oral lichen planus, including MMP, pemphigus vulgaris, and chronic discoid lupus erythematosus.[10] Deposits of IgM, C3, IgG, and IgA are seen in exclusively in cytoid/colloid bodies. Indirect immunofluorescence is negative in lichen planus.

MUCOUS MEMBRANE PEMPHIGOID

Overview

MMP is an autoimmune chronic blistering mucocutaneous disease characterized by subepithelial bullae. The disease is most common in the sixth to eighth decade but can affect all age groups.

Pitfalls
ORAL LICHEN PLANUS

! Ulceration or a candidal superinfection may alter the histology, making diagnosis difficult. Reactive, regenerative, or reparative epithelial changes may be seen in these cases.

! Epithelial dysplasia should not be seen and precludes the diagnosis of lichen planus.

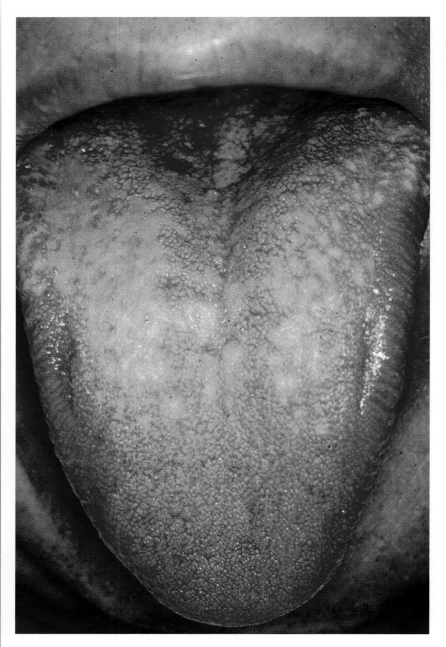

Fig. 2. When lichen planus involves the dorsal tongue, it often presents as thickened white plaques. Erythema and ulcerations can also be present.

The etiology of MMP is unknown, but many target antigens in the hemidesmosomes are associated with MMP. These include bullous pemphigoid antigen 1 or 2 (BPAG1/BPAG2), integrin β4 subunit, and laminin 5 and 6 as well as other antigens with unknown identity.[11] Any mucosal site can be affected in MMP but the oral and ocular mucosae are most commonly involved. Oral MMP can clinically mimic erosive LP, which is the major clinical differential diagnosis, particularly when presenting as desquamative gingivitis (**Fig. 7**). Gingival involvement is seen in more than 60% of cases of oral MMP. The buccal mucosa, palate, alveolus, tongue, and lower lip

Fig. 3. Oral lichen planus presenting as desquamative gingivitis with diffuse erythema and ulcerations of the maxillary and mandibular gingiva. This is associated with significant pain and bleeding.

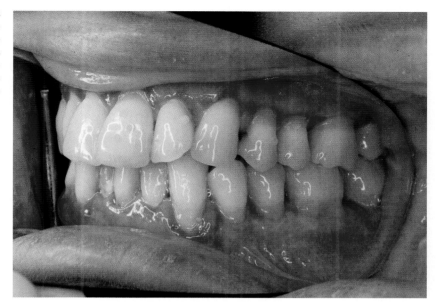

can also be involved. A positive Nikolsky sign (induced trauma can elicit a blister on clinically normal mucosa) is commonly seen in MMP but can also be present in the bullous form or erosive lichen planus. Although uncommon, intact vesicles or blisters can be seen in oral MMP.

Postinflammatory atrophy can mimic the reticular form of lichen planus.[11]

Ocular lesions occur in up to 37% of patients with oral MMP characterized by chronic conjunctival irritation, ulceration, and subsequent scarring.[11] Adhesions (symblepharons) develop that

Fig. 4. Basal cell degeneration (*black arrows*) is the hallmark of lichen planus and leads to a subepithelial separation from the underlying connective tissue, as pictured, resulting in ulceration (erosive lichen planus). A cytoid body (*white arrow*) is near the epithelium–connective tissue interface.

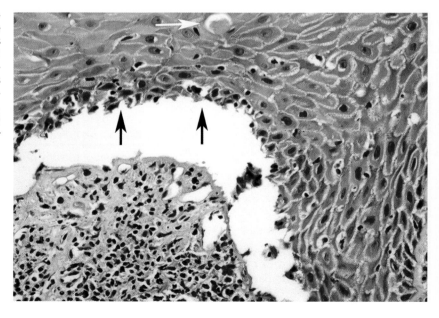

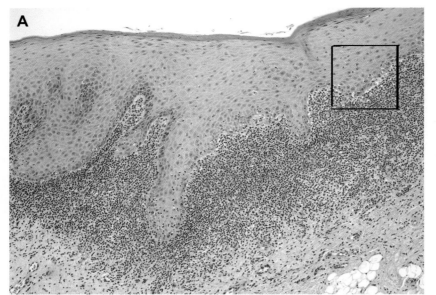

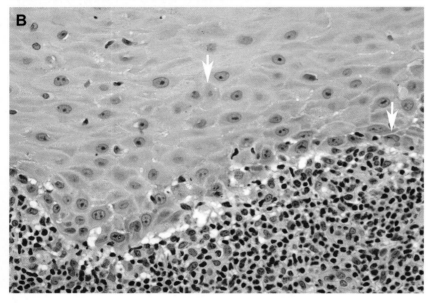

Fig. 5. (*A*) Low-power photomicrograph of lichen planus showing a dense, band-like lymphocytic infiltrate in the superficial lamina propria. The epithelium is acanthotic with saw-toothed rete. (*B*) High-power photomicrograph of the highlighted box area in (*A*) shows the basal cell vacuolar degeneration and scattered dyskeratotic keratinocytes (*arrows*).

Key Features
MUCOUS MEMBRANE PEMPHIGOID

1. Perilesional tissue demonstrates subepithelial clefting.

2. Unlike oral lichen planus, a sparse mixed inflammatory cell infiltrate, is present subjacent to the basal cells.

3. Basal cell liquefaction is absent or minimal.

4. Direct immunofluorescence shows a continuous linear band of IgG or C3 at basement membrane zone. This finding useful in distinguishing cases from oral lichen planus.

---

fuse the scleral and palpepral conjunctiva, which can lead to blindness if left untreated (**Fig. 8**).

Microscopic Features

The histopathology of MMP classically shows subepithelial clefting.[11–13] At times the epithelium is completely detached from the lamina propria, or no lamina propria is even submitted with the biopsy specimen (**Fig. 9**). On closer examination, the basal cells do not exhibit hydropic degeneration typical for lichen planus (**Fig. 10**). Dyskeratosis is not a feature of MMP, which is present in lichen planus. The subepithelial inflammatory infiltrate of MMP is variable and consists of a mixed population of lymphocytes and plasma cells. At times,

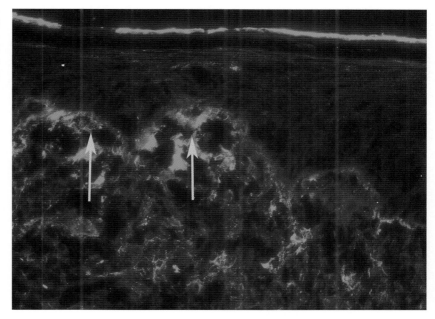

Fig. 6. Direct immunofluorescent microscopy of oral lichen planus demonstrated shaggy deposits of fibrin (*arrows*) in a linear pattern at the basement membrane zone.

however, the microscopic appearance of erosive lichen planus and MMP are similar and direct immunofluorescence is necessary to arrive at a diagnosis.

Immunopathology

The majority of patients with MMP (80%–100%) have a positive direct immunofluorescence. Direct immunofluorescence of perilesional mucosa reveals continuous linear deposits of IgG or complement (C3) along the basement membrane zone (**Fig. 11**).[11,12] Less commonly, both IgA and IgM can be seen. Indirect immunofluorescence using salt-split skin can detect circulating antibodies binding to either the roof or the floor of the split depending on which antibody is used. Not all patients have circulating antibodies,

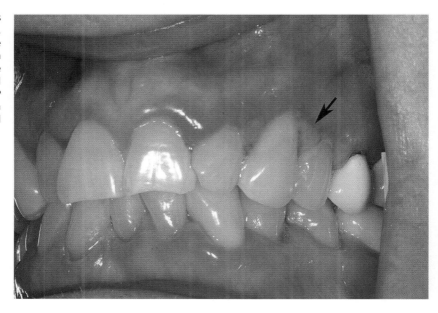

Fig. 7. MMP presenting as desquamative gingivitis. The blisters often collapse leaving a necrotic area (*arrow*). This is one of the most common clinical presentations of MMP but can also be seen in pemphigus vulgaris and lichen planus.

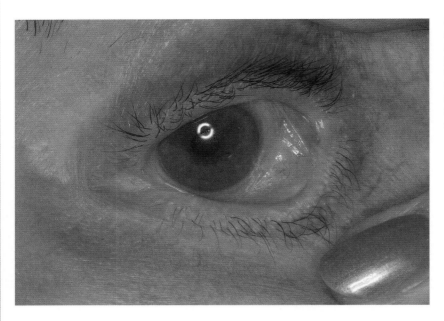

Fig. 8. A patient with ocular involvement of MMP showing symblepharon formation. These fibrous adhesions fuse the bulbar and palpebral conjunctivae and can result in entropion and corneal abrasions.

however, and unlike pemphigus vulgaris, antibody titer does not correlate with disease activity.

GRAFT-VERSUS-HOST DISEASE
Overview

Oral cavity manifestations of chronic GVHD (cGVHD) after allogeneic bone marrow transplantation can be seen in 80% of patients.[14] cGVHD, a major cause of morbidity and mortality, has a median onset of 6 months post-transplantation. This is in contrast to acute GVHD, which appears within the first 100 days post–bone marrow transplantation. In the acute form, the skin, liver, and gastrointestinal tract are most commonly involved. cGVHD has a variable clinical presentation, including skin, ocular, liver, pulmonary, and gastrointestinal manifestations. Lichenoid lesions can present throughout the oral cavity and can present as lacy reticulations, thickened plaques, or erosions.[15] An uncommon site for

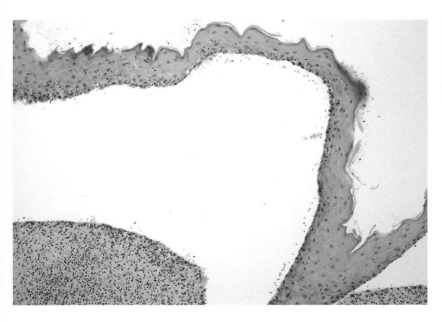

Fig. 9. Biopsies of epithelium, which are cleanly detached from the underlying lamina propria or do not contain any connective tissue, should raise the suspicion for MMP.

Fig. 10. MMP with characteristic subepithelial clefting. Unlike lichen planus, the basal cells are intact and the superficial lamina propria contains a sparse to moderate inflammatory cell infiltrate consisting predominately of lymphocytes and plasma cells.

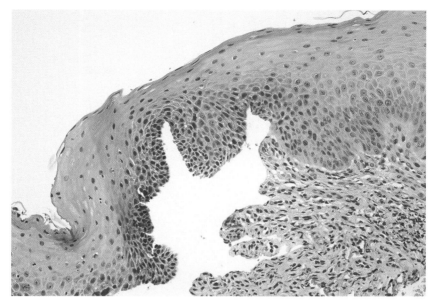

oral lichen planus, the palate can be affected in cGVHD (**Fig. 12**).

Microscopic Features

The microscopic features of cGVHD share many similarities with oral lichen planus and require appropriate clinical history for diagnosis.[14,15]

Basal cell degeneration, dyskeratosis, and a lymphocytic infiltration in the subjacent mucosa are present (**Figs. 13** and **14**). The lymphocytic infiltrate is not as intense as in lichen planus and may have a few plasma cells and eosinophils. The lymphocyte population is a mixture of CD4 and CD8 T lymphocytes in the same ratio as found in lichen planus.[16,17] Because of the

Fig. 11. Direct immunofluorescence of perilesional tissue from a patient with MMP demonstrates a continuous linear band of IgG at the basement membrane zone.

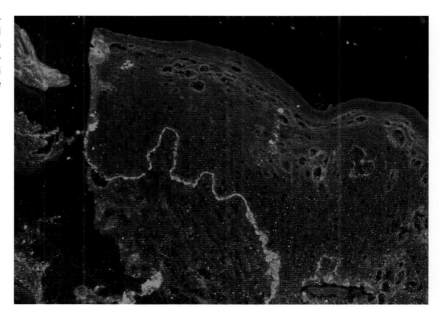

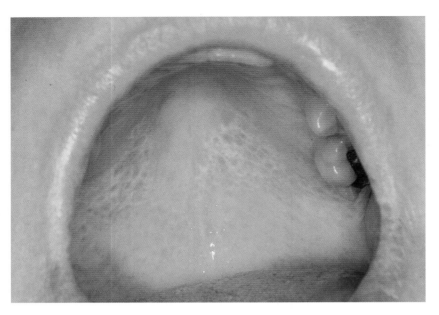

Fig. 12. GVHD involving the hard palate in a patient who underwent a bone marrow transplant for chronic myelogenous leukemia. Note the lace-like reticulations that resemble lichen planus; however, the hard palate is an unusual location for lichen planus.

varied clinical presentations, the diagnosis of cGVHD is based on both the microscopic and clinical findings.

DRUG-RELATED ORAL LICHENOID LESIONS
Overview

Many systemic medications can cause oral lichenoid reactions.[1–3] Both reticular and erosive patterns can be seen and oral lesions can present with or without cutaneous lesions. Rarely reported in the pediatric population, oral lichenoid lesions is common in adults, although the exact incidence is unknown.[18] The interval between the onset of drug-related lichenoid reactions and initial medication use can vary widely, from weeks to more than a year.[19] Unlike lichen planus, which is multifocal and bilateral, drug-related lichenoid lesions may present as a single lesion. The most commonly reported offending medications include

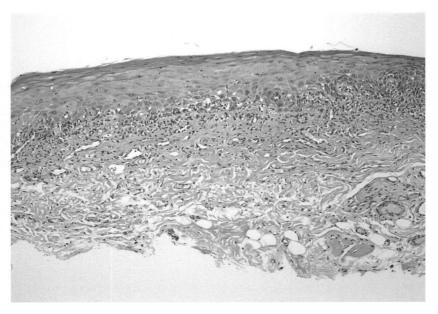

Fig. 13. Low-power photomicrograph of GVHD from the oral mucosa showing a lichenoid pattern of the epithelium with hydropic degeneration of the basal cells overlying a moderate lymphocytic infiltrate.

Fig. 14. The epithelium in oral GVHD often shows intracellular edema, basal cell liquefaction, dyskeratosis (*arrows*), and inflammatory cell exocytosis.

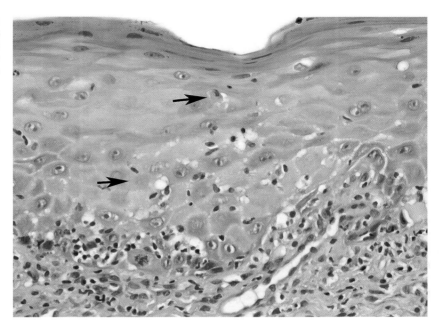

antihypertensives, nonsteroidal inflammatory drugs, antimalarials, and HIV antiretrovirals.[20,21] The pathogenesis of drug-related lichenoid reactions is unclear. No standardized criteria for the diagnosis exist. If a temporal relationship can be identified, then the obvious treatment is discontinuing the offending medication. The lesions may, however, take many months or longer to resolve.

Microscopic Features

The microscopic features of drug-related lichenoid lesions share many similarities to oral lichen planus, although there are some differences. A more diffuse lymphocytic infiltrate is often encountered and both plasma cells and eosinophils may be seen.[2,20] The inflammation is often deeper into the lamina propria rather than the band-like infiltrate present in lichen planus (**Fig. 15**). A higher number of dyskeratotic keratinocytes (colloid or Civatte bodies) may be present than in oral lichen planus. Frequently, a perivascular chronic inflammatory cell infiltrate is seen in drug-related lichenoid lesions. Again, the microscopic findings are not specific and require clinical information, including a temporal association with any systemic medications.

Immunopathology

Direct immunofluorescence of perilesional tissue in oral lichenoid drug reaction is similar to oral lichen planus with a shaggy deposition of fibrin at the basement membrane zone and IgM-positive colloid or cytoid bodies.[22] Using patient sera, indirect immunofluorescence may detect circulating antibodies directed to the basal cells in an annular fluorescent pattern, called a string of pearls pattern.[23] This finding is not seen in oral lichen planus and may aid in making the diagnosis of oral lichenoid drug reactions.

Key Features
ORAL LICHENOID CONTACT REACTIONS

1. Typically unilateral lesion most commonly associated with a large amalgam restoration; however, other dental materials or flavoring agents may be causative

2. Share similarities to oral lichen planus but often have a deeper inflammatory infiltrate with plasma cells and neutrophils along with lymphocytes

3. Perivascular inflammation seen

4. Tertiary lymphoid follicle formation, especially in amalgam reactions

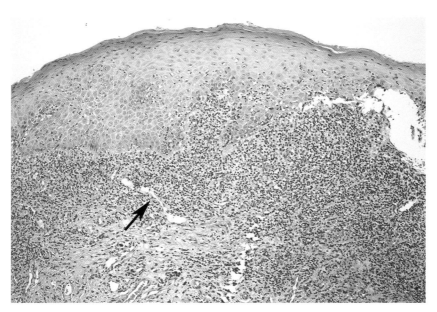

Fig. 15. Drug-related oral lichenoid lesions share overlapping microscopic features to lichen planus, including a subepithelial separation. The inflammatory infiltrate is mixed and extends deeper into the connective tissue than in lichen planus. In addition, there is perivascular inflammation (*arrow*), which is not a usual feature of lichen planus.

ORAL LICHENOID CONTACT REACTION
Overview

There are a variety of agents that are known to cause a lichenoid contact reaction. These include metals, composites, and glass ionomers used in dental restorations.[24,25] Older and/or large amalgam restorations can cause lichenoid lesions and are found on the buccal mucosa or the tongue in direct contact with the amalgam (**Fig. 16**). Although similar in appearance to lichen planus, these lesions are unilateral. On removal of the amalgam, the lesions generally resolve. Flavoring agents, such as cinnamon, menthol, eugenol, and peppermint, have also been associated with

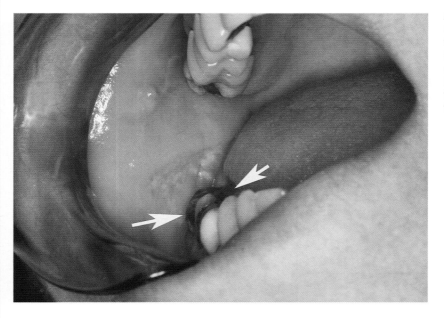

Fig. 16. Oral lichenoid contact reaction to dental amalgam presenting as areas of erythema and white plaques. The large amalgam restoration (*arrows*) directly contacts the affected mucosa.

Fig. 17. Oral lichenoid contact reaction to cinnamon-flavored chewing gum. Within 10 days of discontinuing the gum, the lesion completely resolved.

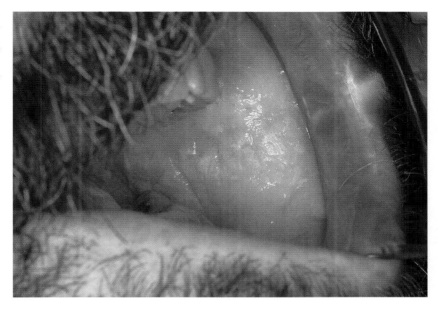

oral lichenoid lesions and occur at the site of contact, most often on the lateral border of the tongue or buccal mucosa (**Fig. 17**).[1,3] Cinnamon or cinnamic aldehyde can induce a cinnamon stomatitis that has a characteristic histology. When the offending agent is removed, the lesions quickly resolve.

Microscopic Features

The microscopic features of oral lichenoid contact reactions are not specific and overlap greatly with oral lichen planus. In amalgam-associated lichenoid reactions, however, the lymphocytic infiltrate may be so dense that lymphoid follicles, called tertiary follicles, may form (**Fig. 18**).[24] Biopsies

Fig. 18. Oral lichenoid contact reaction to dental amalgam often has a dense lymphocytic infiltrate, which can form tertiary follicles (*arrows*). Although not always present, postinflammatory hyperpigmentation can occur and can be seen in the superficial submucosa and basal cells.

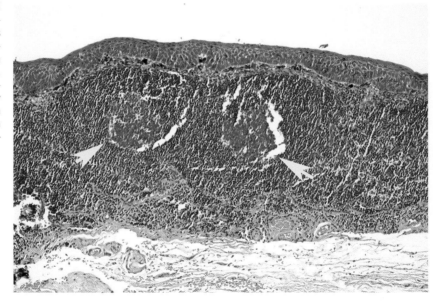

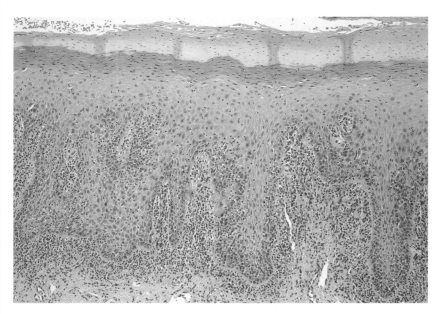

Fig. 19. The microscopic features of oral lichenoid contact reaction to cinnamon show marked epithelial acanthosis with elongation of the rete. A dense inflammatory cell infiltrate is seen in the superficial lamina propria.

from cinnamon-induced lichenoid lesions demonstrate marked epithelial acanthosis with elongated rete ridges (**Fig. 19**). Unlike oral lichen planus, the inflammatory infiltrate is mixed, containing lymphocytes, plasma cells, histiocytes, and eosinophils.[26] Interface mucositis may be evident and a deep perivascular infiltrate is seen (**Fig. 20**).

LUPUS ERYTHEMATOSUS

Overview

Both systemic and discoid (chronic cutaneous) lupus erythematosus can affect the oral mucosa in 25% of cases.[27,28] Oral lesions typically affect the hard palate, buccal mucosa, and gingiva

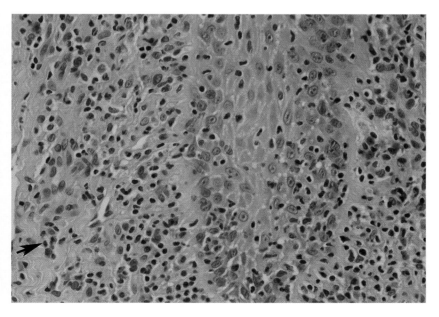

Fig. 20. High-power photomicrograph of oral lichenoid contact reaction to cinnamon showing the inflammatory cell infiltrate to be mixed, including plasma cells and eosinophils (*arrow*).

Key Features
LUPUS ERYTHEMATOSUS

1. May be difficult to distinguish oral lichen planus, particularly when associated systemic or skin lesions are absent
2. Atrophy of the epithelial rete, keratin plugging, and a thickened basement membrane often seen, not typical for oral lichen planus
3. Deep inflammatory infiltrate often in a perivascular location
4. Edema of the lamina propria

Microscopic Features

The histology of oral lupus erythematosus can vary depending on the age of the lesion as well as biopsy site. The microscopic features are not specific and overlap with lichen planus, lichenoid drug reactions, and lichenoid contact reactions.[3,27] The epithelium may exhibit either atrophy or pseudoepitheliomatous hyperplasia (**Fig. 22**). Hyperkeratosis with keratin plugging is often observed as well as a thickened basement membrane with periodic acid–Schiff–positive material. The lamina propria is edematous and incontinent melanin may be seen. The inflammatory cell infiltrate subjacent to the basal cells can range from paucicellular to a lymphocyte rich. Superficial and deep perivascular inflammatory infiltrate is seen.

Immunopathology

Direct immunofluorescence of lesional tissue in both systemic and chronic lupus erythematosus shows granular or shaggy deposits of IgG, IgM, or C3 at the basement membrane zone (**Fig. 23**).[10] These findings are helpful in differentiating lichen planus from lupus erythematosus, particularly in systemic lupus erythematosus where immunoglobulin deposits are found in virtually all cases. This finding is in contrast to discoid lupus in which approximately 70% of biopsies show positivity on direct immunofluorescence.

(**Fig. 21**). Clinically, the oral presentation of systemic lupus erythematosus cannot be distinguished from oral chronic cutaneous lupus erythematosus. Often a central area of ulceration or erythema surrounded by white radiating striae is seen. Palatal lesions may be purely erythematous and patchy in distribution. The clinical presentation can mimic oral lichen planus, in particular erosive lichen planus. Unlike oral lichen planus, however, which often occurs only in the oral cavity, lupus erythematosus does not present solely in the oral cavity and patients will have cutaneous disease or other systemic disease associated with lupus.[3]

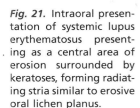

Fig. 21. Intraoral presentation of systemic lupus erythematosus presenting as a central area of erosion surrounded by keratoses, forming radiating stria similar to erosive oral lichen planus.

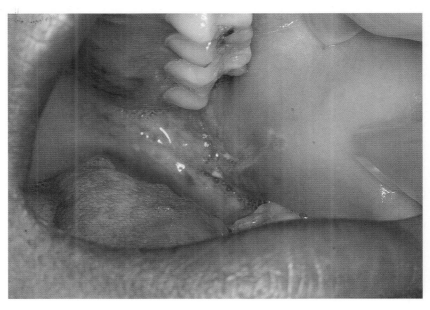

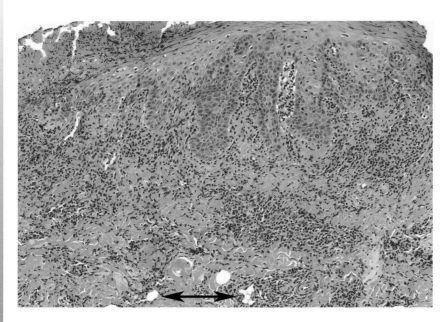

Fig. 22. Biopsy of an oral lesion of lupus erythematosus showing acanthotic epithelium with a patchy inflammatory cell infiltrate in the lamina propria. Unlike lichen planus, perivascular inflammation (*arrows*) is seen in lupus erythematosus.

LICHENOID DYSPLASIA: ORAL DYSPLASIA AND PROLIFERATIVE VERRUCOUS LEUKOPLAKIA

Overview

Malignant transformation of oral lichen planus to squamous cell carcinoma has been reported.[4,7,29–32]

The exact incidence is unclear, most likely because some reported cases of malignant transformation of oral lichen planus were never biopsied initially and the diagnosis of lichen planus was based on clinical features alone.[4] There have been a few well-documented cases of malignant transformation, however, in long-standing lichen planus,

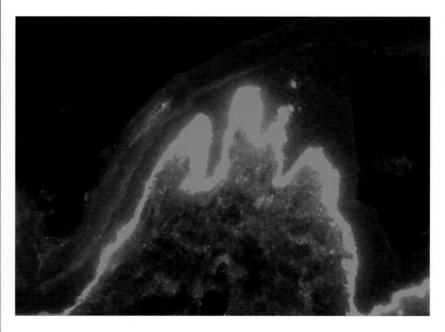

Fig. 23. Direct immunofluorescent microscopy of lesional tissue in lupus erythematosus showing shaggy deposits of IgM at the basement membrane zone.

Key Features
ORAL DYSPLASIA
WITH A LICHENOID PATTERN

1. Pathologists should avoid making the diagnosis of lichen planus with dysplasia. This can result in inappropriate patient treatment and follow-up.

particularly in the erosive or atrophic form, which has been poorly controlled (**Fig. 24**). It is the author's opinion that the presence of dysplasia in a lichenoid lesion should not be diagnosed as lichen planus. In addition, an otherwise lichenoid lesion that is not clinically bilateral or multifocal should not be diagnosed as lichen planus.

An unusual form of leukoplakia that can mimic oral lichen planus both clinically and microscopically is

Fig. 24. (*A*) A 50-year-old woman with a greater than 10-year history of biopsy confirmed oral erosive lichen planus. The patient had poorly controlled erosive lesions on the dorsal tongue and buccal mucosa. (*B*) The patient subsequently developed squamous cell carcinoma arising on the lateral border of the tongue (*arrows*).

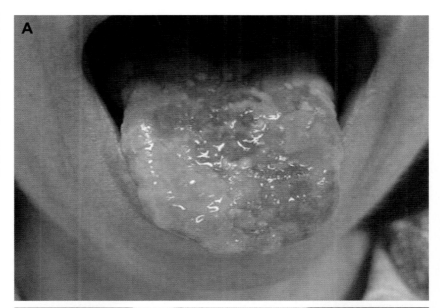

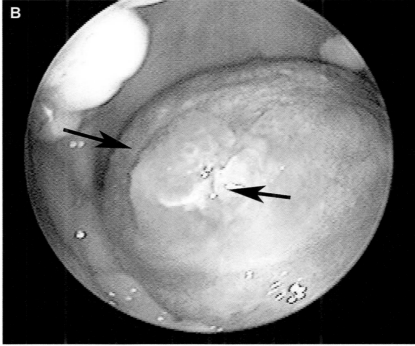

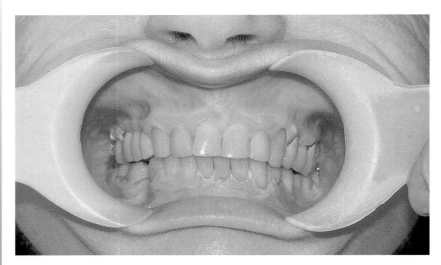

Fig. 25. Typical clinical presentation of proliferative verrucous leukoplakia of the gingiva in a 72-year-old nonsmoking woman. Thickened, keratotic areas are on the gingiva of the maxilla and mandible. This patient developed squamous cell carcinoma of the gingiva within a year of this photograph.

proliferative verrucous leukoplakia. First described in 1985 by Hansen and colleagues,[5] this type of precancerous lesion can be difficult to diagnose, especially in its early presentation, and often it is a diagnosis made in retrospect. The lesions typically grow slowly over a few years to several decades. The patients are typically older women, many without history of tobacco or alcohol abuse.[33,34] The lesions are multifocal similar to oral lichen planus. The lesions have a propensity for the gingiva, palate, tongue, and buccal mucosa (**Figs. 25** and **26**).[33] The hard palate can also be involved but ventral tongue and floor of mouth is uncommon. The lesions may appear as hyperkeratotic plaques and may show erythematous atrophic areas or frank ulceration.

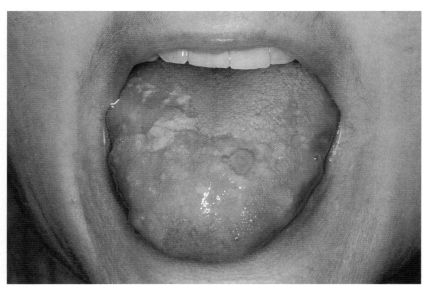

Fig. 26. Proliferative verrucous leukoplakia of the tongue mimicking erosive lichen planus. Note the similarities of this presentation to that in **Fig. 24A**. This patient had lesions involving the palate and gingiva as well and developed squamous cell carcinoma of the gingiva.

Microscopic Features

Microscopically, oral dysplasia can sometimes exhibit a band-like inflammatory infiltrate, which on low power can mimic lichen planus (**Fig. 27A**).[35] This type of dysplasia has sometimes been called lichenoid dysplasia, although the use of this term is discouraged.[4,7] The inflammatory infiltrate is typically mixed, composed of both lymphocytes and plasma cells. Migration of inflammatory cells can be observed through the epithelium and varying degrees of cytologic atypia are present (see **Fig. 27B**).[33] Oral lichenoid lesions that do not have all the typical clinical and histologic features of oral lichen planus have a reportedly higher rate of malignant transformation than oral lichen planus which emphasizes the importance of both clinical and pathologic correlation in making the diagnosis of oral lichen planus.[21]

Biopsies of lesions in patients with proliferative verrucous leukoplakia can exhibit a wide range of histologic features, from hyperkeratosis without dysplasia, to more lichenoid features with a band-like lymphocytic infiltrate, to dysplasia, verrucous carcinoma, or conventional type squamous cell carcinoma (**Fig. 28**).[33] Often the site of malignant transformation is not in the typical location for

Fig. 27. (*A*) A biopsy of moderate dysplasia from the floor of the mouth that on low microscopic power has a lichenoid appearance with a band-like inflammatory cell infiltrate. (*B*) On higher microscopic power, hyperchromatic, pleomorphic nuclei are evident. These cellular features are not a component of oral lichen planus. The diagnosis of lichenoid dysplasia should be avoided because it may lead to undertreatment.

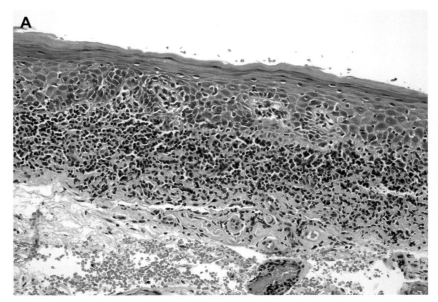

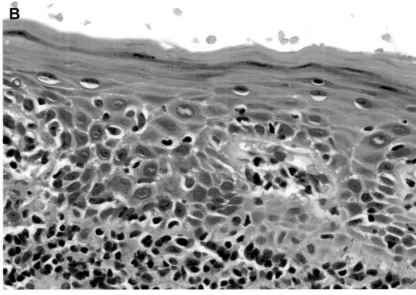

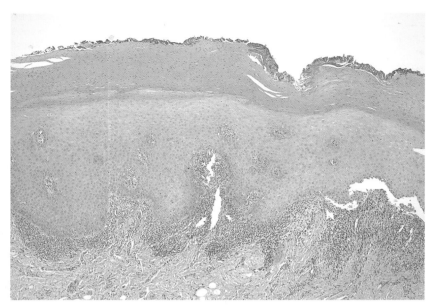

Fig. 28. Photomicrograph of atypical verrucous hyperplasia in a patient with proliferative verrucous leukoplakia. Marked parakeratosis is evident and corresponds to the clinical presentation of thickened, keratotic mucosa. An inflammatory cell infiltrate is present subjacent to the basal cells as well as a subepithelial separation mimicking lichen planus.

△△ Differential Diagnosis
OF ORAL LICHENOID LESIONS

Differentials	Differs from Oral Lichenoid Lesions by the Following
Oral lichen planus	
MMP	• Can clinically mimic erosive lichen planus. • Histologically shows subepithelial clefting; basal cells do not exhibit hydropic degeneration typical for lichen planus. • Immunologically, majority of patients with MMP have positive direct immunofluorescence.
cGVHD	• Clinically, the palate can be affected in cGVHD, uncommon site for oral lichen planus. • Because microscopic features of cGVHD share many similarities with oral lichen planus, appropriate clinical history is required for diagnosis.
Lichenoid drug reactions	• Microscopic findings not specific and require clinical information: more diffuse lymphocytic infiltrate is often encountered; inflammation is often deeper into the lamina propria; higher number of dyskeratotic keratinocytes may be present than in oral lichen planus; perivascular chronic inflammatory cell infiltrate is seen in drug-related lichenoid lesions. • Indirect immunofluorescence may detect circulating antibodies directed to the basal cells in pattern, called a string of pearls pattern, not seen in oral lichen planus.
Lichenoid contact hypersensitivity reactions	• Share similarities to oral lichen planus but often have a deeper inflammatory infiltrate with plasma cells and neutrophils along with lymphocytes with perivascular inflammation. • Tertiary lymphoid follicle formation, especially in amalgam reactions can be seen.
Lupus erythematosus	• May be difficult to distinguish oral lichen planus, particularly when associated systemic or skin lesions are absent. • Histologically can see atrophy of the epithelial rete, keratin plugging, a thickened basement membrane and a deep inflammatory infiltrate often in a perivascular location which is not typical for oral lichen planus.
Lichenoid dysplasia	• The presence of any dysplasia in a mucosal lesion should negate the diagnosis of lichen planus.

Pitfalls
ORAL DYSPLASIA WITH
A LICHENOID PATTERN

! Oral epithelial dysplasia can exhibit a band-like inflammatory cell infiltrate that mimics lichen planus on low power magnification. Closer examination shows mixed inflammation rather than lymphocyte predominance.

! Cytologic atypia, including hyperchromatic and pleomorphic nuclei, is seen and the degree of dysplasia should be graded accordingly.

oral squamous cell carcinoma but arises in the attached gingiva, palate, or dorsal tongue.

SUMMARY: LICHENOID TISSUE REACTIONS

Lichenoid tissue reactions can be challenging for pathologists due to the tremendous overlap in the clinical and pathologic presentation of many inflammatory, reactive, and immune-mediated disorders that commonly involve the oral mucosa. An accurate diagnosis cannot be made in a vacuum and it is essential that good clinical information accompanies the biopsy, including site, presentation, and other relevant information. In addition, adjuvant studies, including direct and indirect immunofluorescence, may be required to arrive at a diagnosis. Dysplastic changes in a lichenoid lesion should not be overlooked and be diagnosed appropriately as dysplasia rather than lichen planus with dysplasia to ensure appropriate treatment for the patient.

REFERENCES

1. Schlosser BJ. Lichen planus and lichenoid reactions of the oral mucosa. Dermatol Ther 2010;23:251–67.
2. van der Waal I. Oral lichen planus and oral lichenoid lesions; a critical appraisal with emphasis on the diagnostic aspects. Med Oral Patol Oral Cir Bucal 2009;14(3):E310–4.
3. Farthing PM, Speight PM. Problems and pitfalls in oral mucosal pathology. Curr Diagn Pathol 2006; 12:66–74.
4. Eisenberg E, Krutchkoff DJ. Lichenoid lesions of oral mucosa. Diagnostic criteria and their importance in the alleged relationship to oral cancer. Oral Surg Oral Med Oral Pathol 1992;73:699–704.
5. Hansen LS, Olson JA, Silverman S Jr. Proliferative verrucous leukoplakia. A long-term study of thirty patients. Oral Surg Oral Med Oral Pathol 1985; 60:285.
6. Thornhill MH. Immune mechanisms in oral lichen planus. Acta Odontol Scand 2001;59(3):174–7.
7. Eisen D. The clinical features, malignant potential, and systemic associations of oral lichen planus: a study of 723 patients. J Am Acad Dermatol 2002;26:207–14.
8. Van der Meij EH, Reibel J, Slootweg PJ, et al. Interobserver and intraobserver variability in the histologic assessment of oral lichen planus. J Oral Pathol Med 1999;28:274–7.
9. Van der Meij EH, van der Waal I. Lack of clinicopathologic correlation in the diagnosis of oral lichen planus based on the presently available diagnostic criteria and suggestions for modifications. J Oral Pathol Med 2003;32:507–12.
10. Schiodt M, Holmstrup P, Dabelsteen E, et al. Deposits of immunoglobulins, complement, and fibrinogen in oral lupus erythematosus, lichen planus, and leukoplakia. Oral Surg Oral Med Oral Pathol 1981;51: 603–8.
11. Bruch-Gerharz P, Hertl M, Ruzicka T. Mucous membrane pemphigoid: clinical aspects, immunopathological features and therapeutics. Eur J Dermatol 2007;17(3):191–200.
12. Scully C, LoMuzio L. Oral mucosal diseases: mucous membrane pemphigoid. Br J Oral Maxillofac Surg 2008;46:358–66.
13. Sollecito TP, Prisis E. Mucous membrane pemphigoid. Dent Clin North Am 2009;49:91–106.
14. Demarosi F, Lodi G, Carrassi A, et al. Clinical and Histopathological features of the oral mucosa in allogeneic haematopoietic stem cell transplantation patients. Exp Oncol 2007;29:304–8.
15. Imanguli MM, Alevizos I, Brown R, et al. Oral graft-versus-host disease. Oral Dis 2008;14(5):396–412.
16. Shulman HM, Kleiner D, Lee SJ, et al. Histopathologic diagnosis of chronic graft versus host disease: National Institutes of Health Consensus Development Project on Criteria for Clinical Trials in chronic graft versus host disease: II Pathology Working Group Report. Biol Blood Marrow Transplant 2006; 34:368–73.
17. Soares AB, Faria PR, Magna LA, et al. Chronic GVHD in minor salivary glands and oral mucosa: histopathological and immunohistochemical evaluation of 25 patients. J Oral Pathol Med 2005;34: 368–82.
18. Woo V, Bonks J, Borukhova L, et al. Oral lichenoid drug eruption: a report of a pediatric case and review of the literature. Pediatr Dermatol 2009;26: 458–64.
19. McCartan BE, McCreary CE. Oral lichenoid drug eruption. Oral Dis 1997;3:58–63.
20. Al-Hashimi I, Schifter M, Lockhart PB, et al. Oral lichen planus and oral lichenoid lesions: diagnostic

and therapeutic considerations. Oral Surg Oral Med Oral Pathol Oral Radiol Endod 2007;103(Suppl S25): e1–12.

21. Van den Haute V, Antoine JL, Lachapell JM. Histopathological discriminant criteria between lichenoid drug eruption and idiopathic lichen planus: retrospective study on selected samples. Dermatologica 1989;179:10–3.

22. Watanabe C, Hayashi T, Kawada A. Immunofluorescence study of drug-induced lichen planus-like lesions. J Dermatol 1981;8:473–7.

23. McQueen A, Behan WM. Immunofluorescence microscopy. The "string of Pearls" phenomenon—an immunofluorescent serological finding in patients screened for adverse drug reactions. Am J Dermatopathol 1982;4:155–9.

24. Thornhill MH, Sankar V, Xu XJ, et al. The role of histopathological characteristics in distinguishing amalgam-associated oral lichenoid reactions and oral lichen planus. J Oral Pathol Med 2006;35:233–40.

25. Issa Y, Duxbury AJ, Macfarlane TV, et al. Oral lichenoid lesions related to dental restorative materials. Br Dent J 2005;198:361–6.

26. Miller RL, Gould AR, Bernstein ML. Cinnamon-induced stomatitis venenata. Clinical and characteristic histopathologic features. Oral Surg Oral Med Oral Pathol 1992;73(6):708–16.

27. Schiodt M. Oral discoid lupus erythematosus. III. A histopathologic study of sixty-six patients. Oral Surg Oral Med Oral Pathol 1984;57:281–93.

28. Orteu CH, Buchanan JA, Hutchison I, et al. Systemic lupus erythematosus presenting with oral mucosal lesions: easily missed? Br J Dermatol 2001;144: 1219–23.

29. Van der Meij EH, Schepman KP, van der Waal I. The possible premalignant character of oral lichen planus and oral lichenoid lesions: a prospective study. Oral Surg Oral Med Oral Pathol Oral Radiol Endod 2003;96:164–71.

30. Roosaar A, Yin L, Sandborgh-Englund G, et al. On the natural course of oral lichen lesions in a Swedish population-based sample. J Oral Pathol Med 2006; 35:257–61.

31. Van der Meij EH, Mast H, van der Waal I. The possible premalignant character of oral lichen planus and oral lichenoid lesions: a prospective five-year follow-up study or 192 patients. Oral Oncol 2007;43:742–8.

32. van der Waal I. Potentially malignant disorders of the oral and oropharyngeal mucosa; terminology, classification and present concepts of management. Oral Oncol 2009;45:317–23.

33. Bagan JV, Murillo J, Poveda R, et al. Proliferative verrucous leukoplakia: unusual locations of oral squamous cell carcinomas, and field cancerization as shown by the appearance of multiple OSCCs. Oral Oncol 2004;40:440–3.

34. Silverman S Jr, Gorsky M. Proliferative verrucous leukoplakia: a follow-up study of 54 cases. Oral Surg Oral Med Oral Pathol Oral Radiol Endod 1997;84:154–7.

35. Krutchkoff DJ, Eisenberg E. Lichenoid dysplasia: a distinct histopathologic entity. Oral Surg Oral Med Oral Pathol 1985;60:308–15.

ODONTOGENIC CYSTS AND TUMORS

Angela C. Chi, DMD*, Brad W. Neville, DDS

KEYWORDS

• Odontogenic • Cyst • Tumor • Jaws • Mandible • Maxilla

ABSTRACT

This article presents various odontogenic cysts and tumors, including periapical cysts, dentigerous cysts, odontogenic keratocysts, orthokeratinized odontogenic cysts, lateral periodontal cysts, glandular odontogenic cysts, ameloblastomas, clear cell odontogenic carcinomas, adenomatoid odontogenic tumors, calcifying epithelial odontogenic tumors, squamous odontogenic tumors, ameloblastic fibromas, ameloblastic fibro-odontomas, odontomas, calcifying cystic odontogenic tumors, and odontogenic myxomas. The authors provide an overview of these cysts and tumors, with microsopic features, gross features, differential diagnosis, prognosis, and potential diagnostic pitfalls.

OVERVIEW

The embryogenesis of teeth involves a complex interaction between specialized epithelial cells and connective tissue elements (odontogenic ectomesenchyme). For each tooth, a group of epithelial cells (dental lamina) proliferates downward from the surface mucosa into the developing alveolar bone to form the enamel organ. This epithelium induces the differentiation of ectomesenchymal cells, which form the central dental papilla and surrounding connective tissue follicle. Specialized epithelial cells (ameloblasts) from the enamel organ are responsible for enamel formation; the dental papilla is destined to become the tooth pulp and gives rise to the odontoblasts, which form the dentin of the tooth. Later in tooth formation, cells from the surrounding dental follicle differentiate into cementoblasts to form a thin layer of bone-like cementum on the outer root surface.

A wide variety of odontogenic cysts and tumors may arise from these diverse cellular elements. Odontogenic cysts may develop de novo or from stimulation of epithelial remnants by odontogenic infections. Tumors of odontogenic origin may arise from the epithelial cells, the ectomesenchymal component, or a combination of both cell lines. The purpose of this article is to review some of the more significant and problematic odontogenic cysts and tumors (**Boxes 1** and **2**).

ODONTOGENIC CYSTS

PERIAPICAL CYST (RADICULAR CYST, APICAL PERIODONTAL CYST)

Periapical cysts are the most common odontogenic cyst, accounting for more than half of all cysts of the jaws.[2] The lesion is inflammatory in origin and arises in association with the root of a nonvital tooth.

When a tooth is affected by dental caries or physical trauma, the central pulp can become inflamed and undergo necrosis. Subsequently, an inflammatory reaction, known as a *periapical granuloma*, may develop within the bone surrounding the tooth root. (Although the inflammation is termed, *granuloma*, it should be understood that this lesion is not a true granuloma but simply a focus of granulation tissue.) This periapical inflammation has the potential to stimulate remnants of odontogenic epithelium (rests of Malassez) within the periodontal ligament space, which may proliferate to form a cyst in this area.

Periapical cysts most often occur at the apex of the tooth where the pulp receives its vascular supply (**Fig. 1**), although some can develop along the lateral root surface if a lateral pulpal canal is

Division of Oral Pathology, Department of Stomatology, College of Dental Medicine, Medical University of South Carolina, MSC 507, 173 Ashley Avenue, Charleston, SC 29425, USA
* Corresponding author.
E-mail address: chi@musc.edu

Surgical Pathology 4 (2011) 1027–1091
doi:10.1016/j.path.2011.07.003

present (lateral radicular cyst). Often the lesion is asymptomatic and is discovered during routine dental radiographic examination. Some periapical cysts may be associated with pain, infection, root resorption, or overlying bony expansion.

Periapical Cyst: Gross Features

Some periapical cysts are removed as well-circumscribed sac-like structures that may contain dark fluid or cholesterol deposits (**Fig. 2**). Most, however, are friable and are curetted out as multiple smaller fragments.

Periapical Cyst: Microscopic Features

A well-formed periapical cyst shows a central lumen that is lined by stratified squamous epithelium.[2,3] This epithelium is often irregular in thickness with hyperplasia of the rete ridges due to the effect of inflammation in the cyst wall (**Fig. 3**). Long-standing periapical cysts may lose most of this inflammation, however, and be lined by a thinner and more regular layer of squamous epithelium (**Fig. 4**). Sometimes the cystic lining includes areas with mucin-producing cells or ciliated columnar epithelium.[4–6] On occasion, the epithelial lining contains curvilinear or polygonal calcifications, known as *Rushton bodies* (**Fig. 5**); such structures may also be found in other odontogenic cysts, especially the dentigerous cyst.[7,8]

The cyst wall is composed of fibrous connective tissue that contains variable amounts of acute and chronic inflammation, including neutrophils, plasma cells, lymphocytes, histiocytes, and (rarely) eosinophils and mast cells. Many periapical cysts also exhibit areas of hemorrhage and hemosiderin deposits (see **Fig. 4**). It is also common to observe deposits of cholesterol within the cyst wall or cyst lumen, which appear as cleft-like slits surrounded by foreign-body type giant cells (**Fig. 6**).

Because many periapical lesions are friable, they are submitted as multiple granulation tissue fragments that are not grossly suggestive of a cystic lesion. If a focal epithelial lining can be identified microscopically, a diagnosis of periapical cyst usually is made. If no epithelial lining is identified, such a lesion is classified as a periapical granuloma. Admittedly, this distinction between a periapical cyst with only focal epithelial lining versus a periapical granuloma is arbitrary. Because these two entities represent variants of the same basic inflammatory process, the choice of names should not affect treatment or prognosis.

Periapical Cyst: Differential Diagnosis

Although the presence of significant inflammation in a jaw cyst may suggest the diagnosis, the

Fig. 1. Periapical cyst. Well-circumscribed unilocular radiolucency located at the apex of the left maxillary lateral incisor.

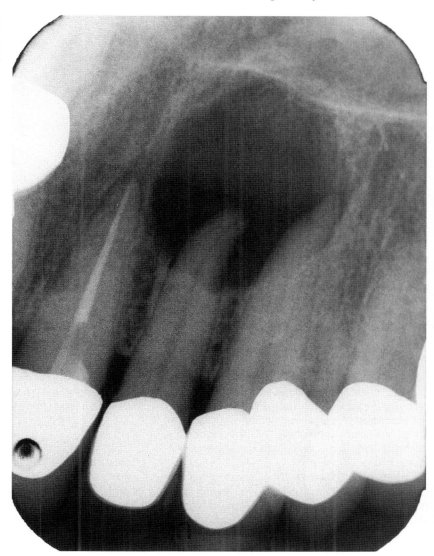

Fig. 2. Periapical cyst. Well-circumscribed sac-like structure that contains yellowish cholesterol debris in the cyst lumen.

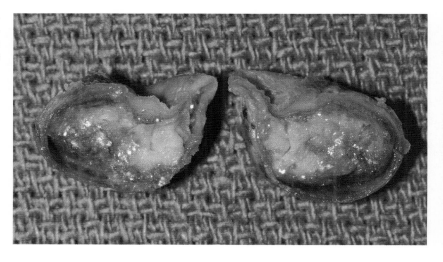

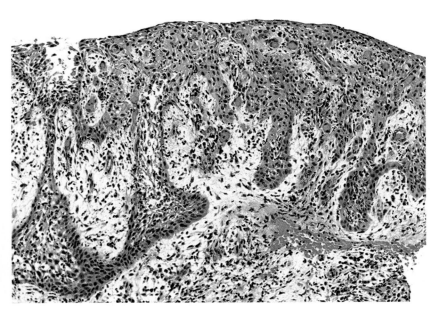

Fig. 3. Periapical cyst. Non-specific stratified squamous epithelial lining that shows irregular hyperplasia of the rete ridges.

microscopic appearance of a periapical cyst is not specific; therefore, a pathologist usually must rely on a good clinical/radiographic history to support the diagnosis. An inflamed dentigerous cyst can show irregular hyperplasia of the squamous epithelial lining that is indistinguishable from a periapical cyst.

Likewise, an inflamed odontogenic keratocyst (OKC) may lose its characteristic features in areas of inflammation. Usually, however, typical features of OKC can still be identified in some areas, including

(1) uniform thickness of approximately 5 to 8 cells, (2) cuboidal/columnar basal cells with nuclear palisading, and (3) wavy, corrugated parakeratin surface.

Periapical Cyst: Prognosis

Periapical cysts can be treated either by conventional root canal therapy or by extraction of the associated tooth with curettage of the lesion. Although root canal therapy is successful in most cases, some lesions persist and require

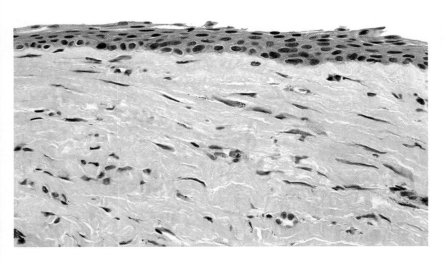

Fig. 4. Periapical cyst. Non-inflamed areas of the cyst may be lined by thinner stratified squamous epithelium. Scattered brown hemosiderin deposits can be seen in the cyst wall.

Fig. 5. Periapical cyst. Bright red curvilinear Rushton bodies within the epithelial lining.

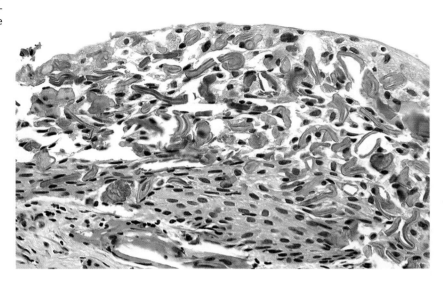

retreatment, surgical endodontic therapy, or extraction of the tooth.

If a tooth is extracted but the lesion is not curetted from the socket, a periapical cyst may persist within the alveolar bone as a well-circumscribed radiolucent defect. Such a lesion, known as *residual cyst*, is microscopically similar to the periapical cyst and should be treated by surgical curettage.

Fig. 6. Periapical cyst. The cyst wall contains multiple cholesterol clefts that are surrounded by foreign-body giant cells.

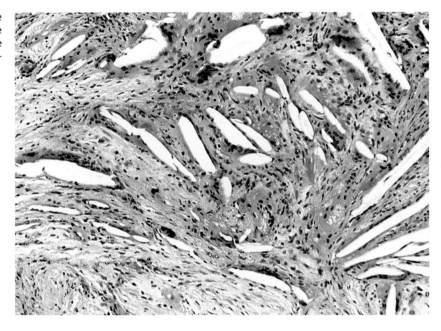

DENTIGEROUS CYST (FOLLICULAR CYST)

After formation of the tooth enamel is completed, the enamel organ epithelium remains as a thin layer of cells (reduced enamel epithelium) surrounding the crown of the unerupted tooth. If normal eruption occurs, the reduced enamel epithelium merges with the surface alveolar mucosal epithelium to form the initial gingival crevicular lining surrounding the tooth. If the tooth is impacted and cannot erupt, then fluid may accumulate between the reduced enamel epithelium and tooth crown to form a dentigerous cyst (**Fig. 7**).

As logic dictates, dentigerous cysts develop around those teeth that are most frequently impacted. The most commonly involved tooth is the mandibular third molar, followed by the maxillary canine, mandibular premolars, and the maxillary third molar.[9] They can occur in association, however, with any unerupted tooth.

Dentigerous cysts are the second most common odontogenic cyst, accounting for 18% to 24% of jaw cysts submitted for microscopic examination.[10,11] Dentigerous cysts can occur at any age, although they are most frequently discovered in teenagers and young adults. Most are asymptomatic and discovered during routine dental radiographic examination. On rare occasions, a large dentigerous cyst may cause visible bony expansion or result in secondary pain and infection.

Dentigerous Cyst: Gross Features

By definition, a dentigerous cyst develops around the crown of an unerupted tooth. In most instances, the tooth is removed in conjunction with the surrounding cyst. If a tooth is submitted as part of the specimen, the cyst typically is attached to the tooth at the junction of the enamel crown and the root (cementoenamel junction), with the crown protruding into the cyst lumen (**Fig. 8**). Frequently, however, an impacted tooth must be surgically sectioned to facilitate its removal, and no tooth or only small fragments of tooth structure may be submitted with the specimen. In such cases, a good clinical history or radiograph may be necessary to allow definitive diagnosis.

Dentigerous Cyst: Microscopic Features

Dentigerous cysts show a variable microscopic appearance depending on whether any secondary inflammation is present.[9,12] A noninflamed dentigerous cyst is usually lined by a thin layer of nonkeratinizing epithelium that is 2 to 4 cells thick (**Fig. 9**). The interface between the epithelium and cyst wall is flat and devoid of rete ridges. The cyst wall is composed of loose to moderately dense fibrous connective tissue, which often includes scattered, small odontogenic epithelial rests that represent remnants of the dental lamina epithelium. Sometimes, these rests undergo dystrophic calcification. Although the dentigerous cyst is considered developmental in nature, many contain a mild to sometimes heavy chronic inflammatory cell infiltrate in the cyst wall—especially those cases that are associated with a partially erupted tooth. In such instances, the

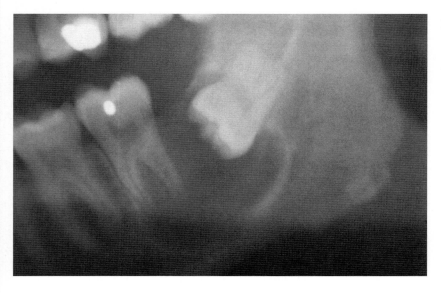

Fig. 7. Dentigerous cyst. Well-circumscribed unilocular radiolucency surrounding the crown of the impacted left mandibular third molar.

Fig. 8. Dentigerous cyst. The cyst surrounds the crown of the tooth and is attached at the cementoenamel junction.

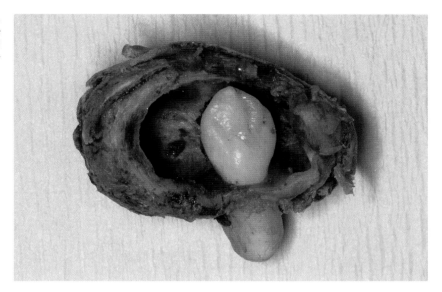

epithelial lining often demonstrates irregular hyperplasia of rete ridges (**Fig. 10**).

The epithelial lining may also include scattered mucin-producing cells, which are indicative of the pluripotentiality of the odontogenic epithelium (**Fig. 11**).[6,13] In rare instances, cilia and sebaceous glands have even been reported. Finding mucous cells in a dentigerous cyst lining is not thought clinically significant, although some investigators have pointed out that the ability to undergo glandular differentiation suggests that odontogenic epithelium may be the source of rare cases of intraosseous mucoepidermoid carcinomas of the jaws.

Occasional dentigerous cysts exhibit irregular linear and polygonal calcifications within the

Fig. 9. Dentigerous cyst. The cyst is lined by a thin layer of stratified squamous epithelium.

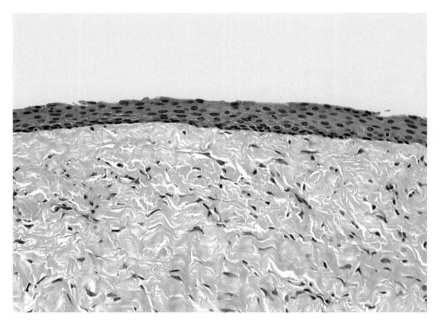

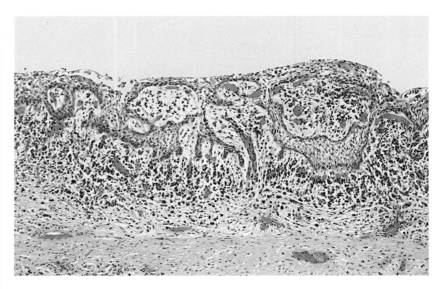

Fig. 10. Dentigerous cyst. The presence of inflammation may result in irregular hyperplasia of the epithelial lining.

epithelial lining (Rushton bodies).[7,8] These structures are not specific, however, for dentigerous cysts and they may be found in other odontogenic cysts, especially the periapical cyst (see **Fig. 5**).

Dentigerous Cyst: Differential Diagnosis

OKCs often occur in association with an impacted tooth and must be distinguished from a simple dentigerous cyst. OKCs show a more uniform epithelial lining ranging from approximately 5 to 8 cells in thickness. The basal cell layer is characterized by a palisaded row of hyperchromatic cuboidal/columnar cells. The epithelial surface produces parakeratin that typically demonstrates a wavy, corrugated appearance. Desquamated keratin may be found in the cyst lumen.

OOCs are another keratinizing jaw cyst often associated with an impacted tooth. They can be

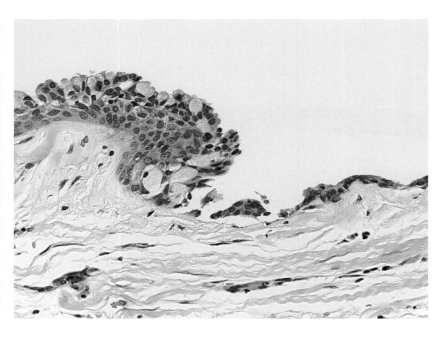

Fig. 11. Dentigerous cyst. Scattered mucin-producing cells are present within the epithelial lining.

distinguished by the presence of surface orthokeratin production associated with a prominent granular cell layer. Unlike odontogenic keratocysts, the basal layer does not exhibit a regular palisaded arrangement.

Inflamed dentigerous cysts may be impossible to distinguish microscopically from other inflamed odontogenic cysts, such as the common periapical (radicular) cyst that arises at the apex of a nonvital tooth. The presence of scattered small rests of dental lamina epithelium in the cyst wall may suggest that the lesion was associated with the pericoronal tooth follicle, thereby favoring a diagnosis of dentigerous cyst. The final diagnosis in such cases often relies, however, on a good clinical history and radiograph indicating the exact source of the tissue.

Because a unicystic ameloblastoma may be associated with an impacted tooth, it is important to distinguish this tumor from the more common dentigerous cyst. At low power, the most suggestive feature of ameloblastoma is nuclear hyperchromatism of the basal cell layer of the cystic lining. These basilar cells exhibit a columnar shape and frequently show reverse nuclear polarization, in which the nuclei are pulled away from the basement membrane. The cytoplasm beneath the nuclei often exhibits a vacuolated appearance. The spinous cell layer may exhibit a loosely cohesive pattern that resembles the stellate reticulum of the enamel organ epithelium.

Dentigerous Cyst: Diagnosis

The microscopic features of the dentigerous cyst may not necessarily be pathognomonic. Therefore, a good clinical history and radiographic correlation are often important to confirm the association of the lesion with the crown of an impacted tooth and allow a definite diagnosis.

One dilemma is trying to distinguish a small dentigerous cyst microscopically from an enlarged dental follicle around an unerupted tooth crown.[14] When the dental follicle around an unerupted tooth is examined microscopically, it is lined by remnants of a thin, and often fragmented, layer of flattened cuboidal and eosinophilic columnar cells that represent part of the reduced enamel epithelium. A pathologist is often unable to determine if an actual cystic space was present between this lining and the tooth crown. This distinction is often an academic exercise, however, that does not affect patient treatment or prognosis. The most important consideration is the ability to rule out potentially more aggressive odontogenic lesions, such as OKC and ameloblastoma.

Dentigerous Cyst: Prognosis

A dentigerous cyst is treated by surgical removal, which usually includes extraction of the associated unerupted tooth. Recurrence is exceedingly rare.

ODONTOGENIC KERATOCYST (KERATOCYSTIC ODONTOGENIC TUMOR)

OKCs are common developmental odontogenic cysts, which are known for locally aggressive potential and high recurrence rate. They are thought to arise from remnants of the dental lamina epithelium. In recent years, some investigators have suggested that OKCs should be reclassified as cystic neoplasms based on increased expression of proliferating cell nuclear antigen, Ki-67, and p53 protein in comparison with other odontogenic cysts.[15,16] In addition, evidence of PTCH gene mutation has been demonstrated in OKCs associated with nevoid basal cell carcinoma syndrome (NBCCS) and some sporadic OKCs. Accordingly, the most recent World Health Organization (WHO) classification uses the term, keratocystic odontogenic tumor, as the preferred designation.[1] The term, odontogenic keratocyst, however, is well established and remains the name favored by the authors.

OKCs can occur at any age, although more than half of all cases develop in the second through fourth decades of life.[16–18] Approximately two-thirds of all cases occur in the mandible, with a predilection for the molar/ramus region. Maxillary cases also are more common in the posterior area of the jaw. Rare peripheral OKCs have been reported in the gingival soft tissues.[19,20]

Small OKCs are usually asymptomatic lesions that are discovered on routine dental radiographic examination. Larger OKCs may be associated with bony expansion, although some large OKCs can produce significant bone destruction without obvious clinical swelling. On rare occasions, pain and drainage may occur. Radiographically, OKCs can present as either a unilocular or multilocular radiolucency, usually with a smooth, well-defined border (**Fig. 12**).

The clinical and radiographic appearance of OKCs can mimic a variety of other odontogenic cysts and tumors. From 25% to 40% are associated with an impacted tooth and may resemble a dentigerous cyst (**Fig. 13**). Interradicular cysts are indistinguishable from the lateral periodontal cyst.[21] OKCs of the maxillary midline region may be clinically mistaken for nasopalatine duct cysts.[22] Sometimes a cyst developed at the site where a tooth failed to develop (usually a mandibular third molar). Although these lesions historically were called *primordial*

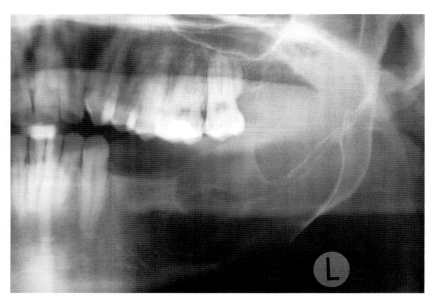

Fig. 12. Odontogenic keratocyst. Destructive multilocular radiolucency of the left posterior mandible.

cysts, such lesions almost always prove to be OKCs microscopically and they should be classified as such.

Odontogenic Keratocyst: Gross Features

OKCs usually have a thin, friable wall, which may make it difficult for surgeons to enucleate the lesion intact. The cyst lumen is often filled with creamy or cheesy keratin debris but may contain clear liquid (**Fig. 14**).

Odontogenic Keratocyst: Microscopic Features

OKCs are lined by a uniform layer of stratified squamous epithelium that is approximately 5 to 8 cells thick.[23–25] The interface between the epithelium and cyst wall is usually flat without rete ridges. The regular, uniform nature of the epithelial lining usually allows the diagnosis to be suspected at low-power examination (**Fig. 15**). It is not unusual for the epithelial lining to separate from the connective tissue wall.

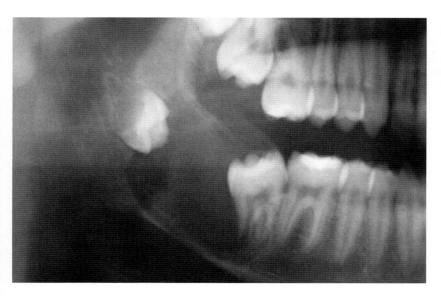

Fig. 13. Odontogenic keratocyst. Well-circumscribed radiolucent lesion associated with two impacted teeth. (*Courtesy of* Dr Kevin Riker.)

Fig. 14. Odontogenic keratocyst. The cyst aspirate may contain cheesy keratin debris.

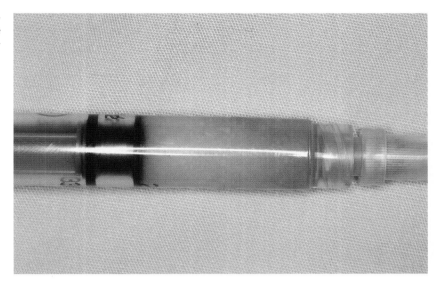

The basal epithelial layer is composed of cuboidal to columnar cells that tend to be palisaded and hyperchromatic (**Fig. 16**). A thin, flattened, corrugated layer of parakeratin is produced on the epithelial surface. Desquamated keratin may also be found in the cyst lumen. In spite of its name, some OKCs exhibit only a minimal amount of luminal keratin production. Occasional OKCs also produce areas of orthokeratin in association with a subjacent granular cell layer; however, wavy surface parakeratin production should predominate.

The fibrous cyst wall often contains scattered small odontogenic epithelial rests consistent with remnants of dental lamina epithelium. Some of these epithelial islands may proliferate to form smaller keratin-filled daughter cysts adjacent to the main cystic lining. Rarely, cartilage formation has been described in the wall of an OKC.[26]

Although OKCs are a developmental cyst, many still are characterized by a significant amount of chronic inflammation in the cyst wall.[27] The epithelium in these inflamed areas may lose its

Fig. 15. Odontogenic keratocyst. The cyst is lined by a uniform layer of stratified squamous epithelium that may range from 5 to 8 cells in thickness. Note the separation of epithelium from the cyst wall.

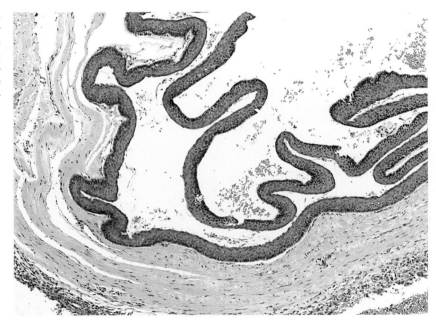

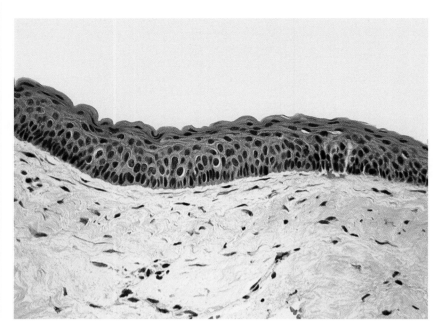

Fig. 16. Odontogenic keratocyst. The basal layer consists of a palisaded row of hyperchromatic columnar cells. A thin, corrugated layer of parakeratin is produced on the epithelial surface.

characteristic features, becoming irregular and hyperplastic (**Fig. 17**). Therefore, if the tissue sample comes from an inflamed part of the lesion, it may be indistinguishable from other inflamed odontogenic cysts.

Odontogenic Keratocyst: Differential Diagnosis

Because OKCs often develop in association with an impacted tooth, they may be confused clinically

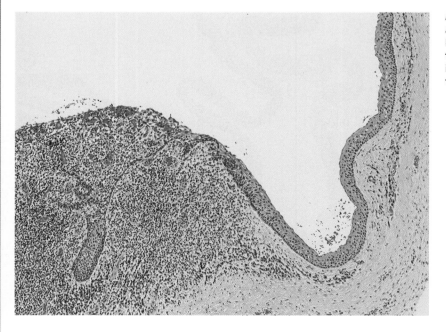

Fig. 17. Odontogenic keratocyst. The epithelial lining may lose its characteristic microscopic features in areas of chronic inflammation.

with dentigerous cysts. Dentigerous cysts, however, do not exhibit the regular, palisaded arrangement of cuboidal/columnar basilar cells or the corrugated surface layer of parakeratin. Although OOCs also produce keratin, this keratin consists of orthokeratin that is associated with a subjacent granular cell layer. In addition, the basilar layer of OOCS do not exhibit nuclear palisading.

Cystic ameloblastomas demonstrate a palisaded layer of columnar basal cells that could mimic an OKC. The basilar cells of the ameloblastoma, however, usually are more hyperchromatic and demonstrate areas with reverse polarization, in which the nuclei are pulled away from the basement membrane. Also, upper epithelial layers of a cystic ameloblastoma are loosely arranged, reminiscent of the stellate reticulum of the enamel organ.

Odontogenic Keratocyst: Prognosis

OKCs are locally aggressive lesions that may be difficult to remove intact because of the thin, friable nature of the lining. The overall prognosis is generally good, although it is estimated that 25% to 30% of OKCs recur. Sometimes such recurrences may not be noted until 10 years or longer after initial removal, so long-term follow-up is necessary. In rare instances, aggressive maxillary OKCs have been reported to extend up to the base of the skull.[28]

Most OKCs are treated by surgical enucleation. If a surgeon suspects or already knows that the lesion is a keratocyst, then more aggressive curettage or peripheral ostectomy with a bone bur often

is attempted to reduce the chance of recurrence. On rare occasions, en bloc resection may be performed for larger, more-aggressive OKCs.

Larger cysts also can often be managed effectively by decompression, in which a polyethylene tube is inserted into the cyst lumen, allowing for a gradual reduction in the size of the lesion before surgery.[29] This technique also results in a thicker cystic lining that is easier to curette from the bony cavity. Pathologists should be aware, however, that decompression also induces more inflammation in the cyst wall, which may alter the characteristic diagnostic features of OKCs.

Most OKCs occur as isolated lesions unrelated to any other problems. Some OKCs may be associated, however, with a hereditary condition— NBCCS or Gorlin syndrome.[30–32] NBCCS is inherited as an autosomal dominant trait caused by a mutation of patched, a tumor suppressor gene that has been mapped to chromosome 9q22.3-q31. This condition may be associated with a wide range of clinical features, including multiple basal cell carcinomas of the skin, frontoparietal bossing, pitting defects of the palms and soles, calcification of the falx cerebri, and bifid ribs. The presence of multiple OKCs in any patient

Key Features
ODONTOGENIC KERATOCYST

1. Uniform stratified squamous epithelial lining that is approximately 5–8 cells thick

2. Interface of the epithelium with the cyst wall is flat and devoid of rete ridges

3. Epithelium may separate from the cyst wall

4. Cuboidal/columnar basal cells with palisading of nuclei

5. Wavy, corrugated surface parakeratin layer

6. Desquamated keratin may be found in cyst lumen

7. Smaller daughter cysts may be found in cyst wall

Pitfalls
ODONTOGENIC KERATOCYST

! Not all OKCs produce significant amounts of keratin in the cyst lumen.

! Not all odontogenic cysts that produce keratin are OKCs (eg, orthokeratinized odontogenic cyst).

! Characteristic diagnostic features of OKC (eg, palisaded cuboidal/columnar basilar layer and corrugated parakeratin surface) may be lost in areas of inflammation.

! Noninflamed dentigerous cysts can also exhibit a regular, uniform epithelial lining that might be confused with an OKC; however, such cysts do not demonstrate other characteristic features of OKC (eg, palisaded cuboidal/columnar basilar layer and corrugated parakeratin surface).

! The columnar basilar cells and nuclear palisading of OKCs could be confused with a cystic ameloblastoma; however, these basilar cells are not as intensely hyperchromatic as ameloblastic epithelium nor do they typically demonstrate reverse polarization of nuclei.

is highly suspicious for NBCCS. Any patient with an OKC should be evaluated clinically for the possibility of NBCCS, especially because these cysts are often the first sign leading to diagnosis of this condition.

ORTHOKERATINIZED ODONTOGENIC CYST

When originally described, orthokeratinized odontogenic cysts (OOCs) were viewed as a microscopic variant of the more common OKCs. It was soon recognized, however, that this cyst exhibits different clinical and microscopic features that warrant its separation from OKCs.[33–35]

From 66% to 90% of OOCs occur in the mandible, and the lesion shows a predilection for the posterior area of both jaws. Approximately two-thirds of cases are associated with an impacted tooth and, therefore, resemble a dentigerous cyst radiographically. The lesion usually appears as a well-circumscribed unilocular radiolucency but can be multilocular.

Orthokeratinized Odontogenic Cyst: Gross Features

The gross features of OOCs are similar to other odontogenic cysts, such as dentigerous cysts or odontogenic keratocysts. Because of the keratinizing features, the lumen may be filled with creamy or thickened keratinaceous material.

Orthokeratinized Odontogenic Cyst: Microscopic Features

OOCs are lined by a thin layer of stratified squamous epithelium that produces a variable amount of

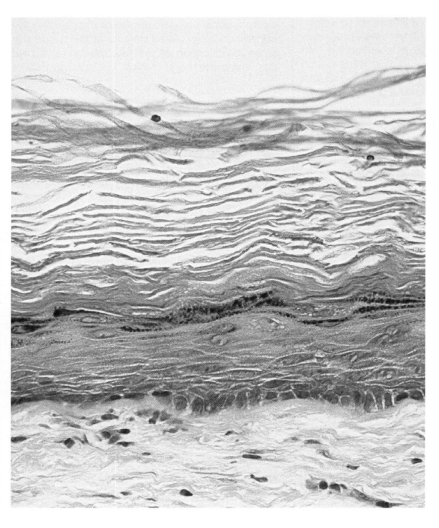

Fig. 18. Orthokeratinized odontogenic cyst. The epithelium produces orthokeratin with an associated granular cell layer. In contrast to odontogenic keratocysts, the basilar cells do not exhibit a palisaded arrangement.

orthokeratin on the surface.[33-35] This orthokeratin production is typically associated with a prominent granular cell layer (**Fig. 18**). Rarely, sebaceous differentiation has been reported.[36]

Orthokeratinized Odontogenic Cyst: Differential Diagnosis

OOCs are most likely to be confused microscopically with OKCs. OKCs, however, exhibit a corrugated parakeratin surface without a subjacent granular cell layer. In addition, the basal cell layer of OKCs typically consists of a palisaded row of cuboidal/columnar cells—a feature not observed in the OOC. When compared with OKCs, immunohistochemical analysis of OOCs shows less expression of Ki-67 and p53.[35]

Orthokeratinized Odontogenic Cyst: Prognosis

OOCs are usually treated by surgical enucleation. Approximately 2% of these lesions have been reported to recur, which is markedly lower than the 25% to 30% recurrence rate for OKCs.[34] The distinction between these two types of lesions is also supported by the observation that OOCs have not been found associated with NBCCS.

LATERAL PERIODONTAL CYST/GINGIVAL CYST OF THE ADULT (BOTRYOID ODONTOGENIC CYST)

Lateral periodontal cysts are uncommon developmental cysts that occur within bone between the roots of the teeth. Gingival cysts of the adult are essentially the same lesion, except that they occur within the gingival soft tissues. Although these cysts are traditionally given separate names, they both arise from remnants of the dental lamina epithelium and represent the same entity, differing only in clinical location.[37] Some cysts occur partially within bone and partially in soft tissue, making exact designation somewhat arbitrary. Neither is related to gingival or periodontal inflammation.

Although these cysts are considered developmental in nature, they usually do not occur until middle age or older.[37-40] Both cysts show a striking predilection for the canine/premolar region of the mandible, accounting for nearly two-thirds of all cases. Maxillary cysts show a similar site predilection. Most other cysts occur farther anterior in the incisor region of both jaws. It is rare for this lesion to develop in the molar region.

Many lateral periodontal cysts are discovered during routine dental radiographic examination as a well-circumscribed unilocular radiolucency between the roots of two teeth (**Fig. 19**). If the teeth have already been extracted, it is possible for the lesion to develop in an edentulous location. Most cysts measure less than 1 cm in diameter, although some cysts can become larger and result in painless clinical expansion of the alveolar bone. Less frequently, the lesion may be polycystic, resulting in a multilocular radiographic appearance (botryoid odontogenic cyst).[41-43]

The gingival cyst of the adult usually appears as a tense, fluid-filled nodule on the facial gingiva or alveolar mucosa (**Fig. 20**). Because of the fluid contents, the lesion may exhibit a bluish discoloration.

Lateral Periodontal Cyst/Gingival Cyst of the Adult: Gross Features

If a lateral periodontal cyst is removed intact, it appears as a round, well-circumscribed, fluid-filled mass. On bisection, watery fluid is released, revealing a thin membranous wall (**Fig. 21**). Botryoid cases may show a bosselated surface resembling a cluster of grapes with a polycystic internal structure.

Gingival cysts of the adult are usually removed as a mucosal wedge that includes the overlying surface epithelium. On bisection, a central cystic cavity may be appreciated, although it may rupture and collapse on surgical removal.

Lateral Periodontal Cyst/Gingival Cyst of the Adult: Microscopic Features

Both variants are lined primarily by a thin, flattened layer of epithelium that is only 1 to 3 cells thick.[37-39] This epithelium, often demonstrates occasional nodular, plaque-like thickenings composed of cells that may show a somewhat swirling pattern (**Fig. 22**). These thickenings frequently include cells with clear cytoplasm due to the presence of abundant glycogen. The cyst wall often contains similar small nests of glycogen-rich clear cells, which represent remnants of dental lamina epithelium (**Fig. 23**). The microscopic variant, known as the *botryoid odontogenic cyst*, shows multiple cystic spaces with a similar epithelial lining.[41-43]

Lateral Periodontal Cyst/Gingival Cyst of the Adult: Differential Diagnosis

The microscopic appearance of a lateral periodontal cyst or gingival cyst of the adult is characteristic; diagnosis is usually easily made, especially with the support of a good clinical history and radiograph. Glandular odontogenic cysts (GOCs) can exhibit some of the same

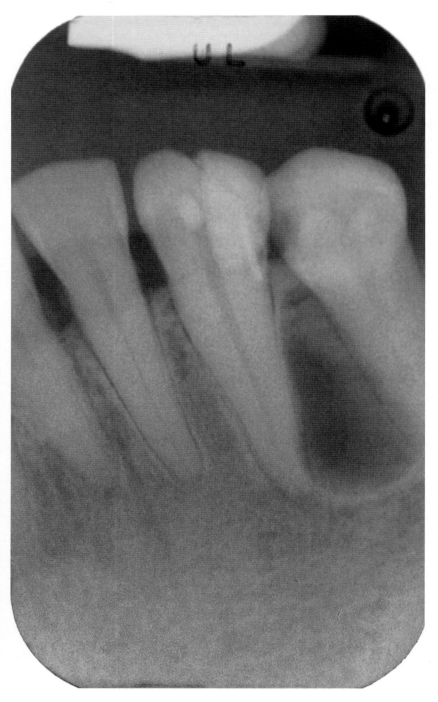

Fig. 19. Lateral periodontal cyst. Dental radiograph showing a well-circumscribed radiolucency between the mandibular canine and first premolar. (*Courtesy of* Dr Ty Sumner.)

Fig. 20. Gingival cyst of the adult. Slightly translucent, fluid-filled nodule on the mandibular gingiva between the canine and first premolar.

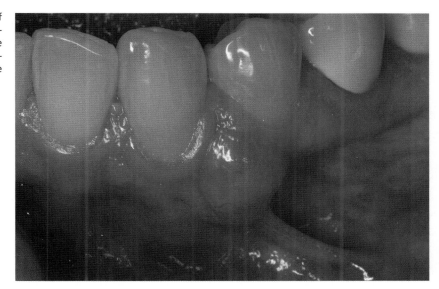

features as a lateral periodontal cyst, including the presence of nodular thickenings of the epithelial lining. GOCs, however, also show surface columnar cells, mucous cells, and intraepithelial gland–like structures.

The gingival cyst of the adult often collapses on removal, releasing its fluid contents. Because the collapsed cyst demonstrates a thin epithelial lining that may be only 1 to 2 cells thick, it is easy to mistake such a cyst for a dilated blood vessel or varix.

Fig. 21. Lateral periodontal cyst. Photograph of a gross specimen demonstrating the thinness of the cyst wall.

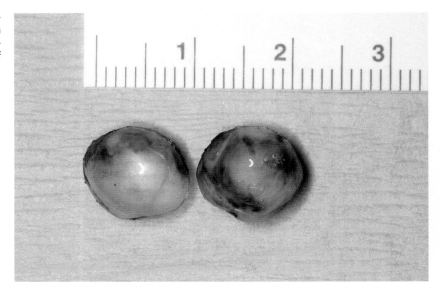

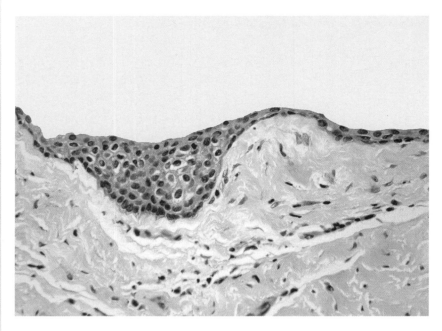

Fig. 22. Lateral periodontal cyst. Thin cystic lining showing a nodular, plaque-like epithelial thickening with clear cells.

Lateral Periodontal Cyst/Gingival Cyst of the Adult: Prognosis

Both lateral periodontal cysts and gingival cysts of the adult are treated with conservative surgical enucleation or excision. Recurrence is rare for simple, isolated lesions. Occasional botryoid odontogenic cysts recur, presumably due to their larger size and multilocular presentation, which makes adequate curettage more difficult.[43]

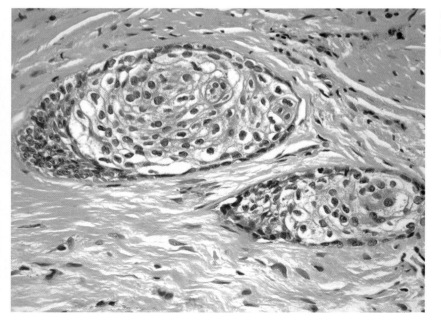

Fig. 23. Lateral periodontal cyst. Nests of glycogen-rich clear cells in the cyst wall.

GLANDULAR ODONTOGENIC CYST (SIALO-ODONTOGENIC CYST)

GOCs are a rare, developmental cyst of odontogenic origin that is characterized by glandular or salivary differentiation. The lesion occurs most frequently in middle-aged adults, with approximately 70% of cases found in the mandible.[44–47] The most common site is the anterior mandible, and the lesion often crosses the midline. The size can vary from small unilocular radiolucencies to large, expansile multilocular lesions that can destroy much of the jaw (**Fig. 24**).

Glandular Odontogenic Cyst: Microscopic Features

GOCs can show a variety of microscopic patterns. The lining consists primarily of stratified squamous epithelium, although the surface layer tends to be composed of cuboidal to columnar cells, which may impart a somewhat papillary or hobnail appearance (**Fig. 25**).[44–46] Scattered mucin-producing cells may be present as well as intraepithelial gland–like spaces that contain mucinous material. On occasion, cilia are observed on the epithelial surface. Many GOCs exhibit focal nodular epithelial thickenings where the cells exhibit a slightly swirling appearance (**Fig. 26**). This pattern is similar to the characteristic plaque-like epithelial thickenings observed in the lateral periodontal cyst, supporting the concept that the GOC is also of odontogenic origin. Usually no significant inflammation is noted.

Glandular Odontogenic Cyst: Differential Diagnosis

Because GOCs are characterized by squamous epithelium, mucin production, and gland-like spaces, distinction from a low-grade central mucoepidermoid carcinoma of the jaws can sometimes be challenging.[47,48] Low-grade mucoepidermoid carcinoma usually exhibits solid tumor islands in addition to cystic spaces. The presence of nodular, plaque-like epithelial thickenings also helps support a diagnosis of GOC versus mucoepidermoid carcinoma. Low-grade mucoepidermoid carcinomas show expression of cytokeratins 18 and 19 more frequently than do GOCs, whereas Ki-67 labeling in low-grade mucoepidermoid carcinomas is lower than in GOCs.[47] Because these markers show a large overlap in expression, their value in any single case is limited.

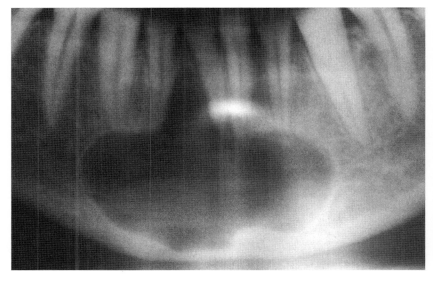

Fig. 24. Glandular odontogenic cyst. Well-defined radiolucent area of bone destruction in the anterior mandible crossing the midline. (*Courtesy of* Dr Carol Gallagher.)

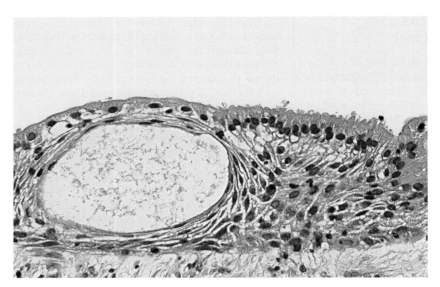

Fig. 25. Glandular odontogenic cyst. The cystic lining is composed primarily of stratified squamous epithelium, although the surface layer is consists of cuboidal/columnar cells. An intraepithelial gland–like space containing mucinous material is noted on the left side.

If a biopsy specimen of a GOC includes only areas of thin epithelial lining with occasional epithelial thickenings, the lesion could easily be confused with a lateral periodontal cyst. Examination of the entire specimen should reveal more typical features, such as surface cuboidal/columnar cells and intraepithelial gland–like spaces.

Glandular Odontogenic Cyst: Prognosis

GOCs have the potential for significant growth and bone destruction. The recurrence rate has been estimated at approximately 30% of all cases, higher in larger multilocular cases. Depending on the size of the lesion, treatment usually consists of either aggressive curettage or en bloc resection.

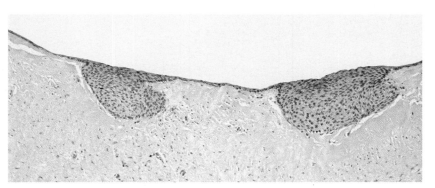

Fig. 26. Glandular odontogenic cyst. Some areas of the epithelial lining may exhibit nodular, plaque-like thickenings similar to the lateral periodontal cyst.

ODONTOGENIC TUMORS

TUMORS OF ODONTOGENIC EPITHELIUM

Ameloblastoma

Ameloblastomas are among the most frequently encountered odontogenic neoplasms. They are well known for characteristic histopathologic features and often locally aggressive behavior. They are tumors of odontogenic epithelium, potentially originating from dental lamina rests, the developing enamel organ, the epithelial lining of an odontogenic cyst, or the basilar epithelial cells of the gingival surface epithelium. The ameloblastoma exhibits a microscopic resemblance to the enamel organ of a developing tooth. In particular, tumor cells within ameloblastomas may mimic the inner enamel epithelium and central stellate reticulum of the enamel organ.

The following major clinicopathologic subtypes are discussed: conventional solid or multicystic, unicystic, and peripheral.

Conventional solid or multicystic ameloblastoma

Approximately 90% of ameloblastomas represent the conventional solid or multicystic type. The average age at diagnosis is 36 years, although the tumor may occur over a broad age range.[49,50] Childhood tumors are rare. There is no strong gender or ethnic predilection, although some studies suggest an increased frequency in blacks. Approximately 85% of conventional ameloblastomas arise in the mandible, particularly in the molar/ascending ramus area. Maxillary tumors also favor the posterior region.[51,52] Additional possible sites of involvement include the maxillary sinus and nasal cavity, with sinonasal lesions exhibiting a predilection for older men.[53]

Patients most commonly present with a bony hard, painless swelling. Pain occasionally may occur. Smaller lesions may be detected incidentally during routine radiographic examination. Conventional ameloblastomas may appear as well-defined, unilocular, or multilocular radiolucencies. Multilocular lesions can exhibit either a soap bubble or honeycomb appearance (large or small loculations) (**Fig. 27**). Many cases are associated with the crowns of unerupted teeth, especially mandibular third molars. Adjacent teeth may exhibit resorption or mobility.

The uncommon desmoplastic variant is unusual in that it tends to arise in the anterior region of the maxilla or mandible and often appears as an ill-defined, mixed radiolucency-radiopacity. Its radiographic appearance may mimic that of a benign fibro-osseous lesion.

Conventional solid or multicystic ameloblastoma:

Gross Features The tumor appears as an intraosseous growth with solid and/or cystic areas in varying proportions.

Conventional solid or multicystic ameloblastoma:

Microscopic features Conventional ameloblastomas are solid infiltrative tumors with a tendency for cyst formation. The amount of cyst formation is variable, and both microcysts and macrocysts are possible. The most common growth patterns are follicular and plexiform. Less common histopathologic variants include acanthomatous, granular cell, desmoplastic, and basal cell types.

Follicular variant There are islands of odontogenic epithelium within a mature fibrous stroma. The islands exhibit a peripheral layer of columnar cells with reverse polarization (nuclei oriented away from the basement membrane) and vacuolated cytoplasm (**Fig. 28**); these features are reminiscent

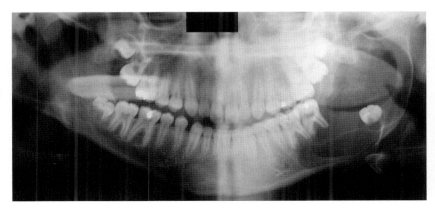

Fig. 27. Ameloblastoma. Large multilocular radiolucency of the posterior mandible. The loculations exhibit a soap bubble appearance, and adjacent teeth exhibit root resorption.

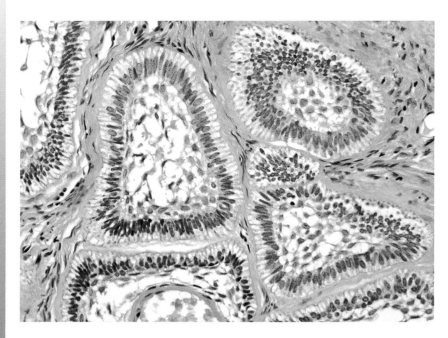

Fig. 28. Conventional ameloblastoma, follicular variant. Islands of odontogenic epithelium. The cells at the periphery of the tumor islands are columnar with reverse polarization of their nuclei and vacuolated cytoplasm. The cells within the center of the tumor islands are angular and loosely arranged, with stellate reticulum–like differentiation.

of ameloblasts. The peripheral cell layer also may include basaloid cuboidal cells without prominent reverse polarization. The central portion of the islands is comprised of loosely arranged, angular cells resembling the stellate reticulum of the enamel organ of a developing tooth. Cyst formation is commonly found within central portions of the epithelial islands.

Plexiform variant There are long, anastomosing cords and sheets of odontogenic epithelium (**Fig. 29**). These cords and sheets exhibit a peripheral layer of columnar to cuboidal cells with reverse polarization. The background stroma is often loosely arranged and vascular. Cyst formation is less common in the plexiform variant compared with the follicular variant.

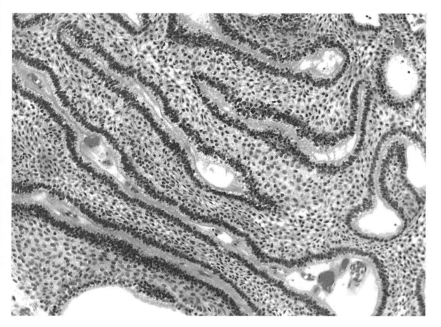

Fig. 29. Conventional ameloblastoma, plexiform variant. Long anastomosing cords of odontogenic epithelium. The peripheral cells are columnar with hyperchromatic nuclei exhibiting reverse polarization.

Acanthomatous variant There is squamous differentiation within the central portions of the tumor islands (**Fig. 30**). Keratin formation, including keratin pearls or individual cell keratinization, may be evident.

In rare cases, referred to as *keratoameloblastoma*, there is extensive keratin-filled cyst formation. Necrotic debris also may be found within these cysts. Additional possible findings within keratoameloblastomas include odontogenic keratocyst–like areas, complex arrangements of epithelial follicles and ribbons with lamellar stacks of parakeratin, and papillary projections within cystic structures (termed, *papilliferous keratoameloblastoma*).[54]

Granular cell variant There are cells with abundant eosinophilic, granular cytoplasm within the center of the tumor islands (**Fig. 31**). Ultrastructural studies have shown this granularity to correlate with high lysosome content. Increased apoptosis of tumor cells and phagocytosis of these apoptotic cells may be the underlying mechanism.[55,56]

Desmoplastic variant The background stroma is densely collagenized, although the stroma immediately surrounding the epithelial component may be more loosely arranged. The epithelial component is relatively sparse and tends to be compressed into strands or small islands (**Fig. 32**). The tumor islands characteristically exhibit irregular, stellate,

or kite-like outlines.[57] It is often difficult to appreciate a peripheral layer of columnar cells with ameloblastic differentiation. Microcysts may be found within the tumor islands.

Basal cell variant This uncommon variant closely resembles basal cell carcinoma of the skin. There are nests or islands of basaloid epithelial cells (**Fig. 33**). The cells at the periphery of the tumor nests and islands may be more cuboidal than columnar, and nuclear palisading and reverse polarization may be less prominent compared with the follicular and plexiform variants. The central portions of the tumor islands do not exhibit stellate reticulum–like differentiation.

Several of the above histopathologic growth patterns may exist within a given tumor; the dominant growth pattern determines the overall microscopic diagnosis. Neither the microscopic variant nor the relative amounts of cystic and solid areas within a conventional ameloblastoma has any bearing on treatment and prognosis.

Conventional solid or multicystic ameloblastoma:

Differential diagnosis Odontogenic epithelial rests within a dental follicle should not be confused with ameloblastoma. The epithelial rests within a dental follicle are usually much smaller than the epithelial islands within an ameloblastoma. Although rests within a follicle occasionally may demonstrate peripheral columnar cells with reverse polarization, these

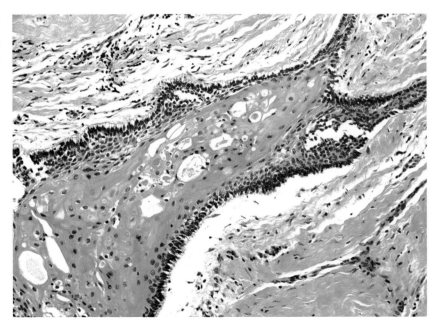

Fig. 30. Conventional ameloblastoma, acanthomatous variant. Tumor island with central squamous differentiation.

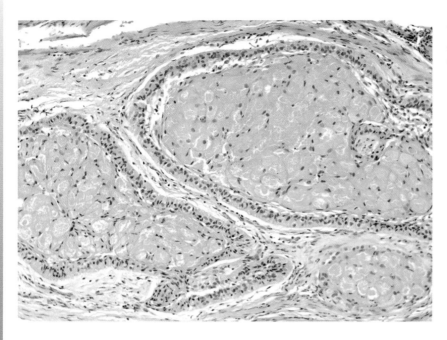

Fig. 31. Conventional ameloblastoma, granular cell variant. Tumor islands with central cells exhibiting abundant eosinophilic, granular cytoplasm.

features are found only focally. Furthermore, it is important to recognize the clinicoradiographic context. A dental follicle appears on a radiograph as a relatively thin radiolucency associated with the crown of an unerupted tooth. Microscopically, a dental follicle is comprised of fibrous connective tissue, with a mixture of dense and myxoid areas. The follicular

tissue may be lined focally by eosinophilic cuboidal to columnar epithelium (reduced enamel epithelium) (**Fig. 34**).

Dentigerous cysts exhibit a nonspecific, nonkeratinizing stratified squamous epithelial lining. Occasionally, there may be a focal suggestion of nuclear palisading within the basilar region of the

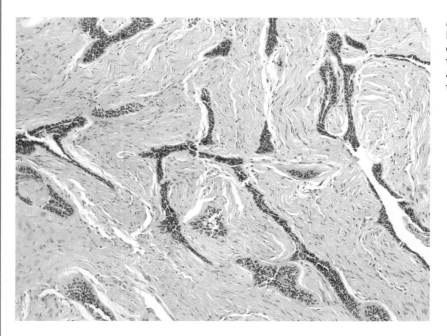

Fig. 32. Desmoplastic ameloblastoma. Compressed cords and islands of odontogenic epithelium within a dense fibrous connective tissue stroma.

Fig. 33. Conventional ameloblastoma, basal cell variant. Nests of uniform basaloid cells. The cells within the center of the nests do not exhibit stellate reticulum–like differentiation.

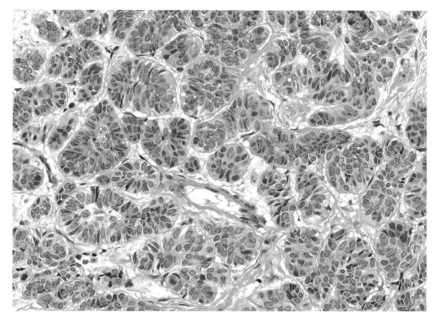

cyst lining. Such changes alone are not sufficient for a diagnosis of ameloblastoma. Additional features that should raise suspicion for ameloblastoma include the following.

1. A basal cell layer with columnar or cuboidal cells exhibiting nuclear hyperchromasia and reverse polarization

2. An edematous (or stellate reticulum–like) appearance of the more superficial epithelial layers
3. Stromal hyalinization directly beneath the epithelium (also known as inductive effect)

Additional types of odontogenic cysts or tumors with epithelium exhibiting ameloblastic differentiation include the calcifying odontogenic cyst,

Fig. 34. Dental follicle. Fibrous connective tissue with scattered odontogenic epithelial rests. A focal fragment of eosinophilic cuboidal epithelium compatible with reduced enamel epithelium also is present. The epithelial rests are small and do not exhibit ameloblastic differentiation. The connective tissue is more fibrous and the epithelium is more abundant compared with an odontogenic myxoma.

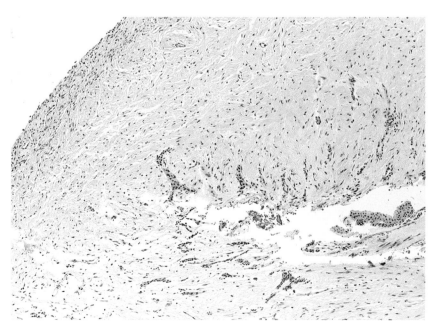

adenomatoid odontogenic tumor, ameloblastic fibroma, ameloblastic fibro-odontoma, and odontoameloblastoma. Distinguishing these entities from ameloblastoma usually is not difficult. The presence of ghost cells, calcifications, and dentinoid differentiate the calcifying odontogenic cyst from ameloblastoma. Although the adenomatoid odontogenic tumor can exhibit ductal or cystic structures lined by columnar cells with polarized nuclei, the recognition of whorled masses of epithelial cells and rosette-like structures within a scant fibrous stroma distinguishes this tumor from ameloblastoma. Also, unlike the ameloblastoma, the adenomatoid odontogenic tumor is typically well-delineated and encapsulated. Furthermore, focal calcifications may be seen in some adenomatoid odontogenic tumors, whereas ameloblastomas should not exhibit any calcifications. The ameloblastic fibroma can be readily distinguished from ameloblastoma by its characteristic primitive stroma. In addition, although the epithelial islands and cords within ameloblastic fibroma exhibit ameloblastic differentiation, the cord-like pattern is often more prominent than what is seen in ameloblastoma. Ameloblastic fibro-odontoma exhibits features similar to ameloblastic fibroma with the additional finding of disorganized tooth material, including dentin, cementum, and enamel. In contrast, by definition, ameloblastoma should not produce any tooth material or other calcified product.

The rare odontoameloblastoma also may be considered in the differential diagnosis. The biologic potential of odontoameloblastoma is similar to that of ameloblastoma. This tumor, however, microscopically exhibits not only an ameloblastoma component but also intermixed odontoma-like elements.

Cyst formation within a conventional ameloblastoma should not be confused with unicystic ameloblastoma (discussed later).

Malignant forms of ameloblastoma include malignant ameloblastoma and ameloblastic carcinoma. A malignant ameloblastoma exhibits the typical bland microscopic features of conventional ameloblastoma in both primary and metastatic components. It is recognized as malignant only by virtue of the fact that it has metastasized. The lung is the most frequent site of metastasis, although cervical lymph nodes, vertebrae, and other locations are possible. Considering that a histopathologically benign-appearing conventional ameloblastoma rarely may metastasize, some investigators prefer to regard ameloblastoma as a low-grade malignancy; however, this point of view has not gained wide acceptance. In contrast to malignant ameloblastoma, ameloblastic carcinoma exhibits microscopic features of malignancy, such as cellular and nuclear pleomorphism, increased nuclear-to-cytoplasmic ratio, hypercellularity, nuclear hyperchromatism, increased mitotic activity, and necrosis (**Fig. 35**).

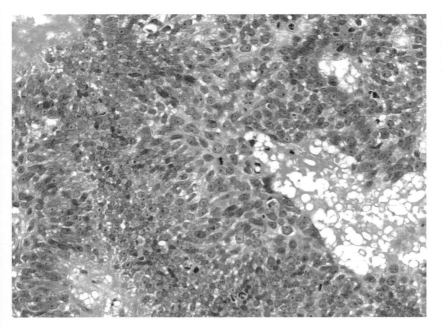

Fig. 35. Ameloblastic carcinoma. Ameloblastic tumor with cytologic atypia, hypercellularity, and frequent mitotic figures.

Conventional solid or multicystic ameloblastoma:

Diagnosis For treatment-planning purposes, it is important for pathologists to convey whether a given lesion represents a conventional solid or multicystic ameloblastoma as opposed to a unicystic or peripheral ameloblastoma. Making this distinction requires correlation of the histopathologic findings with the clinical and radiographic findings.

Conventional solid or multicystic ameloblastoma:

Prognosis Conventional ameloblastomas are benign but infiltrative and locally aggressive. Marginal or en bloc resection is the most widely used treatment. Many surgeons advocate bony margins extending at least 1 cm to 1.5 cm beyond the radiographic limits of a tumor. If there is extension into soft tissue, then there should be at least one soft tissue plane of clearance surrounding a lesion.

Most patients do not die of disease, although the lesion potentially may be fatal if it is allowed to spread to adjacent vital structures. Lesions arising in the posterior maxilla are particularly dangerous, because they may be difficult to resect with adequate margins and may invade through the relatively thin cortical plate into the pterygomaxillary fossa, cranial cavity, sinonasal tract, infratemporal fossa, and orbit.

Reported recurrence rates vary widely. In their large-scale review, Reichart and colleagues[49] reported a recurrence rate of 17% with radical treatment and 35% with conservative treatment. In some series, the recurrence rate after conservative treatment has been as high as 55% to 90%.[58,59] Although most recurrences are detected within 5 years of initial treatment, late recurrences diagnosed after a decade or more are not uncommon. Therefore, lifelong follow-up is recommended. Malignant transformation is rare.

Unicystic ameloblastoma

The unicystic ameloblastoma is a distinct clinicopathologic subtype of ameloblastoma. This subtype accounts for approximately 6% of all ameloblastomas.[49] In their original description of unicystic ameloblastoma, Robinson and Martinez[60] reported a group of cystic lesions with ameloblastic epithelial lining but less aggressive behavior than conventional ameloblastoma. They theorized that these lesions may have arisen de novo, by neoplastic transformation of non-neoplastic odontogenic cyst lining, or by cystic degeneration of a previously solid ameloblastoma.

Compared with conventional ameloblastomas, unicystic ameloblastomas occur in a younger age group, with an average age of approximately 22 years.[49] There is no significant gender predilection. The most common location is the molar-ascending ramus region of the mandible, although maxillary and anterior lesions also are possible. The majority of cases present as a well-circumscribed, unilocular radiolucency associated with the crown of an impacted mandibular third molar (**Fig. 36**). Such lesions mimic dentigerous cysts. Infrequently, the lesions may appear multilocular, develop in an edentulous area, or occur between the roots of

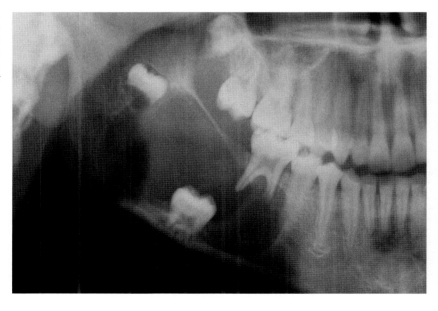

Fig. 36. Unicystic ameloblastoma. Large unilocular radiolucency associated with the crown of an impacted mandibular second molar. (*Courtesy of* Dr Mark Shehan.)

Key Features
AMELOBLASTOMA

1. Three major clinicopathologic types: (1) conventional solid or multicystic, (2) unicystic, and (3) peripheral. Approximately 90% of ameloblastomas represent the conventional solid or multicystic type.

2. The conventional solid or multicystic type includes the following histopathologic variants: follicular, plexiform, acanthomatous, granular cell, desmoplastic, and basal cell. Several of these microscopic variants may be found in a single tumor. These variations have no bearing on treatment or prognosis.

3. Conventional solid or multicystic ameloblastoma
   a. Intraosseous with a predilection for the posterior mandible
   b. Unilocular or multilocular on radiographs, often expansile
   c. Locally aggressive and tends to recur with conservative treatment
   d. Marginal or en bloc resection indicated for most cases

4. Unicystic ameloblastoma
   a. Average age at diagnosis younger compared with the conventional solid or multicystic type (22 years vs 36 years)
   b. Intraosseous with a predilection for the posterior mandible
   c. Most commonly appears as a unilocular radiolucency associated with the crown of an impacted tooth
   d. Grossly appears as a single cystic sac
   e. Microscopically subclassified into luminal, intraluminal, and intramural types
   f. Intramural type exhibits locally aggressive behavior and often is treated by marginal or en bloc resection in a manner similar to conventional ameloblastoma
   g. Luminal and intraluminal types have low recurrence potential and are treated by simple enucleation or curettage with long-term follow-up

5. Peripheral ameloblastoma
   a. Arises within soft tissue
   b. Painless gingival nodule
   c. Treated by conservative excision
   d. Lesser recurrence potential than conventional ameloblastoma

---

teeth. Lesions associated with the crowns of impacted teeth most often arise in the second and third decades, whereas lesions unassociated with impacted teeth most often arise in the fourth and fifth decades.

Unfortunately, there has been a great deal of confusion regarding the unicystic ameloblastoma. One source of confusion is the diverse terminology used to refer to this entity, such as plexiform unicystic ameloblastoma, unilocular and cystic ameloblastoma, and cystogenic ameloblastoma. In addition, the term, *unicystic*, may be confused with the term unilocular. Unicystic refers to the gross and microscopic appearance of a large cystic sac, whereas unilocular refers to the radiographic finding of a single loculus or compartment. Although most unicystic ameloblastomas do appear unilocular on radiographs, a minority of cases may be multilocular. Furthermore, since Robinson and Martinez's original description, several investigators have observed that some unicystic ameloblastomas may be more aggressive than originally thought, especially if there is neoplastic proliferation within the cyst wall. These observations have led to many systems for histopathologic subclassification (eg, simple/intraluminal/intramural, types 1–4, groups 1–3, and so forth).[60–62]

Unicystic ameloblastoma: Gross features If removed intact, a lesion typically appears as a tan or grayish tan, cystic sac attached to the cemento-enamel junction of a tooth. Careful inspection of the inner surface may reveal intraluminal excrescences corresponding to the intraluminal variant (**Fig. 37**). Inspection of either the outer or inner surface may reveal rounded, nodular thickenings corresponding to the intramural variant. The predominant gross finding of a single macrocystic sac differs from the mixture of solid and multicystic areas usually seen in conventional ameloblastoma.

Unicystic ameloblastoma: Microscopic features

There are 3 histopathologic variants of unicystic ameloblastoma:

1. *Luminal unicystic ameloblastoma* consists of a cystic lesion with an ameloblastic epithelial lining (**Fig. 38**). Ameloblastic features include a basal layer of columnar or cuboidal cells with hyperchromatic nuclei exhibiting reverse polarization. The overlying cells are loosely arranged and may resemble stellate reticulum. A dense band of hyalinization may be seen directly beneath the basal layer. No intraluminal or intramural extension of tumor should be present.
2. *Intraluminal unicystic ameloblastoma* exhibits a nodular, often polypoid proliferation of ameloblastoma projecting from the cystic lining into the lumen (**Fig. 39**). This proliferation often exhibits a plexiform growth pattern, characterized by anastomosing epithelial cords within

a delicate fibrovascular stroma. Ameloblastic differentiation of the basal cells may be difficult to appreciate within the intraluminal component.

3. *Intramural unicystic ameloblastoma* exhibits tumor infiltration into the fibrous cyst wall (**Fig. 40**). The infiltrating tumor usually shows features of conventional follicular or plexiform ameloblastoma. Focal or limited tumor invasion may be seen in unicystic ameloblastoma, whereas more extensive invasion into the wall warrants classification as conventional ameloblastoma. Careful examination of multiple levels of sections may be needed to detect intramural involvement.

Unicystic ameloblastoma: Diagnosis The diagnosis of unicystic ameloblastoma requires correlation of the clinical and radiographic findings with the gross and microscopic features. Unicystic ameloblastoma most often appears as a unilocular radiolucency associated with the crown of an impacted tooth in a young patient, although multilocular and/or nondentigerous lesions may occur rarely. On a macroscopic level, the lesion usually appears as a single cystic sac, possibly with focal excrescences or thickenings within the lumen or wall. Microscopically, it is important to rule out intramural involvement, which is associated with more aggressive behavior and greater recurrence potential than the luminal and intraluminal variants. Intramural involvement can be excluded only after thorough examination of the entire lesion. Because a definitive diagnosis of unicystic ameloblastoma requires careful evaluation of the completely

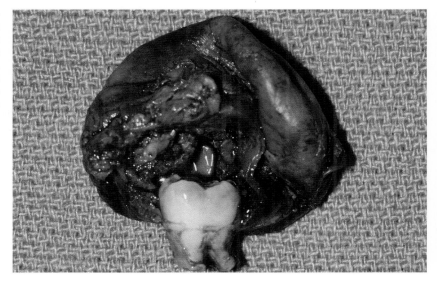

Fig. 37. Unicystic ameloblastoma. Gross specimen appearing as a grayish tan cystic sac surrounding the crown of a molar tooth. The inner surface exhibits excrescences, corresponding to intraluminal proliferation.

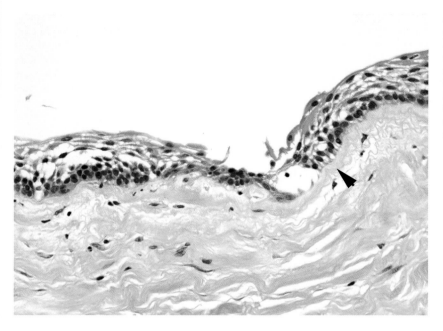

Fig. 38. Luminal unicystic ameloblastoma. The cystic lining has a basal layer of columnar to cuboidal cells with hyperchromatic nuclei. Focal reverse polarization of nuclei is evident (*arrowhead*). The cells overlying the basal layer are loosely arranged.

removed lesion, making such a diagnosis solely based on incisional biopsy material should be avoided.

Unicystic ameloblastoma: Differential diagnosis

The unicystic ameloblastoma must be distinguished from various odontogenic cysts. Both the dentigerous cyst and unicystic ameloblastoma may appear radiographically as a unilocular radiolucency associated with the crown of an impacted tooth. The squamous epithelial lining of a dentigerous cyst, however, does not exhibit ameloblastic features (ie, a basal layer of cuboidal to columnar cells with nuclei exhibiting hyperchromasia and reverse polarization or loosely arranged superficial cells with stellate reticulum–like features). Cysts

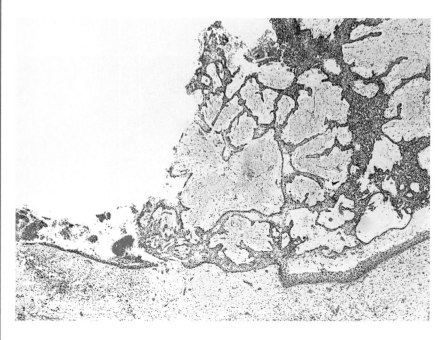

Fig. 39. Intraluminal unicystic ameloblastoma. Nodular epithelial proliferation projecting into the lumen. The epithelial proliferation exhibits a plexiform growth pattern.

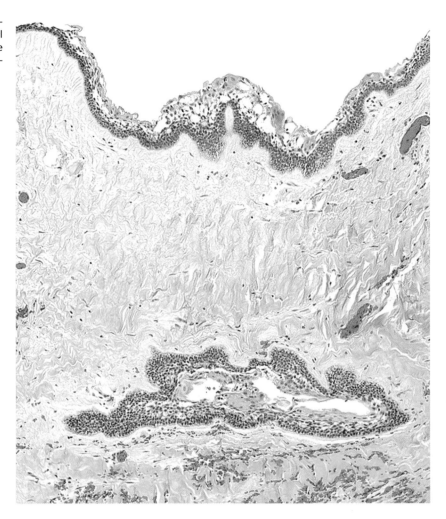

Fig. 40. Intramural unicystic ameloblastoma. Focal tumor island within the wall of a unicystic ameloblastoma.

that are inflamed—such as periapical cysts or secondarily inflamed dentigerous cysts—may exhibit hyperplasia of the epithelial lining. This hyperplasia should not be confused with the intraluminal plexiform proliferation seen in intraluminal unicystic ameloblastoma.

Unicystic ameloblastoma: Prognosis Based on the clinical and radiographic presentation, the majority of unicystic ameloblastomas initially are presumed to represent dentigerous or other odontogenic cysts. Therefore, simple enucleation or curettage usually is performed upfront, and the diagnosis of unicystic ameloblastoma is made in retrospect. The luminal and intraluminal variants have a low recurrence potential, and thus, simple enucleation or curettage should suffice, provided

that long-term follow-up can be performed. In contrast, the intramural variant may exhibit more aggressive behavior. Some surgeons prefer to treat intramural unicystic ameloblastomas by marginal resection, in a manner similar to how a conventional solid and multicystic ameloblastoma is treated. Others prefer to maintain patients under close observation and delay further surgery until there is evidence of recurrence. Alternative treatment methods include primary marsupialization followed by enucleation of any remaining lesion or primary enucleation combined with application of Carnoy solution.[63]

The reported recurrence rate for unicystic ameloblastoma after enucleation or curettage is in the range of 10% to 25%, which is considerably lower than that for conventional ameloblastoma.[62]

Estimates of recurrence have been limited by studies with small numbers of cases, short follow-up periods, and inadequate descriptions of treatment rendered. A few recent studies have suggested that the recurrence rate after enucleation may be higher (30%–35%), especially for cases with intramural involvement.[63,64]

Peripheral ameloblastoma

Peripheral ameloblastoma represents the soft tissue counterpart of intraosseous solid or multicystic ameloblastoma. This subtype comprises approximately 2% to 10% of all ameloblastomas.[49,65] The tumor usually presents as a painless, exophytic gingival growth. The clinical presentation may mimic that of a fibroma, pyogenic granuloma, or papilloma. Extragingival lesions (usually involving the buccal mucosa) are rare and controversial.[66,67] Peripheral ameloblastoma may arise over a broad age range, with an average age of approximately 52 years; the average age is significantly higher than that for central ameloblastoma.[49,65] The mandibular mucosa is more commonly affected than the maxillary mucosa, with a predilection for mandibular premolar and anterior regions.

Peripheral ameloblastoma: Gross features The gross specimen typically consists of a firm to spongy mucosal nodule. The mucosal surface may be smooth, pebbly, papillary, or warty. The size of reported lesions ranges from 0.3 to 4.5 cm, with a mean diameter of 1.3 cm.[65]

Peripheral ameloblastoma: Microscopic features The microscopic features are similar to conventional intraosseous ameloblastoma in terms of growth patterns and cell types. Follicular, plexiform, acanthomatous, and basal cell patterns are possible. The epithelial islands may exhibit a peripheral row of columnar cells with nuclear palisading and reverse polarization. Stellate reticulum–like differentiation may not be prominent. In some cases, the tumor epithelium fuses with the overlying surface epithelium (**Fig. 41**). The surface epithelium may be smooth, pebbly, or papillary.

Peripheral ameloblastoma: Differential diagnosis It is important to distinguish between a peripheral ameloblastoma and an intraosseous ameloblastoma that has penetrated the bone with extension into soft tissue, because the two lesions require different treatment approaches (see discussion of treatment later). Correlation with the clinical and radiographic findings is necessary to make this distinction.

The peripheral odontogenic fibroma (WHO-type) is similar to the peripheral ameloblastoma in that it clinically presents as a slow-growing gingival nodule. Microscopically, islands or strands of odontogenic epithelium are scattered within a background of moderately cellular to myxoid fibrous connective tissue. The epithelium does not exhibit the basal cell layer with reverse polarization characteristic of ameloblastoma. Also, peripheral odontogenic fibromas occasionally produce dysplastic dentin, cementum-like calcifications, or osteoid, whereas no calcified product is seen in peripheral ameloblastomas.

Odontogenic gingival epithelial hamartoma (OGEH), or hamartoma of the dental lamina, originally was described by Baden and colleagues[68] as a transitional stage between a developmental anomaly and a true odontogenic neoplasm. Only 11 cases have been reported to date.[68–74] Similar to the peripheral ameloblastoma, OGEH clinically presents as a small gingival nodule in an adult patient with little recurrence potential. Similar to the peripheral ameloblastoma, there is a proliferation of islands, nests, or cords of basaloid odontogenic epithelial cells. At times there even may be focal ameloblastic differentiation, with a peripheral layer of cuboidal to columnar cells exhibiting reverse nuclear polarization. Clear cell and focal squamous differentiation also are possible. Some investigators have proposed that compared with peripheral ameloblastoma, OGEH should exhibit a more localized nodular growth without communication with the surface epithelium.[70,74] Diagnostic criteria for OGEH are not well established, however, and many investigators now believe reported cases of OGEH actually represent peripheral ameloblastomas or peripheral odontogenic fibromas.[65]

From a practical standpoint, differentiating between a peripheral ameloblastoma, peripheral odontogenic fibroma, and OGEH may be considered an academic exercise. All 3 of these lesions are benign and appropriately treated by conservative excision.

Peripheral ameloblastoma: Diagnosis Diagnosis requires correlation of the microscopic findings with the clinical and radiographic presentation. Clinical and radiographic findings should indicate a tumor of soft tissue origin. Radiographs usually show no bony involvement, although superficial pressure (or cupping) resorption of the underlying bone occasionally may be found.

Peripheral ameloblastoma: Prognosis Conservative excision down to periosteum is the treatment of choice. Peripheral ameloblastoma does not exhibit the locally aggressive behavior and

Fig. 41. Peripheral ameloblastoma. (*A*) A proliferation of ameloblastic epithelium within the gingival mucosa. Some of the tumor islands or cords merge with the surface epithelium. In this case, the surface appears papillary. (*B*) High-power photomicrograph shows tumor islands with features resembling conventional intraosseous ameloblastoma.

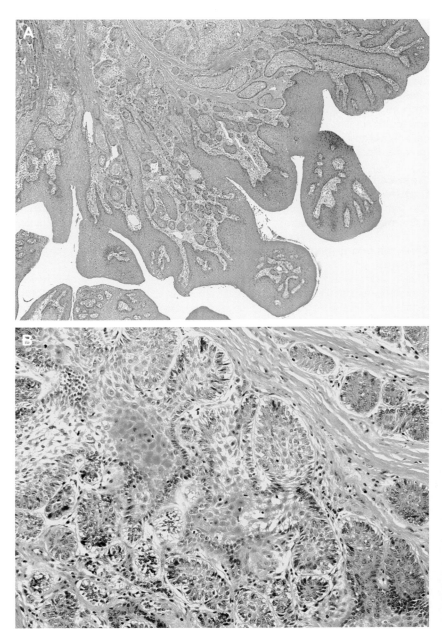

high recurrence rate typical of its intraosseous counterpart. Reported recurrence rates range from 16% to 19%, with most reported "recurrences" likely representing persistence of incompletely excised tumors.[65] Long-term follow-up is recommended because of isolated reports of malignant transformation or dysplastic change developing within a peripheral ameloblastoma.[75–77]

Clear Cell Odontogenic Carcinoma

Clear cell odontogenic carcinomas are rare neoplasms, with approximately 64 cases reported in the literature.[78–82] In the past, these tumors have been referred to as clear cell ameloblastomas or clear cell odontogenic tumors. The term, *clear cell odontogenic carcinoma*, is now preferred by most authorities.

Clear cell odontogenic carcinomas tend to arise in older individuals, with an average age at presentation of 54 years and an age range of 14 to 89 years. There is a female predilection, with a female-to-male ratio of 2:1. The mandible is affected more often than the maxilla by a ratio of 2.8:1.[78–82] Patients often present with a painful jaw swelling and tooth mobility. Radiographic examination typically shows an ill-defined radiolucency with irregular margins. Root resorption is possible.

Clear cell odontogenic carcinoma: Gross features

The tumor grossly appears as a solid mass with a tan, white, or pinkish gray cut surface.

Clear cell odontogenic carcinoma: Microscopic features

Clear cell odontogenic carcinomas most commonly exhibit a biphasic growth pattern, characterized by islands and nests of large clear cells intermixed with small eosinophilic epithelial cells (**Fig. 42**). The large clear cells usually have well-defined cell borders and central nuclei with mild to moderate pleomorphism. The small cells tend to have pale eosinophilic cytoplasm and monomorphic, hyperchromatic nuclei. They may exhibit basaloid, squamoid, or ameloblastic differentiation. The small cells may occupy the periphery of the tumor islands, line focal duct–like structures within the center of the tumor islands, or form separate tumor nests. Ameloblastic differentiation is characterized by peripheral cells with reverse polarization of their nuclei; although not always present, it can be a helpful clue for recognizing an odontogenic origin.

A monophasic growth pattern also is possible. In this pattern, the tumor is comprised entirely of large clear cells arranged in nests, islands, or cords. The monophasic variant may be more difficult to recognize.

In both variants, mitoses and necrosis are usually absent or minimal. The background stroma is fibrous and occasionally may be hyalinized. The tumor is infiltrative and ill-defined. Cortical destruction with extension into soft tissue is common.

The clear cells have high glycogen content; their cytoplasm stains with periodic acid–Schiff (PAS) and is diastase sensitive. Immunohistochemical studies have shown the tumor cells to be positive for cytokeratins (including cytokeratins 8, 13, 14, 18, 19, and AE1/AE3) and epithelial membrane antigen. Immunoreactivity for vimentin, laminin, and collagen type IV is typically restricted to the stroma surrounding the tumor islands. The tumor cells are negative for smooth muscle actin, desmin, CD31, CD34, S-100, and HMB-45.[82,83]

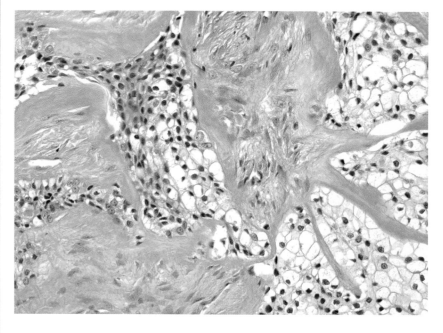

Fig. 42. Clear cell odontogenic carcinoma. Epithelial tumor islands comprised of large clear cells and small eosinophilic cells.

Clear cell odontogenic carcinoma: Differential diagnosis

In addition to clear cell odontogenic carcinoma, the differential diagnosis for clear cell tumors of the jaws includes metastatic renal cell carcinoma, intraosseous salivary neoplasms (such as clear cell mucoepidermoid carcinoma, clear cell acinic cell carcinoma, epithelial-myoepithelial carcinoma, and hyalinizing clear cell carcinoma), ameloblastoma, and the clear cell variant of calcifying epithelial odontogenic tumor.

Immunoreactivity for vimentin and the presence of prominent vascularity aid in distinguishing metastatic renal cell carcinoma from clear cell odontogenic carcinoma. Primary salivary neoplasia generally is rare within the jaws. Mucicarmine or Alcian blue should demonstrate intracytoplasmic mucin production in clear cell mucoepidermoid carcinoma but not clear cell odontogenic carcinoma. In addition, the presence of squamous differentiation, intermediate cells, and/or prominent cyst formation favors a diagnosis of mucoepidermoid carcinoma. In a clear cell acinic cell carcinoma, there should be at least occasional cells with PAS-positive, diastase-resistant intracytoplasmic granules. In contrast, the tumor cells in clear cell odontogenic carcinoma are PAS-positive and diastase sensitive. The presence of biphasic tubules (with central cuboidal to low columnar luminal cells and outer clear myoepithelial cells) and myoepithelial immunoreactivity for S-100 protein help to distinguish epithelial-myoepithelial carcinoma from clear cell odontogenic carcinoma. In hyalinizing clear cell carcinoma, the hyalinized stromal component tends to predominate and may show areas with near obliteration of the epithelial component, which is unusual for clear cell odontogenic carcinoma. Ameloblastic differentiation can be found in both the clear cell odontogenic carcinoma and ameloblastoma. Vacuolar change is typically restricted to the peripheral cells in ameloblastoma, whereas it is more pervasive in the clear cell odontogenic carcinoma. In addition, in clear cell odontogenic carcinoma, there is a lack of stellate reticulum–like differentiation. The absence of amyloid deposition and Liesegang ring calcifications helps to exclude the clear cell variant of calcifying epithelial odontogenic tumor.

Melanoma and the so-called sugar tumors are found only rarely within the jaws but might be included in the differential diagnosis. Immunoreactivity for S-100 protein and HMB-45 helps to distinguish these tumors from clear cell odontogenic carcinoma.

> △△ **Differential Diagnosis**
> CLEAR CELL ODONTOGENIC CARCINOMA
>
> - Metastatic renal cell carcinoma
> - Intraosseous salivary neoplasms: clear cell mucoepidermoid carcinoma, clear cell acinic cell carcinoma, epithelial-myoepithelial carcinoma, and hyalinizing clear cell carcinoma
> - Ameloblastoma
> - Clear cell variant of calcifying epithelial odontogenic tumor
> - Melanoma and sugar tumors

Clear cell odontogenic carcinoma: Prognosis

Marginal resection is the treatment of choice. In some cases, lymph node dissection and adjuvant radiation therapy may be considered as well. Indications for adjuvant radiation therapy include extensive soft tissue invasion, perineural invasion, positive surgical margins, and the presence of lymph node metastasis with or without extracapsular spread. Lymph node metastasis is infrequent on initial presentation but found in approximately one-third of patients with recurrent disease. Distant metastasis to the lung and extragnathic bones also is possible.

Among reported cases, the overall recurrence rate is approximately 55%.[84] In their review of the literature, Werle and colleagues[78] found that out of 21 reported cases with a follow-up period of 5 years or longer, there were 8 patients who died of disease. Long-term follow-up is recommended because of the potential for late recurrence.

Adenomatoid Odontogenic Tumor

More than 1000 cases of adenomatoid odontogenic tumor have been reported in the literature. Most studies have found adenomatoid odontogenic tumors to comprise approximately 2% to 8% of odontogenic tumors, although a recent comprehensive review reveals reported frequencies ranging worldwide from 0.6% to 38%.[85] This benign odontogenic epithelial neoplasm has been theorized to originate from enamel organ epithelium or remnants of dental lamina. Its particularly nonaggressive behavior has prompted some investigators even to regard it as an odontogenic hamartoma.

Adenomatoid odontogenic tumors tend to arise in young individuals, with nearly two-thirds of cases diagnosed in the second decade and more than 90% of cases found before the age of 30. The male-to-female ratio is approximately 1:2. There is a predilection for the tumor to arise in the anterior regions of the jaws, and approximately twice as many cases affect the maxilla than the mandible. The vast majority of cases arise intraosseously, although a rare extraosseous (or peripheral) variant comprises approximately 2% of cases.[85]

Most lesions are painless and grow slowly. Intraosseous tumors often are found incidentally on radiographs or are discovered because of delayed tooth eruption. Larger lesions may produce a noticeable swelling. Radiographic examination shows a well-defined unilocular radiolucency, which in two-thirds of cases may include fine radiopacities (or snowflake calcifications). Periapical radiographs are superior to panoramic radiographs for detecting these radiopacities. Approximately 70% of cases are associated with the crown of an impacted tooth (referred to as the follicular or dentigerous type). The canine teeth are involved most frequently. At times the radiolucency may extend apically past the cementoenamel junction of the associated tooth, which is a feature not typically seen in a dentigerous cyst (**Fig. 43**). Other lesions may arise between the roots of teeth (referred to as the extrafollicular type).[86]

The rare peripheral type usually appears as a small, sessile nodule on the maxillary facial gingiva; radiographic findings may be absent or consist of superficial cupping resorption of the underlying bone.

Adenomatoid odontogenic tumor: Gross features

Intraosseous lesions typically consist of a well-defined soft tissue mass encased by a fibrous capsule. On sectioning, the cut surface may appear either solid or cystic. There may be several small cystic spaces or one large cystic space. Nodular vegetations may be present on the luminal surface. Tumor calcifications often are too fine to be appreciated grossly but may produce a gritty consistency. The crown of an associated impacted tooth may be embedded within the tumor.

Adenomatoid odontogenic tumor: Microscopic features

Microscopic examination shows a well-defined tumor surrounded by a fibrous capsule (**Fig. 44**A). The tumor includes two major epithelial cell types. The first type is characterized by spindle-shaped epithelial cells arranged in sheets, strands, or whorled nodules within a scant fibrous stroma. These epithelial cells occasionally may form rosette-like structures, which surround an empty space or a small amount of amorphous eosinophilic material. This material may stain for amyloid. The second epithelial cell type is cuboidal to columnar and forms tubular or duct-like structures (hence, the term, *adenomatoid*) (see **Fig. 44**B). Such tubular or duct-like structures may vary considerably

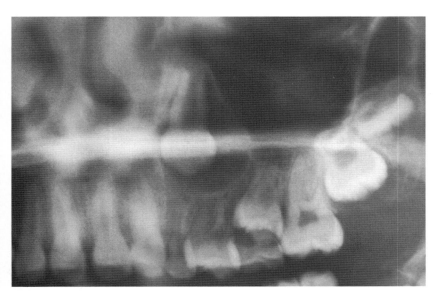

Fig. 43. Adenomatoid odontogenic tumor. Radiolucency associated with the crown of an impacted maxillary canine. In contrast to the typical dentigerous cyst, the radiolucency nearly extends to the apex of the tooth. (*Courtesy of* Dr Tony Traynham.)

Fig. 44. Adenomatoid odontogenic tumor. (*A*) Low-power photomicrograph shows a well-defined, encapsulated tumor mass with a whorled growth pattern and scattered duct-like structures. (*B*) High-power photomicrograph shows variably sized duct-like structures and focal rosette formation within a background of spindle cells. The cuboidal to columnar cells lining the duct-like structures have nuclei polarized away from the lumens.

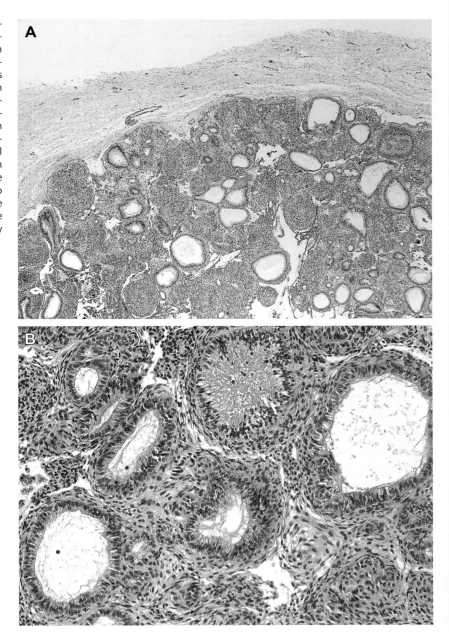

in size and are not always present. They are lined by a single row of cuboidal to columnar epithelial cells. The nuclei of these cells are polarized away from the lumen.

Most lesions also produce varying amounts of calcified material. There may be small basophilic calcifications, which likely represent dystrophic enamel calcifications. Sometimes these calcifications may exhibit a concentric ring pattern. In some cases, there may be larger masses of matrix or calcification. This material has been interpreted as dentinoid, osteodentin, or cementum. Dentinoid seems to result from a metaplastic process, because there is no odontogenic ectomesenchyme present to induce dentin production.

A few cases of adenomatoid odontogenic tumor with focal calcifying epithelial odontogenic tumor-like areas (referred to as *combined epithelial odontogenic tumor*) have been reported.[87–91] The presence of such foci does not seem to influence biologic behavior; thus, these lesions may be regarded as a histopathologic variant of adenomatoid odontogenic tumor.

Adenomatoid odontogenic tumor: Differential diagnosis

Adenomatoid odontogenic tumors display such distinctive features that they usually are not mistaken for other lesions. The cuboidal to columnar epithelial cells lining the duct-like structures in adenomatoid odontogenic tumors bear some resemblance to the peripheral columnar cells with reverse polarization in ameloblastoma. Tumor encapsulation, a whorled growth pattern, and calcifications, however, are not found in ameloblastoma. Distinction between these two entities is crucial because of the more extensive surgical treatment required for ameloblastoma compared with adenomatoid odontogenic tumor.

The duct-like structures in adenomatoid odontogenic tumor might suggest an adenocarcinoma of salivary or other origin. An adenocarcinoma arising within the jaws of an adolescent is rare, however, and recognition of tumor encapsulation, the characteristic whorled growth pattern, and calcifications should make diagnosis straightforward.

Adenomatoid odontogenic tumor: Prognosis

Simple enucleation is appropriate treatment, and recurrence is rare.

Calcifying Epithelial Odontogenic Tumor (Pindborg Tumor)

Calcifying epithelial odontogenic tumors are rare benign neoplasms, comprising approximately 0.4% to 3% of odontogenic tumors. Investigators have suggested an origin from the stratum intermedium of the enamel organ or remnants of dental lamina.[92,93]

These tumors occur over a broad age range (first through tenth decades), with a mean age at diagnosis of 37 years and peak prevalence during the third through sixth decades. The majority of cases are intraosseous, with a predilection for the posterior mandible. Extraosseous lesions (also known as *peripheral calcifying epithelial odontogenic tumors*) comprise only 6% of cases. There is no significant gender predilection.[92]

The usual clinical presentation is a slowly growing, painless mass. Among intraosseous cases, the typical radiographic findings include a unilocular or multilocular radiolucency, often with calcifications of variable size (**Fig. 45**). The radiographic borders may be either well-defined or ill-defined. Approximately half of intrabony cases are associated with an unerupted tooth. The uncommon peripheral calcifying epithelial odontogenic tumor usually appears as a firm,

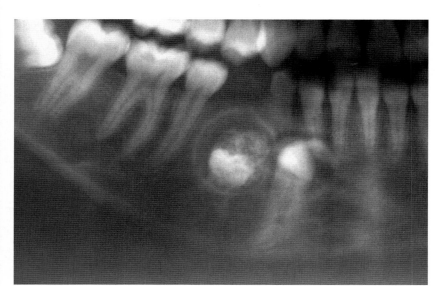

Fig. 45. Calcifying epithelial odontogenic tumor. Radiograph showing a well-defined, mixed radiolucent-radiopaque lesion surrounding the crown of an impacted deciduous molar. (*Courtesy of* Dr James Lemon.)

painless, sessile gingival mass, which occasionally may be associated with an underlying bony depression (or cupping erosion).

Calcifying epithelial odontogenic tumor: Gross features

Intraosseous tumors typically are enucleated easily. If a tumor is associated with an impacted tooth, then the gross specimen may consist of a soft tissue mass attached to the cemento-enamel junction of the tooth. On sectioning, calcifications may be evident. The tumor may appear grayish white, yellow, or tan-pink.

Calcifying epithelial odontogenic tumor: Microscopic features

There is a proliferation of polyhedral, eosinophilic epithelial cells arranged in islands, sheets, or cords (**Fig. 46**). The epithelial cells have distinct cell borders, and intercellular bridging may be evident with high-power magnification.

In some cases, cellular and nuclear pleomorphism, prominent nucleoli, scattered multinucleated cells, and rare mitoses may be observed; however, such features are not indicative of malignancy. Malignant transformation has been reported only rarely. Histopathologic features associated with malignancy include significant mitotic activity, atypical mitotic figures, necrosis, perineural invasion, and vascular invasion.[94–96]

A hallmark feature of the calcifying epithelial odontogenic tumor is deposition of homogeneous eosinophilic material that exhibits apple-green birefringence with Congo red staining. This amyloid-like material may form pools or globules within the background stroma or may occupy cribriform spaces within the epithelium. Recent investigations have shown this amyloid-like material to represent N-terminal fragments of the odontogenic ameloblast-associated protein.[97] In some cases, this material may form basophilic calcifications with concentric laminations (Liesegang ring calcifications) (see **Fig. 46**A). The proportion of epithelium to amyloid-like material and calcification is highly variable. Tumors with abundant matrix and only occasional epithelial nests and cords may be more difficult to recognize than those tumors with a pronounced epithelial component (see **Fig. 46**B).

Uncommon histopathologic variants include the clear cell variant, noncalcifying Langerhans cell–rich variant, and combined epithelial odontogenic tumor. The clear cell variant is characterized by epithelial cells with clear cytoplasm, often accompanied by zones of more classic eosinophilic tumor cells (**Fig. 47**). The clear cells contain PAS-positive, diastase-sensitive glycogen granules. In a few cases, investigators have found the clear cells to exhibit immunohistochemical and ultrastructural features of Langerhans cells. These rare cases have been reported as the noncalcifying Langerhans cell–rich variant and mainly have arisen in the anterior-premolar region of the maxilla.[98–100] The combined epithelial odontogenic tumor represents an adenomatoid odontogenic tumor with focal calcifying epithelial odontogenic tumor–like areas.

Calcifying epithelial odontogenic tumor: Differential diagnosis

Diagnosis typically is straightforward. In cases that exhibit marked pleomorphism, however, the tumor potentially may be mistaken for a primary or metastatic malignant neoplasm. Pleomorphic epithelial cells with intercellular bridging may bear some resemblance to primary intraosseous carcinoma or metastatic squamous cell carcinoma. A cribriform growth pattern may prompt consideration of the remote possibility of a metastatic adenoid cystic carcinoma. Amyloid-like material and basophilic lamellar calcifications, however, are not produced by such tumors.

The diagnosis may not be obvious in cases where the epithelial component consists of widely scattered nests and cords with little amyloid-like material. Such cases might bear some resemblance to an odontogenic fibroma, and careful examination for focal production of amyloid-like material may aid diagnosis.

The clear cell variant of calcifying epithelial odontogenic tumor must be distinguished from other clear cell tumors, such as metastatic renal cell carcinoma, clear cell odontogenic carcinoma, clear cell mucoepidermoid carcinoma, clear cell acinic cell carcinoma, or epithelial-myoepithelial carcinoma. None of these other tumor types produces amyloid, however. Furthermore, careful examination in most cases of clear cell calcifying epithelial odontogenic tumor reveal at least some areas with characteristic eosinophilic, polyhedral tumor cells.

Calcifying epithelial odontogenic tumor: Prognosis

Early descriptions suggested the calcifying epithelial odontogenic tumor to be locally aggressive with biologic behavior similar to that of ameloblastoma. Subsequent reviews have reported, however, a recurrence rate of only approximately 15%, which mainly has been attributed to inadequate treatment.[101] The clear cell variant has been regarded by some investigators as particularly aggressive because of its tendency for cortical perforation; however, the recurrence

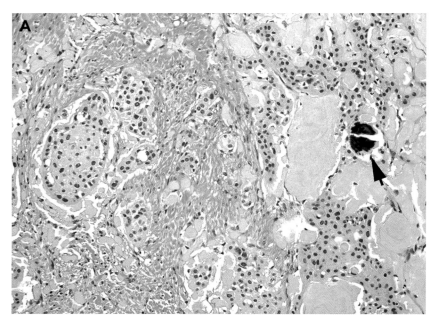

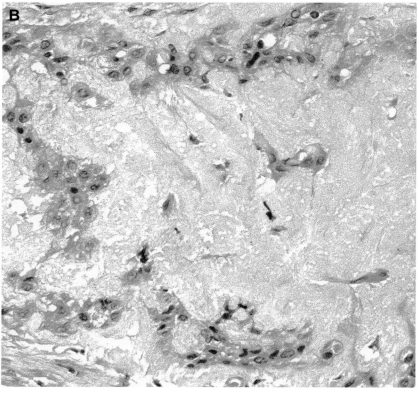

Fig. 46. Calcifying epithelial odontogenic tumor. (*A*) Islands and sheets of eosinophilic epithelial cells with pools of amyloid-like material. A focal basophilic, lamellar calcification (Liesegang ring calcification) also is present (*arrow*). (*B*) In some cases, there may be abundant amyloid matrix and only scant strands of epithelium.

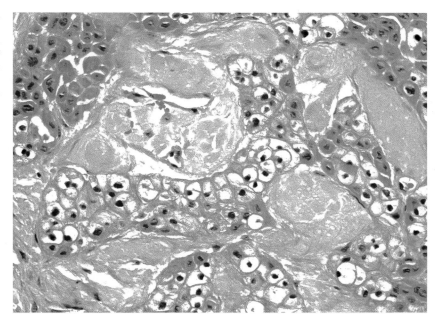

Fig. 47. Calcifying epithelial odontogenic tumor, clear cell variant. Epithelial cords comprised of clear cells as well as more classic eosinophilic cells. Pools of amyloid-like material are present within the background.

rate of the clear cell variant is not significantly higher than that of the conventional type.[102]

For mandibular tumors, the treatment of choice is conservative excision with a narrow rim of normal tissue. Maxillary lesions may require more aggressive treatment, because they tend to grow rapidly and often do not remain well confined.

Pitfalls
CALCIFYING EPITHELIAL
ODONTOGENIC TUMOR

! Cellular and nuclear pleomorphism, prominent nucleoli, scattered multinucleated cells, and rare mitoses may be present in some cases. Such features, however, are not indicative of malignancy.

! The clear cell variant of calcifying epithelial odontogenic tumor must not be confused with clear cell carcinomas (eg, metastatic renal cell carcinoma, clear cell odontogenic carcinoma, clear cell mucoepidermoid carcinoma, clear cell acinic cell carcinoma, or epithelial-myoepithelial carcinoma). Misdiagnosis may be avoided by recognition of amyloid and focal areas with characteristic eosinophilic, polyhedral tumor cells.

Long-term follow-up is recommended for intraosseous lesions. Conservative enucleation is sufficient for peripheral lesions, which exhibit minimal recurrence potential.

Squamous Odontogenic Tumor

Squamous odontogenic tumors are rare, benign epithelial odontogenic neoplasms. The tumors represent a proliferation of mature squamous epithelium originating from the rests of Malassez or remnants of dental lamina. The rests of Malassez are epithelial remnants of Hertwig's epithelial root sheath found within the periodontal ligament; therefore, the tumor typically arises intraosseously in association with the lateral root surfaces of teeth. The uncommon peripheral variant seems to arise from remnants of the dental lamina.

Squamous odontogenic tumors occur over a broad age range, from childhood to the eighth decade, with most cases arising in adulthood. There is no gender predilection, and cases are equally distributed between the maxilla and mandible. Maxillary lesions tend to arise in the anterior region, whereas mandibular lesions tend to arise in the posterior region. A few rare cases of multifocal squamous odontogenic tumors have been reported, which at times have been familial.[103–105] The lesion typically presents as a mildly painful or painless gingival swelling. Tooth mobility may be evident. Radiographic examination typically shows a unilocular radiolucency associated with the lateral root surface of an erupted tooth. Less commonly, the lesion may be found within an edentulous area or surrounding the crown of an unerupted tooth. The radiolucency may be either well-defined or ill-defined and is often triangular (with the base located between the apices of adjacent tooth roots), semicircular, or oval. The tumor may splay the roots of the adjacent teeth. Most lesions are small and measure less than 1.5 cm in greatest diameter.

Squamous odontogenic tumor: Gross features

The tumor grossly appears as pink to grayish-tan, firm, solid tissue.

Squamous odontogenic tumor: Microscopic features

Microscopic examination shows a proliferation of bland squamous epithelium arranged in islands and nests within a fibrous stroma (**Fig. 48**). The islands may be round, oval, or irregular in shape. Unlike ameloblastoma, the peripheral cells are flattened without nuclear reverse polarization, and the central cells do not exhibit stellate reticulum–like differentiation. Individual cell keratinization is common. Infrequent findings include multicystic vacuolization, clear cells, laminated calcified bodies, and eosinophilic globular structures. Mitotic activity is absent or scant.

Squamous odontogenic tumor: Differential diagnosis

It is important to distinguish between ameloblastoma and squamous odontogenic tumor, because the former requires more extensive surgical treatment compared with the latter. In squamous odontogenic tumor, the epithelial cells at the periphery of the islands are flattened rather than columnar and do not exhibit reverse polarization of their nuclei. In addition, the cells within the center of the tumor islands do not exhibit stellate reticulum–like differentiation as might be seen in ameloblastoma.

Hyperplastic squamous epithelial islands resembling squamous odontogenic tumor occasionally may be found within the walls of radicular cysts and dentigerous cysts. This phenomenon is referred to as a *squamous odontogenic tumor–like proliferation* and does not have any impact on the clinical behavior of the cyst. Clinical, radiographic, and histopathologic correlation should allow one to recognize that the proliferation is occurring within the wall of an odontogenic cyst and to avoid misdiagnosis as a squamous odontogenic tumor.

Intraosseous squamous cell carcinoma also may be considered in the differential diagnosis.

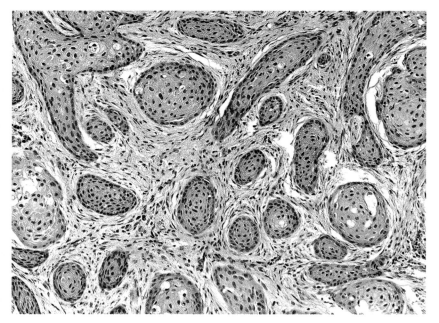

Fig. 48. Squamous odontogenic tumor. Islands of bland squamous epithelium within a fibrous stroma. Unlike ameloblastoma, the cells at the periphery of the epithelial islands are flattened without nuclear reverse polarization, and the central cells do not exhibit stellate reticulum–like differentiation.

The lack of cytologic atypia differentiates the squamous odontogenic tumor from squamous cell carcinoma. Other features that favor squamous cell carcinoma include frequent mitoses and peripheral, infiltrative small cords. Malignant transformation of squamous odontogenic tumor into squamous cell carcinoma has been reported in only a single case.[106]

There has been confusion in the literature regarding gingival lesions reported as oral pseudoepitheliomatous hyperplasia versus peripheral squamous odontogenic tumor. Oral pseudoepitheliomatous hyperplasia often arises in young patients and presents as a gingival nodule with a smooth or warty surface. Microscopic examination shows budding islands of bland squamous epithelium with a broad, pushing front; keratin-filled crypts or cyst formation also may be found. The epithelial islands in pseudoepitheliomatous hyperplasia are often interconnected, whereas in squamous odontogenic tumor they are usually separate from one another.[107]

Squamous odontogenic tumor: Prognosis
Curettage, enucleation, or local excision is usually adequate treatment. Recurrence has been reported in only a few cases.[105,108,109] Malignant transformation is rare.

TUMORS OF ODONTOGENIC EPITHELIUM AND ODONTOGENIC ECTOMESENCHYME (MIXED ODONTOGENIC TUMORS)

Ameloblastic fibromas, ameloblastic fibrodentinomas, ameloblastic fibro-odontomas, and odontomas comprise a spectrum of mixed odontogenic tumors. Within this spectrum, odontomas represent a benign hamartoma rather than a true neoplasm. There has been controversy regarding the nature of the remaining tumor types. Some investigators have theorized that they merely represent progressive stages in the formation of an odontoma.[110] Nevertheless, these lesions often behave as true neoplasms, with significant growth potential and—particularly in the case of ameloblastic fibroma—appreciable recurrence potential. Furthermore, the average age at diagnosis is somewhat older for the ameloblastic fibroma compared with the ameloblastic fibro-odontoma and odontoma, which does not support the concept of the ameloblastic fibroma representing the earliest stage in the evolution of an odontoma. Some investigators have attempted to reconcile these disparate observations by hypothesizing that tumors within this group may develop along either a neoplastic line or a hamartomatous line.[111] Unfortunately, this issue remains largely unresolved, and in practice it may not always be possible to predict whether a given lesion within this spectrum will behave as a neoplasm or a hamartoma.

Ameloblastic Fibroma

Most authorities regard ameloblastic fibromas as a benign odontogenic neoplasm in which both the epithelial and ectomesenchymal elements are neoplastic. A few investigators also have hypothesized that at least some cases of ameloblastic fibroma may represent the earliest stage in the development of an odontoma.[110] The ameloblastic fibroma is uncommon and comprises approximately 1.5% to 4.5% of odontogenic tumors.[111]

This tumor usually arises in young patients, with a mean age at diagnosis of 16 years and more than 70% of cases diagnosed in the first and second decades.[112] There is a slight male predilection. Ameloblastic fibroma almost exclusively arises within the jawbones; however, a few rare cases involving the gingival soft tissue (peripheral ameloblastic fibroma) have been reported.[113–116] The most common location is the posterior mandible. Most patients present with jaw swelling, although occasionally the lesion may be discovered incidentally during radiographic examination. The lesions typically are painless and grow slowly. Ulceration, pain, tenderness, and drainage have been described in some cases. Radiographs typically show a well-defined, unilocular or multilocular radiolucency (**Fig. 49**). There is often a sclerotic margin, and many cases are associated with the crown of an unerupted tooth. Lesion size is variable (0.7–16 cm), with many cases diagnosed only after reaching extensive proportions.[112]

Ameloblastic fibroma: Gross features
The tumor grossly appears as a solid soft tissue mass. A fibrous capsule may or may not be present.

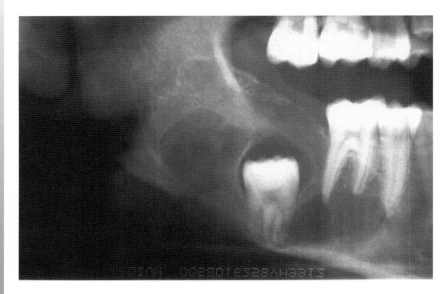

Fig. 49. Ameloblastic fibroma. Radiograph showing a well-defined, multilocular radiolucency associated with the crown of an impacted mandibular second molar. (*Courtesy of* Dr Mark Chishom.)

Ameloblastic fibroma: Microscopic features
Histopathologic examination shows cords and islands of odontogenic epithelium within a primitive mesenchymal stroma (**Fig. 50**). The epithelial cords are long, narrow, and anastomosing with a bilayer of cuboidal to columnar cells. The epithelial islands exhibit a peripheral layer of columnar cells and a central zone of loosely arranged, stellate reticulum–like cells. In contrast to follicular ameloblastoma, these islands tend to be relatively small without cyst formation. The mesenchymal component is richly cellular and comprised of stellate to ovoid fibroblasts within a delicate, myxoid background. The stroma resembles the dental papilla (pulp of a developing tooth).

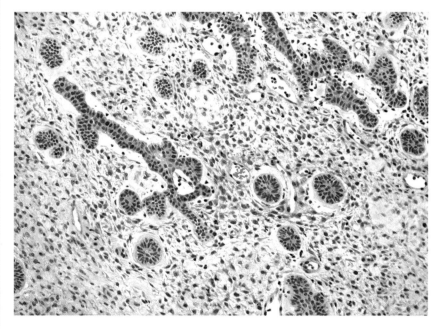

Fig. 50. Ameloblastic fibroma. Cords and islands of odontogenic epithelium within a primitive mesenchymal stroma. The cords are bilayered with an anastomosing growth pattern.

Ameloblastic fibroma: Differential diagnosis

Ameloblastic fibroma may be mistaken for ameloblastoma; however, the characteristic primitive mesenchymal component of the ameloblastic fibroma is not found in ameloblastomas. In addition, in contrast to ameloblastoma, the epithelial islands in ameloblastic fibroma tend to be relatively small and lack cyst formation.

By definition, an ameloblastic fibroma should not produce any dental hard tissue. A lesion with features of ameloblastic fibroma as well as dentin formation is referred to as ameloblastic fibrodentinoma. A lesion with features of ameloblastic fibroma as well as enamel and dentin formation may represent an ameloblastic fibro-odontoma or a developing odontoma.

The stroma in ameloblastic fibroma is bland with minimal to absent mitotic activity. If the stroma exhibits hypercellularity, cytologic atypia, and significant mitotic activity, then a diagnosis of ameloblastic fibrosarcoma should be considered (**Fig. 51**). Ameloblastic fibrosarcoma may arise either de novo or by malignant transformation of a pre-existing ameloblastic fibroma.

Rarely, a tumor with an ameloblastic fibroma–like pattern but both sarcomatous and carcinomatous elements may arise. Such lesions may be referred to as odontogenic carcinosarcomas.

Ameloblastic fibroma: Prognosis

Initial treatment generally consists of enucleation, curettage, or local excision, with more aggressive surgery reserved for large or recurrent lesions. A recent review of well-documented cases in the literature found an overall recurrence rate of 33%, with 5-year and 10-year recurrence rates of 42% and 69%, respectively. Malignant transformation of recurrent ameloblastic fibroma into an ameloblastic fibrosarcoma or a fibrosarcoma was reported in 11% of cases.[112] Long-term follow-up is recommended because of the risk of recurrence and malignant transformation.

Ameloblastic Fibro-Odontoma

Ameloblastic fibro-odontomas are a benign tumor that exhibits features of an ameloblastic fibroma but also produces enamel and dentin. The tumor mainly arises in children and adolescents, with a mean age of approximately 9 years and a slight male predilection.[111] The most commonly involved site is the posterior mandible. All reported cases have been intraosseous. The lesion is usually painless and slowly growing. Occasionally these tumors may become extremely large and cause marked facial disfigurement. Smaller lesions may be discovered during radiographic examination for delayed tooth eruption, whereas larger lesions produce noticeable swelling. Radiographs show a well-defined, unilocular, or multilocular radiolucency with associated radiopacity. There is often a sclerotic border. The radiopaque component may range from several small, scattered calcifications to a single, large calcified mass. Many cases

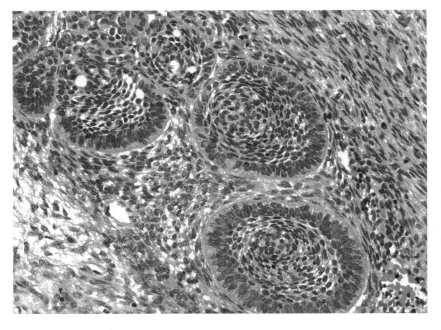

Fig. 51. Ameloblastic fibrosarcoma. Ameloblastic tumor islands within a hypercellular, atypical fibrous stroma.

are associated with the crown of an unerupted tooth.

Ameloblastic fibro-odontoma: Gross features

Ameloblastic fibro-odontomas usually appear as a firm, solid mass with a smooth surface. The crown of an associated impacted tooth may be embedded within the tumor. The cut surface may exhibit granular or nodular hard tissue deposits.

Ameloblastic fibro-odontoma: Microscopic features

The tumor includes both soft and hard tissue components. The soft tissue component exhibits features of ameloblastic fibroma (ie, anastomosing cords and small islands of odontogenic epithelium within a primitive mesenchymal stroma). The hard tissue component includes enamel and dentin, which may appear as focal calcifications, larger disorganized masses, or rudimentary teeth (**Fig. 52**). Dentin formation can vary from immature dentinoid or dysplastic dentin to more mature, tubular dentin. Cementum also may be present in some cases, usually on the outer surfaces of rudimentary tooth structures.

The term, *ameloblastic fibrodentinoma*, may be applied to cases in which the hard tissue component only includes dentinoid or tubular dentin. Enamel is absent. Some investigators have regarded ameloblastic fibrodentinoma as a distinct entity, whereas others have preferred to regard it as a variant of ameloblastic fibro-odontoma or ameloblastic fibroma.

Ameloblastic fibro-odontoma: Differential diagnosis

Histopathologic distinction between an ameloblastic fibro-odontoma and a developing odontoma may be virtually impossible. Practically speaking, lesions that seem to represent true neoplasms due to progressive growth are best classified as ameloblastic fibro-odontomas, whereas lesions with more limited growth consistent with a hamartoma may be classified as developing odontomas.

The epithelium within the ameloblastic fibro-odontoma resembles that of ameloblastoma. Enamel, dentin, and primitive mesenchymal stroma, however, readily distinguish ameloblastic fibro-odontoma from ameloblastoma.

Careful examination of the stromal component is necessary to differentiate between ameloblastic fibro-odontoma and ameloblastic fibro-odontosarcoma (or between ameloblastic fibrodentinoma and ameloblastic fibrodentinosarcoma). Sarcomatous transformation is rare and evidenced by cytologic atypia, nuclear pleomorphism, and significant mitotic activity.

Ameloblastic fibro-odontoma: Prognosis

The prognosis is excellent. Curettage is the most common treatment, and recurrence is rare.

Odontoma

Odontomas are hamartomas comprised of tooth-like elements. Odontomas represent one of the most common types of odontogenic tumors. Among various large-scale surveys, the reported

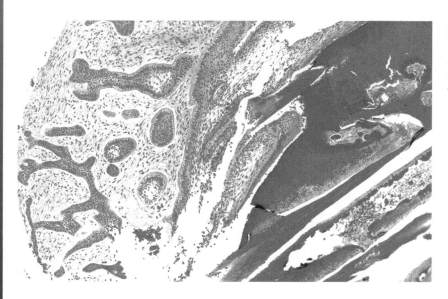

Fig. 52. Ameloblastic fibro-odontoma. The tumor includes an ameloblastic fibroma–like component (*left*) as well as an odontoma-like component (*right*).

frequency ranges from 4% to 67% of all odontogenic tumors, with higher frequencies generally reported in the Americas and Europe and lower frequencies in Asia and Africa.[117–121] It is uncertain whether this variation reflects differences in types of specimens submitted for histopathologic diagnosis rather than true differences in prevalence.

There are two types of odontomas—compound and complex. The distinction between these two types is somewhat subjective and of little clinical relevance. Compound odontomas are comprised of fairly organized tooth-like structures (denticles or toothlets), whereas complex odontomas are comprised of haphazard conglomerates of dental tissues.

Odontomas tend to arise in young patients, with the majority of cases diagnosed in the first and second decades. Compound odontomas most commonly involve the anterior maxilla, whereas complex odontomas most commonly involve the posterior mandible. The lesions usually are painless and slow-growing. Most cases are discovered either during routine radiographic examination or when radiographs are obtained to determine the cause of failed tooth eruption. The compound odontoma is readily recognized radiographically as a cluster of dwarfed, malformed tooth–like structures surrounded by a radiolucent zone (**Fig. 53**). In contrast, the complex odontoma appears as an amorphous mass of calcified material with a narrow radiolucent rim; this radiographic presentation may mimic that of other intraosseous lesions, such as the osteoma, ossifying fibroma, or cemento-osseous dysplasia. Many odontomas are associated with impacted teeth. In addition, in some instances, small odontomas may be found between the roots of erupted teeth.

In unusual cases, odontomas may arise entirely within the gingival soft tissues without bony involvement. Rare cases of patients with multiple odontomas involving both jaws (so-called odontoma syndrome) also have been reported.[122] Multiple odontomas may arise in association with Gardner syndrome.

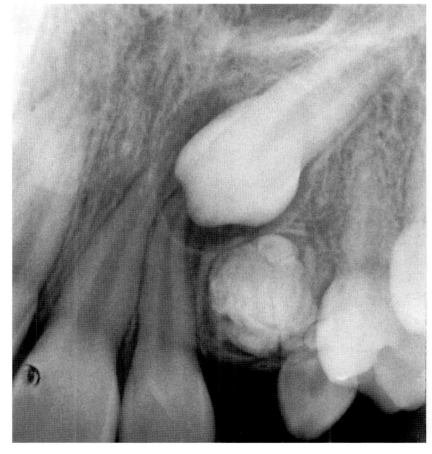

Fig. 53. Compound odontoma. Radiograph showing a cluster of dwarfed, malformed tooth–like structures surrounded by a radiolucent zone. The mass is blocking eruption of the maxillary canine. (*Courtesy of* Dr Dirk Anderson.)

Odontoma: Gross features

A compound odontoma is comprised of a variable number of denticles. Denticles grossly appear as malformed tooth–like structures, which typically are smaller than normal teeth (**Fig. 54**). In a complex odontoma, the dental hard tissue may exhibit a nonspecific ovoid, rounded, or irregular morphology. Parts of a dental follicle also may be seen grossly in association with an odontoma. Most odontomas are small, but giant lesions and lesions comprised of hundreds of denticles are possible.

Odontoma: Microscopic features

In a compound odontoma, there are several tooth-like structures comprised of enamel, dentin, cementum, and pulp tissue (**Fig. 55**). In contrast, a complex odontoma is characterized by more haphazard conglomerates of dental tissue (**Fig. 56**). On decalcification, what remains of the enamel is the matrix, which appears basophilic with a hexagonal pattern when cut en face. Dentin appears as eosinophilic tubules or more poorly organized, amorphous dentinoid. A cementum layer is typically found overlying dentin. The pulp appears as fibrous connective tissue occupying a chamber surrounded by dental hard tissue; it may be possible to observe odontoblasts lining the periphery of the chamber.

Other elements may include fragments of reduced enamel epithelium (appearing as eosinophilic cuboidal epithelium) and dental follicle (appearing as loosely arranged fibrous connective tissue). Formation of a dentigerous cyst from the follicular tissue associated with an odontoma is possible. In addition, focal aggregates of ghost cells occasionally may be found within odontomas; these ghost cells appear as eosinophilic epithelial cells, which have lost their nuclei but retain their nuclear outlines. Approximately 24% of calcifying odontogenic cysts have been reported to occur in association with odontomas.[123]

Odontoma: Differential diagnosis

The microscopic diagnosis usually is straightforward. The distinction between a developing odontoma and an ameloblastic fibro-odontoma, however, may be difficult (discussed previously). If a compound odontoma were comprised of a single denticle, then alternative classification as a supernumerary tooth could be considered.

Odontoma: Prognosis

The treatment of choice is conservative enucleation. In cases associated with an impacted tooth, odontoma removal may allow for tooth eruption. The lesions do not recur.

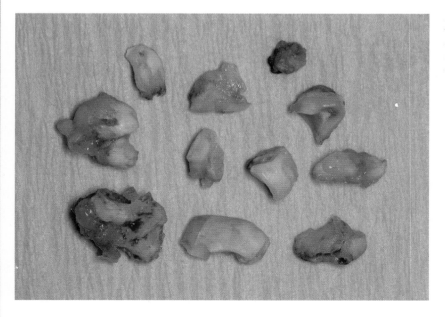

Fig. 54. Compound odontoma. Gross specimen consisting of multiple, malformed tooth–like structures (denticles).

Fig. 55. Compound odontoma. (*A*) Malformed tooth–like structures (or denticles). (*B*) Detail from a denticle in (*A*) shows tubular dentin, dentinoid, enamel, and a fragment of odontogenic epithelium.

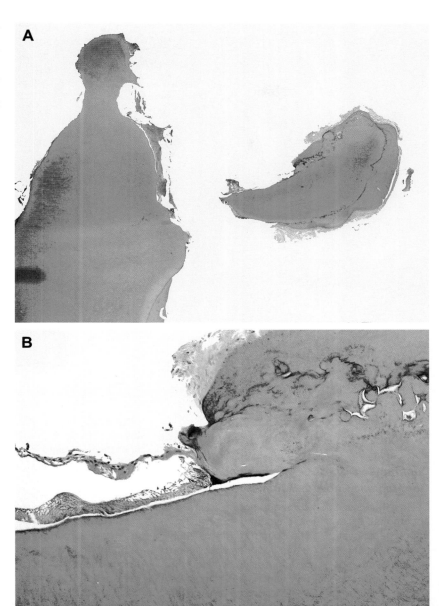

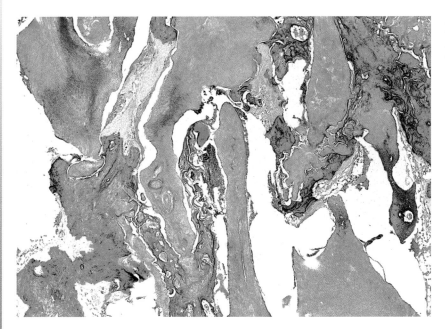

Fig. 56. Complex odontoma. Haphazard mass of dentin, dentinoid, cementum, and dystrophic enamel.

Calcifying Cystic Odontogenic Tumor (Calcifying Odontogenic Cyst, Keratinizing and Calcifying Odontogenic Cyst, Gorlin Cyst, Dentinogenic Ghost Cell Tumor, and Epithelial Odontogenic Ghost Cell Tumor)

Calcifying cystic odontogenic tumors (CCOTs) are uncommon lesions first described as calcifying odontogenic cysts.[124] The spectrum of this entity, however, includes those that occur as solid lesions with little attempt at cyst formation, which were subsequently classified as dentinogenic ghost cell tumors (DGCTs).[125] Over the years, several different terms have been used to describe microscopic variations of this pathologic process.[126] The most recent WHO classification considers this spectrum to be neoplastic, identifying two separate entities: CCOT and DGCT.[127,128] These lesions are undoubtedly related—one occurring as primarily a cystic process (CCOT) and the other occurring as a more aggressive solid tumor (DGCT). In addition, a malignant counterpart (ghost cell odontogenic carcinoma) is also recognized.[129]

CCOTs can occur anywhere in the jaws, but the most common location is the anterior maxilla. The lesion most often develops within bone, although 5% to 30% of cases have been reported to occur within the gingival soft tissues. CCOTs may occur at any age, but most cases are diagnosed during the second to fourth decades of life. The lesion sometimes occurs in association with other odontogenic tumors, especially the odontoma.

Small CCOTs may be discovered as incidental findings on dental radiographs, but larger lesions can present as slowly enlarging, painless swellings. Radiographically, these lesions often appear as a well-circumscribed unilocular radiolucency although they can be multilocular. From one-third to one-half of all cases also demonstrate irregular radiopaque calcifications within the lesion, especially those cases that are associated with odontoma formation. Approximately one-third of cases are associated with an impacted tooth.

Solid DGCTs occur less frequently, comprising 5% to 14% of odontogenic ghost cell lesions. Intraosseous DGCTs have the potential for more significant growth and destruction, although peripheral DGCTs within the gingival soft tissues behave less aggressively.

Calcifying cystic odontogenic tumor: Gross features

The gross appearance of a CCOT is usually indistinguishable from other odontogenic cysts and tumors. The presence of calcified material within the lesion may suggest the possibility of a CCOT in the differential diagnosis, although it may be difficult to distinguish such calcifications from incidental bone fragments or the mineralized product formed within other jaw lesions.

Calcifying cystic odontogenic tumor: Microscopic features

CCOTs are cystic lesions that are lined by odontogenic epithelium ranging from 4 to 10 cells in thickness. This epithelium often exhibits ameloblastic differentiation with a hyperchromatic, palisaded layer of cuboidal to columnar basal cells, sometimes with reverse nuclear polarization (**Fig. 57**). The upper layers may be loosely arranged and reminiscent of the stellate reticulum of the enamel organ. The hallmark of a CCOT is the presence of scattered eosinophilic ghost cells in the epithelial lining, which show loss of nuclei but preservation of the nuclear outlines. This ghost cell change was originally thought to be an abnormal form of keratinization, although some investigators believe that it represents necrosis or accumulation of enamel protein material. The ghost cells frequently undergo calcification, first appearing as small basophilic granules that may increase in size to produce larger masses of calcified material. Sheets of ghost cells may also be found in the cyst wall or cyst lumen, sometimes in association with the formation of dysplastic dentin (dentinoid) (**Fig. 58**). Solid DGCTs have similar microscopic features, albeit with little or no attempt at cyst formation. Some

CCOTs are associated with adjacent odontoma formation, characterized by the presence of tubular dentin and enamel matrix.

Calcifying cystic odontogenic tumor: Differential diagnosis

The basic microscopic appearance of a CCOT mimics an ameloblastoma. Both lesions are characterized by (1) hyperchromatic, palisaded, columnar basilar cells with reverse nuclear polarization consistent with ameloblasts and (2) loosely arranged cells in the spinous layer consistent with the stellate reticulum of the enamel organ. Although rare ghost cells have been reported in ameloblastomas, significant numbers of ghost cells should always be found in CCOTs. Also, an ameloblastoma should not be associated with the elaboration of a dentinoid product, as may be observed in a CCOT.

Calcifying cystic odontogenic tumor: Prognosis

Most CCOTs are treated by surgical enucleation and have an excellent prognosis with only a small chance of recurrence. Peripheral CCOTs and DGCTs in the gingival soft tissues also have a good prognosis after local excision. Occasionally, larger DGCTs in bone may require more significant surgical management, such as local resection.

Fig. 57. Calcifying odontogenic cyst. The basal epithelial layer is composed of hyperchromatic, palisaded columnar cells with reverse nuclear polarization. Scattered eosinophilic ghost cells can be seen in the epithelial lining.

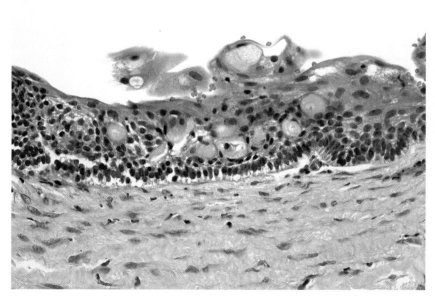

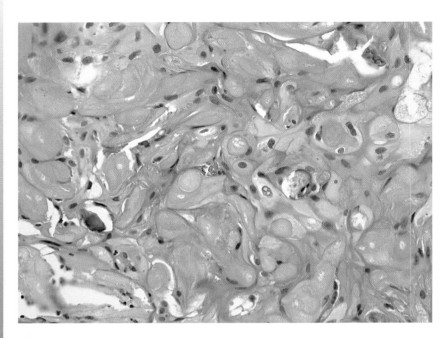

Fig. 58. Calcifying odontogenic cyst. Sheets of ghost cells within the cyst wall. Focal dystrophic calcification can be seen.

Rare cases of malignant transformation have been reported (ghost cell odontogenic carcinoma). Recurrences are more common with these malignant tumors, and a few have metastasized. Although few cases have been documented, a 5-year survival rate of 73% has been estimated.

TUMORS OF ODONTOGENIC ECTOMESENCHYME

Central Odontogenic Fibroma

The central odontogenic fibroma is a rare benign odontogenic neoplasm, characterized by a proliferation of odontogenic ectomesenchyme, with or without odontogenic epithelium. Unfortunately, there has been much confusion in the literature regarding this tumor. In the past, well-circumscribed fibrous masses associated with the crowns of unerupted teeth were reported as odontogenic fibromas; most authorities now agree that these lesions should be classified as enlarged dental follicles rather than true neoplasms.[130] Another source of confusion has been the considerable histopathologic variation among these tumors; the so-called simple type, WHO-type, and giant cell variants are described later. The peripheral odontogenic fibroma and central granular cell odontogenic tumor (granular cell odontogenic fibroma) are discussed separately.

The central odontogenic fibroma occurs over a broad age range (4–80 years), with a peak in the second and third decades.[131] Approximately 70% of cases have occurred in females.[132] The mandible and maxilla are involved with equal frequency. In the maxilla, the anterior region is most commonly involved, whereas in the mandible, the posterior region is most commonly involved. The usual clinical presentation is a painless swelling. Pain and paresthesia are infrequent findings. On radiographic examination, small lesions typically appear as well-defined unilocular radiolucencies, whereas large lesions tend to be multilocular or exhibit a scalloped border. Root resorption and divergence of adjacent teeth are possible. A periapical or interradicular relationship with adjacent teeth is found most often; however, a few rare cases of pericoronal lesions radiographically mimicking dentigerous cysts have been reported.[132,133]

Central odontogenic fibroma: Gross features

Gross examination typically shows white or tan, firm to rubbery, solid tissue.

Central odontogenic fibroma: Microscopic features

There are two histopathologic variants: the simple type and the WHO type. The simple type is comprised of evenly spaced, stellate to ovoid fibroblasts set within an abundant ground substance (**Fig. 59**). The fibroblasts may be arranged in

Fig. 59. Central odonto-genic fibroma, simple type. Dense fibrous con-nective tissue. Odonto-genic epithelial rests are absent in this example.

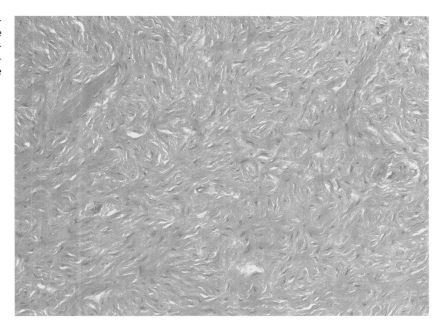

a whorled or interlacing pattern, and the collagen fibrils may be either delicate or dense. Odontogenic epithelial rests are absent or minimally present. Isolated dystrophic calcifications may be identified. In contrast, the WHO type is characterized by more cellular fibrous connective tissue with scattered nests or strands of odontogenic epithelium (**Fig. 60**). The cellular areas of the connective tissue may be intermixed with less cellular zones with numerous capillaries. The epithelial component may be sparse or abundant, and the connective tissue may range from myxoid to hyalinized. Dentinoid, cementum-like calcifications or osteoid occasionally may be present. In some cases, the

Fig. 60. Central odonto-genic fibroma, WHO type. Moderately cellular fib-rous connective tissue with numerous strands and nests of odontogenic epi-thelium.

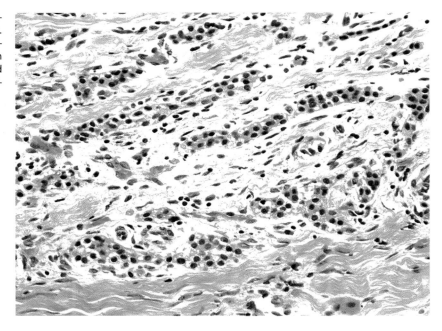

central odontogenic fibroma may be accompanied by a giant cell granuloma–like component.

Central odontogenic fibroma: Differential diagnosis

The simple type of central odontogenic fibroma potentially may be confused with a hyperplastic dental follicle. A dental follicle is always associated with the crown of an unerupted tooth; in contrast, the central odontogenic fibroma more often is found in an interradicular or periapical relationship to teeth than in a pericoronal location. In addition, hyperplastic dental follicles tend to be smaller than central odontogenic fibromas.

There is histopathologic similarity between the simple type of central odontogenic fibroma and the myxofibroma. Some investigators have suggested that the simple odontogenic fibroma belongs within the spectrum of odontogenic myxoma, which includes not only entirely myxoid lesions but also the more collagenized myxofibroma or fibromyxoma.[130,134] Unlike the myxofibroma, the central odontogenic fibroma is not infiltrative and tends to have a more limited growth potential.

Differentiating between a central odontogenic fibroma and a desmoplastic fibroma may be especially difficult in some cases; this distinction is clinically relevant because the latter is infiltrative and requires more extensive surgery. Central odontogenic fibromas with abundant ground substance, odontogenic epithelium, and/or calcified product do not pose much diagnostic difficulty. However, cases with dense connective tissue in the absence of odontogenic epithelium and calcification may appear similar to desmoplastic fibroma. In such cases, correlation with the clinical and radiographic features is essential. Local infiltration and cortical destruction, particularly in young patients, favor a desmoplastic fibroma. In addition, the collagen fibers tend to be arranged in broader, longer bands in a desmoplastic fibroma. Nevertheless, considering the potential difficulty in distinguishing between these tumors, treatment should be determined on an individual basis with respect to the extent of a given lesion.

Central odontogenic fibromas with an epithelial component should not be confused with ameloblastomas. Unlike the epithelium in an ameloblastoma, the epithelium in a central odontogenic fibroma appears inactive. There is no peripheral layer of columnar cells with reverse polarization of their nuclei, and there is no central stellate reticulum–like differentiation. Furthermore, inductive effect (a zone of hyalinization directly surrounding the epithelium) should not be found in a central odontogenic fibroma.

Central odontogenic fibroma: Prognosis

Enucleation with vigorous curettage is the preferred treatment. Recurrence is infrequent. There is no difference in clinical behavior between the simple type and WHO type of central odontogenic fibroma. There is an increased likelihood of recurrence, however, among central odontogenic fibromas with an associated giant cell granuloma–like component.

Peripheral Odontogenic Fibroma

Peripheral odontogenic fibromas are the extraosseous counterpart of central odontogenic fibromas. More than 380 cases have been reported in the literature.[135,136] According to two large case series, they represent the most common type of peripheral odontogenic tumor.[74,137] Furthermore, they are the only peripheral odontogenic tumor more frequently found than its central counterpart, with an approximate 1.4:1 peripheral-to-central ratio.[137]

The peripheral odontogenic fibroma exclusively occurs on the gingiva or alveolar mucosa. The typical clinical presentation is a firm, slowly growing, painless, sessile nodule. The clinical findings are nonspecific and mimic those of a fibroma, peripheral ossifying fibroma, pyogenic granuloma, or peripheral giant cell granuloma. Among reported cases, there is a broad age range (newborn to 83 years), with an average age of approximately 37 to 40 years. The lesion is slightly more common in females than males (female-to-male ratio of 1:0.8). The mandibular and maxillary mucosae are involved with similar frequency, and there is a predilection for the incisor-canine region. Reported lesion size ranges from 0.3 to 4.5 cm, with most lesions measuring less than 3 cm.[135,136] Radiographic examination shows either no bony involvement or cupping resorption of the underlying alveolar bone. In some cases, calcified flecks may be evident radiographically.

Peripheral odontogenic fibroma: Gross features

The lesion grossly appears as a firm, tan nodule. On sectioning, a gritty texture may be evident if the lesion has produced calcification. Lesions with considerable calcification may require decalcification before sectioning.

Peripheral odontogenic fibroma: Microscopic features

The histopathologic findings are similar to the WHO-type central odontogenic fibroma. Microscopic examination shows a nodular tumor mass.

The surface epithelium overlying the lesion often has slender, elongated rete ridges. The tumor is characterized by a variable amount of odontogenic epithelium scattered within a fibrous to myxoid stroma (**Fig. 61**). The odontogenic epithelium may be either scant or prominent and is arranged in cords, nests, or islands. In approximately half of cases, calcification is present, including osteoid, dysplastic dentin, cementum-like calcifications, and/or dystrophic calcifications. Hyalinization or calcification may be evident surrounding the odontogenic epithelium (so-called inductive effect). Unusual variants include peripheral odontogenic fibromas with multinucleated giant cells (or giant cell granuloma–like areas) and peripheral odontogenic fibromas with stromal granular cells (peripheral granular cell odontogenic fibroma or peripheral granular cell odontogenic tumor).

Fig. 61. Peripheral odontogenic fibroma. (*A*) Low-power photomicrograph shows a nodule surfaced by squamous epithelium. (*B*) High-power photomicrograph shows moderately cellular fibrous connective tissue with scattered nests of odontogenic epithelium.

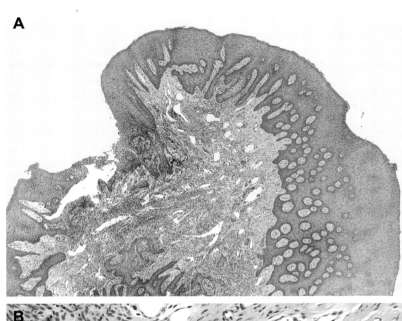

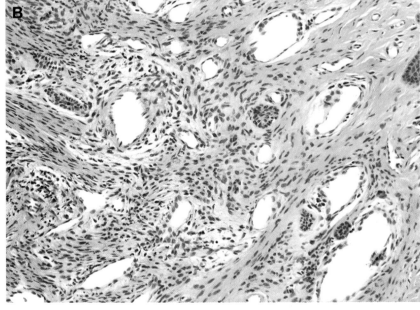

Peripheral odontogenic fibroma: Differential diagnosis

Peripheral ossifying fibromas may be confused with peripheral odontogenic fibromas, because of similarity in clinical presentation and terminology. In addition, both types of lesions may exhibit a moderately cellular fibroblastic proliferation with associated calcification. Unlike peripheral odontogenic fibromas, peripheral ossifying fibromas do not exhibit a significant odontogenic epithelial component.

Peripheral odontogenic fibromas also are similar to peripheral ameloblastomas. Both lesions present as slow-growing gingival nodules and microscopically are characterized by islands or strands of odontogenic epithelium within a moderately cellular fibrous to myxoid stroma. The odontogenic epithelium within peripheral odontogenic fibromas, however, does not exhibit the characteristic basal layer with reverse polarization seen in ameloblastoma. Also, peripheral odontogenic fibromas occasionally produce dysplastic dentin, cementum-like calcifications, or osteoid, whereas no calcified product is seen in peripheral ameloblastomas.

OGEH also exhibits clinical and microscopic similarities to the peripheral odontogenic fibroma (see previous discussion of differential diagnosis for peripheral ameloblastoma). Many investigators now believe that OGEH represents the same lesion as either the peripheral odontogenic fibroma or peripheral ameloblastoma.

Peripheral odontogenic fibroma: Prognosis

Conservative surgical excision is the preferred treatment. Clinical follow-up is recommended, because some cases have been reported to recur. In one study, the presence of budding hyperplasia of the overlying surface epithelium was associated with an increased recurrence rate.[135]

Central Granular Cell Odontogenic Tumor

The central granular cell odontogenic tumor is a rare odontogenic neoplasm, with only 35 cases reported in the literature.[138–143] This tumor also has been referred to as granular cell ameloblastic fibroma, central granular cell odontogenic fibroma, and central granular cell tumor of the jaws. Because of the uncertain histogenesis of the granular cells in this lesion, the authors prefer the noncommittal term, central granular cell odontogenic tumor.

Among reported cases, the average age at diagnosis is 45 years, and there is a female predilection (approximate female-to-male ratio of 3:1). The most common location is the mandibular molar-premolar region. The lesions range in size from 0.5 to 8.0 cm, with an average size of 3.5 cm.[138–140] A painless, expansile mass is often clinically evident, although pain, tenderness, and lack of expansion also are possible. Radiographic examination typically shows a well-defined, unilocular or multilocular radiolucency. Focal calcifications may be seen in some cases. Tooth displacement and root resorption also are possible.

Central granular cell odontogenic tumor: Gross features

The lesion typically appears as a firm, solid tumor mass, which may separate cleanly from the surrounding bone. On sectioning, a grainy texture and/or calcified flecks may be evident.

Central granular cell odontogenic tumor: Microscopic features

Microscopic examination shows sheets and lobules of plump, eosinophilic granular cells. These granular cells exhibit abundant granular cytoplasm and either eccentric or centrally located nuclei (**Fig. 62**). Thin fibrovascular connective tissue septa intervene between tumor lobules. Scattered among the granular cells are cords and nests of odontogenic epithelium. The epithelial cells exhibit lightly eosinophilic to clear cytoplasm. At the periphery of the nests, the epithelial cells tend to be cuboidal to low columnar. The central epithelial cells do not exhibit stellate reticulum–like differentiation. A zone of hyalinization surrounding the epithelial cords and nests (inductive effect) may be observed. In addition, small basophilic cementum–like calcifications, dystrophic calcifications, or dentinoid may be found in some lesions. The calcifications most often are associated with the granular cells, although occasionally they may be associated with tumor epithelium.[139]

The granular cells are PAS-positive and diastase resistant. Immunohistochemical studies typically show the granular cells to be positive for CD68 and negative for S-100. The granular cells also may be positive for α_1-antichymotrypsin, α_1-antitrypsin, lysozyme, bcl-2, and vimentin. Negativity for glial fibrillary acidic protein, CD1a, muscle-specific actin, and cytokeratins has been reported. On an ultrastructural level, the cytoplasmic granules are consistent with lysosomes.[139,140,142] Based on immunohistochemical and ultrastructural findings, the granular cells are likely mesenchymal in origin with a possible histiocytic lineage, although various other theories on histogenesis have been proposed. It is unclear whether these granular cells are neoplastic, reactive, degenerative, or metabolic in nature.

Fig. 62. Central granular cell odontogenic tumor. Lobules of plump granular cells with nests of odontogenic epithelium.

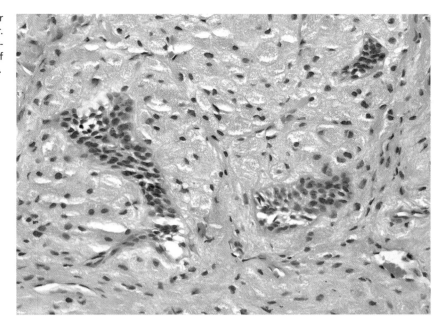

Central granular cell odontogenic tumor: Differential diagnosis

Both the granular cell ameloblastoma and the central granular cell odontogenic tumor are intraosseous tumors with granular cells and odontogenic epithelium. In the granular cell ameloblastoma, the granular cells occupy the central portions of the epithelial tumor islands. In contrast, the granular cells in the granular cell odontogenic tumor represent the mesenchymal component surrounding the epithelium. Accordingly, the granular cells in granular cell ameloblastoma exhibit immunoreactivity for cytokeratins, whereas the granular cells in granular cell odontogenic tumor lack cytokeratin immunoreactivity.

There is a single documented case of a malignant granular cell odontogenic tumor.[143] This tumor consisted of an expansile, polypoid mass involving the palate and maxillary sinus. CT scans showed poorly delineated borders and cortical erosion—features that are unusual for a benign central granular cell odontogenic tumor. Histopathologic examination showed fibroblastic spindle cells and granular cells with strands of odontogenic epithelium and scattered cementicles. The granular cells exhibited atypical features, including hyperchromatic, pleomorphic nuclei, and prominent nucleoli. The spindle cells exhibited modest nuclear pleomorphism as well. Frequent mitoses were evident. Therefore, cytologic atypia and mitotic activity are features that should prompt consideration of malignancy. In this particular case, the tumor recurred after radical excision, although no regional or distant metastasis was reported.

Central granular cell odontogenic tumor: Prognosis

Central granular cell odontogenic tumors usually are treated by conservative enucleation and/or curettage. Recurrence has been reported in only one case.[139]

Odontogenic Myxoma (Myxoma, Fibromyxoma, and Myxofibroma)

Odontogenic myxomas are benign, locally aggressive neoplasms comprised of spindled, round, or stellate cells within an abundant myxoid stroma. The tumors are believed to originate from the primitive ectomesenchyme of a developing tooth or the undifferentiated mesenchymal cells of the periodontal ligament. An odontogenic origin is supported by its predominant occurrence in the tooth-bearing areas of the jaws, frequent association with unerupted or missing teeth, predilection for young individuals, histologic similarity to the papilla or follicle or a developing tooth, and occasional inclusion of inactive odontogenic epithelium.

The mean age among larger reported case series ranges from approximately 24 to 37 years,[144] with the majority of cases diagnosed in the second through fourth decades of life.[145] Most investigators have reported either a slight female predilection or no significant gender predilection.[144] The mandibular molar region and ramus are involved most frequently. Maxillary lesions tend to arise posteriorly also and may invade the maxillary sinus. The tumor is often a slowly enlarging, asymptomatic mass that is only discovered after it has grown to a considerable size. Pain, paresthesia, and tooth mobility occasionally have been reported.[146–148] The radiographic presentation is variable. Small lesions tend to be unilocular, whereas large lesions are frequently multilocular with a honeycomb, soap bubble, wispy, or tennis racket–like pattern (**Fig. 63**). The radiographic borders may be either well-defined or ill-defined.

Odontogenic myxoma is a central lesion of the jaws. Soft tissue myxomas also are possible, although such tumors are not odontogenic and thus not discussed. In addition, there are several examples of cases reported as maxillary myxomas in pediatric patients; however, it is debatable whether such lesions are maxillary odontogenic myxomas versus nonodontogenic, extraosseous sinonasal myxomas.[149–154]

Odontogenic myxoma: Gross features

Lesions that are predominantly myxoid have a gelatinous, translucent appearance. In contrast, lesions with a more collagenized stroma may be firm and opaque.

Odontogenic myxoma: Microscopic features

Microscopic examination shows an unencapsulated, infiltrative mass comprised of loosely arranged spindled, round, or stellate cells within an abundant myxoid stroma. The tumor cells exhibit delicate, slender processes with pale, eosinophilic cytoplasm. Binucleation, nuclear hyperchromatism, mild pleomorphism, and focal mitotic activity are possible but not indicative of greater recurrence potential. The myxoid matrix is rich in hyaluronic acid and chondroitin sulfate and stains strongly with Alcian blue at pH 2.5.[148] Although most cases exhibit only sparse collagen production, the amount of collagen may vary considerably. Lesions with more collagenous stroma may be classified under the alternative terms, *fibromyxoma* or *myxofibroma*. Nests or islands of inactive odontogenic epithelium are an infrequent finding (**Fig. 64**).

Odontogenic myxoma: Differential diagnosis

A well-known pitfall is misdiagnosis of a dental follicle or dental papilla as an odontogenic myxoma. Kim and Ellis[155] reported that among 847 dental follicles and dental papillae submitted to the Armed Forces Institute of Pathology for diagnostic consultation, only 53% of submitting pathologists correctly identified these structures; 20% of cases were misdiagnosed as odontogenic cyst or tumor, and the dental papilla was most commonly misdiagnosed as odontogenic myxoma. The clinicoradiographic context should help distinguish a dental follicle or dental papilla from an odontogenic myxoma. A dental follicle

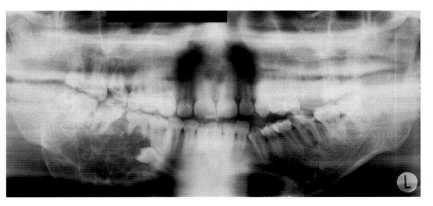

Fig. 63. Odontogenic myxoma. Radiograph showing a large, multilocular radiolucency with a tennis racket–like pattern in the posterior mandible. (*Courtesy of* Dr Brent Klinger.)

Fig. 64. Odontogenic myxoma. Loosely arranged spindle cells with delicate collagen fibrils set within an abundant myxoid stroma. An isolated nest of inactive odontogenic epithelium also is seen.

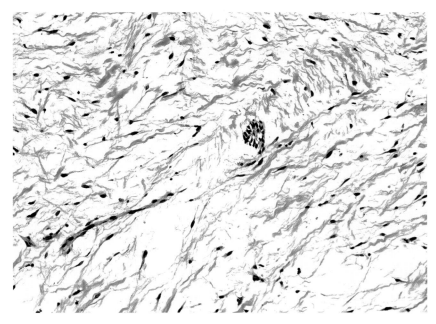

radiographically appears as a lucency surrounding the crown of an unerupted tooth; even when hyperplastic, a dental follicle is typically only a few millimeters in maximum diameter. The follicular tissue is attached to the cemento-enamel junction of the associated tooth or may be submitted as several detached fragments of soft, grayish tan tissue. In contrast, an odontogenic myxoma is generally larger, may appear unilocular or multilocular radiographically, and grossly tends to appear more gelatinous. Both the dental papilla and odontogenic myxoma are

Fig. 65. Dental papilla. Discrete, round mass with a peripheral condensation of mesenchymal cells and primitive odontoblasts. Its myxoid appearance should not be confused with an odontogenic myxoma.

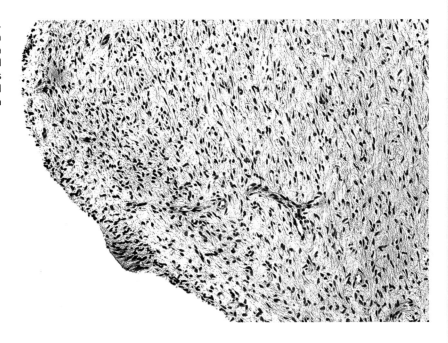

Pitfalls
ODONTOGENIC MYXOMA

! A dental follicle or dental papilla may be confused with an odontogenic myxoma.

! Helpful features for recognizing a dental follicle

- Radiographically appears as a unilocular lucency surrounding the crown of an unerupted tooth. Even when hyperplastic, a dental follicle is typically only a few millimeters in maximum diameter. In contrast, an odontogenic myxoma is generally larger and may be either unilocular or multilocular.

- Macroscopically, the follicular tissue is attached to the cervicoenamel junction of the associated tooth or may be submitted as several detached fragments of soft, grayish tan tissue. In contrast, an odontogenic myxoma grossly appears more gelatinous.

- Microscopically, the dental follicle is usually more collagenous compared with an odontogenic myxoma. A follicle may be focally lined by reduced enamel epithelium. Scattered odontogenic epithelial rests are usually more abundant compared with the scant epithelium that occasionally may be found in an odontogenic myxoma.

! Helpful features for recognizing a dental papilla

- Macroscopically, both the dental papilla and odontogenic myxoma appear gelatinous. The dental papilla, however, is a distinct, round, translucent white disc-like mass with a maximum diameter of approximately 1 cm. Recognition of this distinct tissue mass received separately or attached to the apical aspect of a developing tooth crown should readily distinguish it from an odontogenic myxoma.

- Microscopically, appears as a discrete, round mass with a peripheral condensation of mesenchymal cells/primitive odontoblasts.

grossly gelatinous. The dental papilla is a round, translucent white disc-like mass with a maximum diameter of approximately 1 cm. Recognition of this distinct disc-like mass received separately or attached to the apical aspect of a developing tooth crown should readily distinguish it from an odontogenic myxoma.

On a microscopic level, the dental follicle, dental papilla, and odontogenic myxoma all may appear hypocellular and myxoid. The dental follicle is usually more collagenous compared with an odontogenic myxoma. In addition, the focal presence of reduced enamel epithelium (eosinophilic columnar to cuboidal epithelium) lining a dental follicle may aid in recognition. Furthermore, scattered odontogenic epithelium is usually more abundant in a dental follicle compared with an odontogenic myxoma (see **Fig. 34**). As for the dental papilla, its appearance as a discrete, round mass with a peripheral condensation of mesenchymal cells/primitive odontoblasts should help with proper identification (**Fig. 65**).

Odontogenic myxoma: Prognosis

Because of the infiltrative nature of the odontogenic myxoma, marginal resection is the treatment of choice. Curettage with peripheral ostectomy may be considered for small tumors. Complete removal is especially difficult for maxillary lesions. Reported recurrence rates range from 10% to 33%.[156] Malignant transformation into an odontogenic myxosarcoma has been reported only rarely.[157,158]

REFERENCES

1. Philipsen HP. Keratocystic odontogenic tumour. In: Barnes L, Eveson JW, Reichart P, et al, editors. World Health Organization classification of tumours: pathology and genetics of head and neck tumours. Lyon (France): IARC Press; 2005. p. 306–7.

2. Shear M, Speight PM. Radicular cyst and residual cyst. Cysts of the oral and maxillofacial regions. 4th edition. Oxford (United Kingdom): Blackwell Munksgaard; 2007. p. 123–42.

3. Neville BW, Damm DD, Allen CM, et al. Periapical cyst (radicular cyst; apical periodontal cyst). Oral and maxillofacial pathology. 3rd edition. St Louis (MO): Saunders Elsevier; 2009. p. 130–5.

4. Slabbert H, Shear M, Altini M. Vacuolated cells and mucous metaplasia in the epithelial linings of radicular and residual cysts. J Oral Pathol Med 1995; 24(7):309–12.

5. Nair PN, Pajarola G, Luder HU. Ciliated epithelium-lined radicular cysts. Oral Surg Oral Med Oral Pathol Oral Radiol Endod 2002;94(4):485–93.

6. Takeda Y, Oikawa Y, Furuya I, et al. Mucous and ciliated cell metaplasia in epithelial linings of odontogenic inflammatory and developmental cysts. J Oral Sci 2005;47(2):77–81.

7. Rushton MA. Hyaline bodies in the epithelium of dental cysts. Proc R Soc Med 1955;48(5):407–9.

8. El-Labban NG. Electron microscopic investigation of hyaline bodies in odontogenic cysts. J Oral Pathol 1979;8(2):81–93.

9. Shear M, Speight PM. Dentigerous cyst. Cysts of the oral and maxillofacial regions. 4th edition. Oxford (United Kingdom): Blackwell Munksgaard; 2007. p. 59–75.

10. Daley TD, Wysocki GP, Pringle GA. Relative incidence of odontogenic tumors and oral and jaw cysts in a Canadian population. Oral Surg Oral Med Oral Pathol 1994;77(3):276–80.

11. Jones AV, Craig GT, Franklin CD. Range and demographics of odontogenic cysts diagnosed in a UK population over a 30-year period. J Oral Pathol Med 2006;35(8):500–7.

12. Neville BW, Damm DD, Allen CM, et al. Dentigerous cyst (follicular cyst). Oral and maxillofacial pathology. 3rd edition. St Louis (MO): Saunders Elsevier; 2009. p. 679–82.

13. Browne RM. Metaplasia and degeneration in odontogenic cysts in man. J Oral Pathol 1972;1(4):145–58.

14. Daley TD, Wysocki GP. The small dentigerous cyst. A diagnostic dilemma. Oral Surg Oral Med Oral Pathol Oral Radiol Endod 1995;79(1):77–81.

15. Shear M. The aggressive nature of the odontogenic keratocyst: is it a benign cystic neoplasm? Part 2. Proliferation and genetic studies. Oral Oncol 2002;38(4):323–31.

16. Shear M, Speight PM. Odontogenic keratocyst. Cysts of the oral and maxillofacial regions. 4th edition. Oxford (United Kingdom): Blackwell Munksgaard; 2007. p. 6–58.

17. Brannon RB. The odontogenic keratocyst. A clinicopathologic study of 312 cases. Part I. Clinical features. Oral Surg Oral Med Oral Pathol 1976; 42(1):54–72.

18. Browne RM. The odontogenic keratocyst. Clinical aspects. Br Dent J 1970;128(5):225–31.

19. Chehade A, Daley TD, Wysocki GP, et al. Peripheral odontogenic keratocyst. Oral Surg Oral Med Oral Pathol 1994;77(5):494–7.

20. Chi AC, Owings JR Jr, Muller S. Peripheral odontogenic keratocyst: report of two cases and review of the literature. Oral Surg Oral Med Oral Pathol Oral Radiol Endod 2005;99(1):71–8.

21. Neville BW, Mishkin DJ, Traynham RT. The laterally positioned odontogenic keratocyst. A case report. J Periodontol 1984;55(2):98–102.

22. Neville BW, Damm DD, Brock T. Odontogenic keratocysts of the midline maxillary region. J Oral Maxillofac Surg 1997;55(4):340–4.

23. Browne RM. The odontogenic keratocyst. Histological features and their correlation with clinical behaviour. Br Dent J 1971;131(6):249–59.

24. Payne TF. An analysis of the clinical and histopathologic parameters of the odontogenic keratocyst. Oral Surg Oral Med Oral Pathol 1972;33(4): 538–46.

25. Brannon RB. The odontogenic keratocyst. A clinicopathologic study of 312 cases. Part II. Histologic features. Oral Surg Oral Med Oral Pathol 1977;43(2): 233–55.

26. Kratochvil FJ, Brannon RB. Cartilage in the walls of odontogenic keratocysts. J Oral Pathol Med 1993; 22(6):282–5.

27. Rodu B, Tate AL, Martinez MG Jr. The implications of inflammation in odontogenic keratocysts. J Oral Pathol 1987;16(10):518–21.

28. Jackson IT, Potparic Z, Fasching M, et al. Penetration of the skull base by dissecting keratocyst. J Craniomaxillofac Surg 1993;21(8):319–25.

29. Brøndum N, Jensen VJ. Recurrence of keratocysts and decompression treatment. A long-term follow-up of forty-four cases. Oral Surg Oral Med Oral Pathol 1991;72(3):265–9.

30. Gorlin RJ, Goltz RW. Multiple nevoid basal-cell epithelioma, jaw cysts and bifid rib. A syndrome. N Engl J Med 1960;262:908–12.

31. Cohen MM Jr. Nevoid basal cell carcinoma syndrome: molecular biology and new hypotheses. Int J Oral Maxillofac Surg 1999;28(3):216–23.

32. Gorlin RJ. Nevoid basal cell carcinoma (Gorlin) syndrome. Genet Med 2004;6(6):530–9.

33. Wright JM. The odontogenic keratocyst: orthokeratinized variant. Oral Surg Oral Med Oral Pathol 1981;51(6):609–18.

34. Crowley TE, Kaugars GE, Gunsolley JC. Odontogenic keratocysts: a clinical and histologic comparison of the parakeratin and orthokeratin variants. J Oral Maxillofac Surg 1992;50(1):22–6.

35. Dong Q, Pan S, Sun LS, et al. Orthokeratinized odontogenic cyst: a clinicopathologic study of 61 cases. Arch Pathol Lab Med 2010;134(2): 271–5.

36. Chi AC, Neville BW, McDonald TA, et al. Jaw cysts with sebaceous differentiation: report of 5 cases and a review of the literature. J Oral Maxillofac Surg 2007;65(12):2568–74.

37. Wysocki GP, Brannon RB, Gardner DG, et al. Histogenesis of the lateral periodontal cyst and the gingival cyst of the adult. Oral Surg Oral Med Oral Pathol 1980;50(4):327–34.

38. Cohen DA, Neville BW, Damm DD, et al. The lateral periodontal cyst. A report of 37 cases. J Periodontol 1984;55(4):230–4.

39. Buchner A, Hansen LS. The histomorphologic spectrum of the gingival cyst in the adult. Oral Surg Oral Med Oral Pathol 1979;48(6):532–9.

40. Giunta JL. Gingival cysts in the adult. J Periodontol 2002;73(7):827–31.

41. Weathers DR, Waldron CA. Unusual multilocular cysts of the jaws (botryoid odontogenic cysts). Oral Surg Oral Med Oral Pathol 1973;36(2):235–41.

42. Gurol M, Burkes EJ Jr, Jacoway J. Botryoid odontogenic cyst: analysis of 33 cases. J Periodontol 1995;66(12):1069–73.

43. Greer RO Jr, Johnson M. Botryoid odontogenic cyst: clinicopathologic analysis of ten cases with three recurrences. J Oral Maxillofac Surg 1988; 46(7):574–9.

44. Gardner DG, Kessler HP, Morency R, et al. The glandular odontogenic cyst: an apparent entity. J Oral Pathol 1988;17(8):359–66.

45. Koppang HS, Johannessen S, Haugen LK, et al. Glandular odontogenic cyst (sialo-odontogenic cyst): report of two cases and literature review of 45 previously reported cases. J Oral Pathol Med 1998;27(9):455–62.

46. Qin XN, Li JR, Chen XM, et al. The glandular odontogenic cyst: clinicopathologic features and treatment of 14 cases. J Oral Maxillofac Surg 2005; 63(5):694–9.

47. Kaplan I, Anavi Y, Hirshberg A. Glandular odontogenic cyst: a challenge in diagnosis and treatment. Oral Dis 2008;14(7):575–81.

48. Waldron CA, Koh ML. Central mucoepidermoid carcinoma of the jaws: report of four cases with analysis of the literature and discussion of the relationship to mucoepidermoid, sialodontogenic, and glandular odontogenic cysts. J Oral Maxillofac Surg 1990;48(8):871–7.

49. Reichart PA, Philipsen HP, Sonner S. Ameloblastoma: biological profile of 3677 cases. Eur J Cancer B Oral Oncol 1995;31B(2):86–99.

50. Small IA, Waldron CA. Ameloblastomas of the jaws. Oral Surg Oral Med Oral Pathol 1955;8(3):281–97.

51. Nastri AL, Wiesenfeld D, Radden BG, et al. Maxillary ameloblastoma: a retrospective study of 13 cases. Br J Oral Maxillofac Surg 1995;33(1):28–32.

52. Tsaknis PJ, Nelson JF. The maxillary ameloblastoma: an analysis of 24 cases. J Oral Surg 1980; 38(5):336–42.

53. Schafer DR, Thompson LD, Smith BC, et al. Primary ameloblastoma of the sinonasal tract: a clinicopathologic study of 24 cases. Cancer 1998;82(4): 667–74.

54. Whitt JC, Dunlap CL, Sheets JL, et al. Keratoameloblastoma: a tumor sui generis or a chimera? Oral Surg Oral Med Oral Pathol Oral Radiol Endod 2007;104(3):368–76.

55. Kumamoto H, Ooya K. Immunohistochemical and ultrastructural investigation of apoptotic cell death in granular cell ameloblastoma. J Oral Pathol Med 2001;30(4):245–50.

56. Nasu M, Takagi M, Yamamoto H. Ultrastructural and histochemical studies of granular-cell ameloblastoma. J Oral Pathol 1984;13(4):448–56.

57. Philipsen HP, Reichart PA, Takata T. Desmoplastic ameloblastoma (including "hybrid" lesion of ameloblastoma). Biological profile based on 100 cases from the literature and own files. Oral Oncol 2001; 37(5):455–60.

58. Gardner DG. A pathologist's approach to the treatment of ameloblastoma. J Oral Maxillofac Surg 1984;42(3):161–6.

59. Pogrel MA, Montes DM. Is there a role for enucleation in the management of ameloblastoma? Int J Oral Maxillofac Surg 2009;38(8):807–12.

60. Robinson L, Martinez MG. Unicystic ameloblastoma: a prognostically distinct entity. Cancer 1977;40(5):2278–85.

61. Philipsen HP, Reichart PA. Unicystic ameloblastoma. A review of 193 cases from the literature. Oral Oncol 1998;34(5):317–25.

62. Ackermann GL, Altini M, Shear M. The unicystic ameloblastoma: a clinicopathological study of 57 cases. J Oral Pathol 1988;17(9–10):541–6.

63. Lau SL, Samman N. Recurrence related to treatment modalities of unicystic ameloblastoma: a systematic review. Int J Oral Maxillofac Surg 2006;35(8):681–90.

64. Li TJ, Wu YT, Yu SF, et al. Unicystic ameloblastoma: a clinicopathologic study of 33 Chinese patients. Am J Surg Pathol 2000;24(10):1385–92.

65. Philipsen HP, Reichart PA, Nikai H, et al. Peripheral ameloblastoma: biological profile based on 160 cases from the literature. Oral Oncol 2001;37(1):17–27.

66. Isomura ET, Okura M, Ishimoto S, et al. Case report of extragingival peripheral ameloblastoma in buccal mucosa. Oral Surg Oral Med Oral Pathol Oral Radiol Endod 2009;108(4):577–9.

67. Yamanishi T, Ando S, Aikawa T, et al. A case of extragingival peripheral ameloblastoma in the buccal mucosa. J Oral Pathol Med 2007;36(3):184–6.

68. Baden E, Moskow BS, Moskow R. Odontogenic gingival epithelial hamartoma. J Oral Surg 1968; 26(11):702–14.

69. Baden E, Splaver T. Odontogenic gingival epithelial hamartoma: report of case. J Oral Surg 1973; 31(12):932–5.

70. Sciubba JJ, Zola MB. Odontogenic epithelial hamartoma. Oral Surg Oral Med Oral Pathol 1978; 45(2):261–5.

71. Moskow BS, Baden E. Odontogenic epithelial hamartomas in periodontal structures. J Clin Periodontol 1989;16(2):92–7.

72. Kitano M, Landini G, Urago A, et al. Odontogenic epithelial hamartoma of the gingiva: a case report. J Periodontol 1991;62(7):452–7.

73. Philipsen HP, Reichart PA. An odontogenic gingival epithelial hamartoma (OGEH) possibly derived from remnants of the dental lamina ("dental laminoma"). Oral Oncol Extra 2004;40(4–5):63–7.

74. Ide F, Obara K, Mishima K, et al. Peripheral odontogenic tumor: a clinicopathologic study of 30 cases. General features and hamartomatous lesions. J Oral Pathol Med 2005;34(9):552–7.

75. Wettan HL, Patella PA, Freedman PD. Peripheral ameloblastoma: review of the literature and report of recurrence as severe dysplasia. J Oral Maxillofac Surg 2001;59(7):811–5.

76. Baden E, Dqyle JL, Petriella V. Malignant transformation of peripheral ameloblastoma. Oral Surg Oral Med Oral Pathol 1993;75(2):214–9.

77. Lin SC, Lieu CM, Hahn LJ, et al. Peripheral ameloblastoma with metastasis. Int J Oral Maxillofac Surg 1987;16(2):202–4.

78. Werle H, Blake FA, Reichelt U, et al. Clear-cell odontogenic carcinoma: a new case and long-term follow-up of an old case, and review of the literature. J Oral Maxillofac Surg 2009;67(6):1342–8.

79. Avninder S, Rakheja D, Bhatnagar A. Clear cell odontogenic carcinoma: a diagnostic and therapeutic dilemma. World J Surg Oncol 2006;4:91.

80. Chera BS, Villaret DB, Orlando CA, et al. Clear cell odontogenic carcinoma of the maxilla: a case report and literature review. Am J Otolaryngol 2008;29(4):284–90.

81. Elbeshir EI, Harris M, Barrett AW. Clear cell odontogenic carcinoma of the maxilla: clinical, histological and immunohistochemical features of a case. Oral Oncol Extra 2004;40(8–9):91–4.

82. Xavier FC, Rodini CO, Ramalho LM, et al. Clear cell odontogenic carcinoma: case report with immunohistochemical findings adding support to the challenging diagnosis. Oral Surg Oral Med Oral Pathol Oral Radiol Endod 2008;106(3):403–10.

83. Maiorano E, Altini M, Viale G, et al. Clear cell odontogenic carcinoma. Report of two cases and review of the literature. Am J Clin Pathol 2001;116(1):107–14.

84. Ebert CS Jr, Dubin MG, Hart CF, et al. Clear cell odontogenic carcinoma: a comprehensive analysis of treatment strategies. Head Neck 2005;27(6):536–42.

85. Philipsen HP, Reichart PA, Siar CH, et al. An updated clinical and epidemiological profile of the adenomatoid odontogenic tumour: a collaborative retrospective study. J Oral Pathol Med 2007;36(7):383–93.

86. Philipsen HP, Reichart PA. Adenomatoid odontogenic tumour: facts and figures. Oral Oncol 1999;35(2):125–31.

87. Damm DD, White DK, Drummond JF, et al. Combined epithelial odontogenic tumor: adenomatoid odontogenic tumor and calcifying epithelial odontogenic tumor. Oral Surg Oral Med Oral Pathol 1983;55(5):487–96.

88. Bingham RA, Adrian JC. Combined epithelial odontogenic tumor-adenomatoid odontogenic tumor and calcifying epithelial odontogenic tumor: report of a case. J Oral Maxillofac Surg 1986;44(7):574–7.

89. Siar CH, Ng KH. The combined epithelial odontogenic tumour in Malaysians. Br J Oral Maxillofac Surg 1991;29(2):106–9.

90. Montes Ledesma C, Mosqueda Taylor A, Romero de Leon E, et al. Adenomatoid odontogenic tumour with features of calcifying epithelial odontogenic tumour. (The so-called combined epithelial odontogenic tumour.) Clinico-pathological report of 12 cases. Eur J Cancer B Oral Oncol 1993;29B(3):221–4.

91. Miyake M, Nagahata S, Nishihara J, et al. Combined adenomatoid odontogenic tumor and calcifying epithelial odontogenic tumor: report of case and ultrastructural study. J Oral Maxillofac Surg 1996;54(6):788–93.

92. Philipsen HP, Reichart PA. Calcifying epithelial odontogenic tumour: biological profile based on 181 cases from the literature. Oral Oncol 2000;36(1):17–26.

93. Chomette G, Auriol M, Guilbert F. Histoenzymological and ultrastructural study of a bifocal calcifying epithelial odontogenic tumor. Characteristics of epithelial cells and histogenesis of amyloid-like material. Virchows Arch A Pathol Anat Histopathol 1984;403(1):67–76.

94. Veness MJ, Morgan G, Collins AP, et al. Calcifying epithelial odontogenic (Pindborg) tumor with malignant transformation and metastatic spread. Head Neck 2001;23(8):692–6.

95. Basu MK, Matthews JB, Sear AJ, et al. Calcifying epithelial odontogenic tumour: a case showing features of malignancy. J Oral Pathol 1984;13(3):310–9.

96. Demian N, Harris RJ, Abramovitch K, et al. Malignant transformation of calcifying epithelial odontogenic tumor is associated with the loss of p53 transcriptional activity: a case report with review of the literature. J Oral Maxillofac Surg 2010;68(8):1964–73.

97. Kestler DP, Foster JS, Macy SD, et al. Expression of odontogenic ameloblast-associated protein (ODAM) in dental and other epithelial neoplasms. Mol Med 2008;14(5–6):318–26.

98. Wang YP, Lee JJ, Wang JT, et al. Non-calcifying variant of calcifying epithelial odontogenic tumor with Langerhans cells. J Oral Pathol Med 2007;36(7):436–9.

99. Takata T, Ogawa I, Miyauchi M, et al. Non-calcifying Pindborg tumor with Langerhans cells. J Oral Pathol Med 1993;22(8):378–83.

100. Asano M, Takahashi T, Kusama K, et al. A variant of calcifying epithelial odontogenic tumor with Langerhans cells. J Oral Pathol Med 1990;19(9):430–4.

101. Franklin CD, Pindborg JJ. The calcifying epithelial odontogenic tumor. A review and analysis of 113 cases. Oral Surg Oral Med Oral Pathol 1976; 42(6):753–65.

102. Anavi Y, Kaplan I, Citir M, et al. Clear-cell variant of calcifying epithelial odontogenic tumor: clinical and radiographic characteristics. Oral Surg Oral Med Oral Pathol Oral Radiol Endod 2003;95(3): 332–9.

103. Hopper TL, Sadeghi EM, Pricco DF. Squamous odontogenic tumor. Report of a case with multiple lesions. Oral Surg Oral Med Oral Pathol 1980; 50(5):404–10.

104. Leider AS, Jonker LA, Cook HE. Multicentric familial squamous odontogenic tumor. Oral Surg Oral Med Oral Pathol 1989;68(2):175–81.

105. Pullon PA, Shafer WG, Elzay RP, et al. Squamous odontogenic tumor. Report of six cases of a previously undescribed lesion. Oral Surg Oral Med Oral Pathol 1975;40(5):616–30.

106. Ide F, Shimoyama T, Horie N, et al. Intraosseous squamous cell carcinoma arising in association with a squamous odontogenic tumour of the mandible. Oral Oncol 1999;35(4):431–4.

107. Slater LJ. Squamous odontogenic tumor versus pseudoepitheliomatous hyperplasia. J Oral Maxillofac Surg 2004;62(9):1177.

108. de Oliveira MG, Carrard VC, Danesi CC, et al. Squamous odontogenic tumor: with recurrence and 12 years of follow-up. Rev Cienc Med Campinas 2007;16(1):51–6.

109. Hietanen J, Lukinmaa PL, Ahonen P, et al. Peripheral squamous odontogenic tumour. Br J Oral Maxillofac Surg 1985;23(5):362–5.

110. Cahn LR, Blum T. Ameloblastic odontoma: case report critically analyzed. J Oral Surg 1952;10:169–70.

111. Philipsen HP, Reichart PA, Praetorius F. Mixed odontogenic tumours and odontomas. Considerations on interrelationship. Review of the literature and presentation of 134 new cases of odontomas. Oral Oncol 1997;33(2):86–99.

112. Chen Y, Wang JM, Li TJ. Ameloblastic fibroma: a review of published studies with special reference to its nature and biological behavior. Oral Oncol 2007;43(10):960–9.

113. Abughazaleh K, Andrus KM, Katsnelson A, et al. Peripheral ameloblastic fibroma of the maxilla: report of a case and review of the literature. Oral Surg Oral Med Oral Pathol Oral Radiol Endod 2008;105(5):e46–8.

114. Darling MR, Daley TD. Peripheral ameloblastic fibroma. J Oral Pathol Med 2006;35(3):190–2.

115. Ide F, Shimoyama T, Horie N. Peripheral ameloblastic fibroma. Oral Oncol 2000;36(3):308.

116. Kusama K, Miyake M, Moro I. Peripheral ameloblastic fibroma of the mandible: report of a case. J Oral Maxillofac Surg 1998;56(3):399–401.

117. Lu Y, Xuan M, Takata T, et al. Odontogenic tumors. A demographic study of 759 cases in a Chinese population. Oral Surg Oral Med Oral Pathol Oral Radiol Endod 1998;86(6):707–14.

118. Jing W, Xuan M, Lin Y, et al. Odontogenic tumours: a retrospective study of 1642 cases in a Chinese population. Int J Oral Maxillofac Surg 2007;36(1): 20–5.

119. Ochsenius G, Ortega A, Godoy L, et al. Odontogenic tumors in Chile: a study of 362 cases. J Oral Pathol Med 2002;31(7):415–20.

120. Fernandes AM, Duarte EC, Pimenta FJ, et al. Odontogenic tumors: a study of 340 cases in a Brazilian population. J Oral Pathol Med 2005; 34(10):583–7.

121. Regezi JA, Kerr DA, Courtney RM. Odontogenic tumors: analysis of 706 cases. J Oral Surg 1978; 36(10):771–8.

122. Mani NJ. Odontoma syndrome: report of an unusual case with multiple multiform odontomas of both jaws. J Dent 1974;2(4):149–52.

123. Hirshberg A, Kaplan I, Buchner A. Calcifying odontogenic cyst associated with odontoma: a possible separate entity (odontocalcifying odontogenic cyst). J Oral Maxillofac Surg 1994;52(6):555–8.

124. Gorlin RJ, Pindborg JJ, Odont, et al. The calcifying odontogenic cyst–a possible analogue of the cutaneous calcifying epithelioma of Malherbe. An analysis of fifteen cases. Oral Surg Oral Med Oral Pathol 1962;15:1235–43.

125. Praetorius F, Hjorting-Hansen E, Gorlin RJ, et al. Calcifying odontogenic cyst. Range, variations and neoplastic potential. Acta Odontol Scand 1981;39(4):227–40.

126. Hong SP, Ellis GL, Hartman KS. Calcifying odontogenic cyst. A review of ninety-two cases with reevaluation of their nature as cysts or neoplasms, the nature of ghost cells, and subclassification. Oral Surg Oral Med Oral Pathol 1991;72(1):56–64.

127. Praetorius F, Ledesma-Montes C. Calcifying cystic odontogenic tumor. In: Barnes L, Eveson JW, Reichart P, et al, editors. World Health Organization classification of tumours: pathology and genetics of head and neck tumours. Lyon (France): IARC Press; 2005. p. 313.

128. Praetorius F, Ledesma-Montes C. Dentinogenic ghost cell tumour. In: Barnes L, Eveson JW, Reichart P, et al, editors. World Health Organization classification of tumours: pathology and genetics of head and neck tumours. Lyon (France): IARC Press; 2005. p. 314.

129. Ledesma-Montes C, Gorlin RJ, Shear M, et al. International collaborative study on ghost cell odontogenic tumours: calcifying cystic odontogenic

tumour, dentinogenic ghost cell tumour and ghost cell odontogenic carcinoma. J Oral Pathol Med 2008;37(5):302–8.

130. Gardner DG. Central odontogenic fibroma current concepts. J Oral Pathol Med 1996;25(10):556–61.

131. Ramer M, Buonocore P, Krost B. Central odontogenic fibroma—report of a case and review of the literature. Periodontal Clin Investig 2002;24(1):27–30.

132. Daniels JS. Central odontogenic fibroma of mandible: a case report and review of the literature. Oral Surg Oral Med Oral Pathol Oral Radiol Endod 2004;98(3):295–300.

133. Svirsky JA, Abbey LM, Kaugars GE. A clinical review of central odontogenic fibroma: with the addition of three new cases. J Oral Med 1986;41(1):51–4.

134. Gardner DG. The central odontogenic fibroma: an attempt at clarification. Oral Surg Oral Med Oral Pathol 1980;50(5):425–32.

135. Ritwik P, Brannon RB. Peripheral odontogenic fibroma: a clinicopathologic study of 151 cases and review of the literature with special emphasis on recurrence. Oral Surg Oral Med Oral Pathol Oral Radiol Endod 2010;110(3):357–63.

136. Lin CT, Chuang FH, Chen JH, et al. Peripheral odontogenic fibroma in a Taiwan chinese population: a retrospective analysis. Kaohsiung J Med Sci 2008;24(8):415–21.

137. Buchner A, Merrell PW, Carpenter WM. Relative frequency of peripheral odontogenic tumors: a study of 45 new cases and comparison with studies from the literature. J Oral Pathol Med 2006;35(7):385–91.

138. Lotay HS, Kalmar J, DeLeeuw K. Central odontogenic fibroma with features of central granular cell odontogenic tumor. Oral Surg Oral Med Oral Pathol Oral Radiol Endod 2010;109(2):e63–6.

139. Brannon RB, Goode RK, Eversole LR, et al. The central granular cell odontogenic tumor: report of 5 new cases. Oral Surg Oral Med Oral Pathol Oral Radiol Endod 2002;94(5):614–21.

140. Calvo N, Alonso D, Prieto M, et al. Central odontogenic fibroma granular cell variant: a case report and review of the literature. J Oral Maxillofac Surg 2002;60(10):1192–4.

141. Reichart PA, Philipsen HP, Moegelin A, et al. Central odontogenic fibroma, granular cell variant. Oral Oncol Extra 2006;42(1):5–9.

142. Meer S, Altini M, Coleman H, et al. Central granular cell odontogenic tumor: immunohistochemistry and ultrastructure. Am J Otolaryngol 2004;25(1):73–8.

143. Piatelli A, Rubini C, Goteri G, et al. Central granular cell odontogenic tumour: report of the first malignant case and review of the literature. Oral Oncol 2003;39(1):78–82.

144. Noffke CE, Raubenheimer EJ, Chabikuli NJ, et al. Odontogenic myxoma: review of the literature and report of 30 cases from South Africa. Oral Surg Oral Med Oral Pathol Oral Radiol Endod 2007;104(1):101–9.

145. Kaffe I, Naor H, Buchner A. Clinical and radiological features of odontogenic myxoma of the jaws. Dentomaxillofac Radiol 1997;26(5):299–303.

146. Simon EN, Merkx MA, Vuhahula E, et al. Odontogenic myxoma: a clinicopathological study of 33 cases. Int J Oral Maxillofac Surg 2004;33(4):333–7.

147. MacDonald-Jankowski DS, Yeung R, Lee KM, et al. Odontogenic myxomas in the Hong Kong Chinese: clinico-radiological presentation and systematic review. Dentomaxillofac Radiol 2002;31(2):71–83.

148. Li TJ, Sun LS, Luo HY. Odontogenic myxoma: a clinicopathologic study of 25 cases. Arch Pathol Lab Med 2006;130(12):1799–806.

149. King TJ 3rd, Lewis J, Orvidas L, et al. Pediatric maxillary odontogenic myxoma: a report of 2 cases and review of management. J Oral Maxillofac Surg 2008;66(5):1057–62.

150. Wachter BG, Steinberg MJ, Darrow DH, et al. Odontogenic myxoma of the maxilla: a report of two pediatric cases. Int J Pediatr Otorhinolaryngol 2003;67(4):389–93.

151. Leiberman A, Forte V, Thorner P, et al. Maxillary myxoma in children. Int J Pediatr Otorhinolaryngol 1990;18(3):277–84.

152. James DR, Lucas VS. Maxillary myxoma in a child of 11 months. A case report. J Craniomaxillofac Surg 1987;15(1):42–4.

153. Slater LJ. Infantile lateral nasal myxoma: is it odontogenic? J Oral Maxillofac Surg 2004;62(3):391.

154. Fenton S, Slootweg PJ, Dunnebier EA, et al. Odontogenic myxoma in a 17-month-old child: a case report. J Oral Maxillofac Surg 2003;61(6):734–6.

155. Kim J, Ellis GL. Dental follicular tissue: misinterpretation as odontogenic tumors. J Oral Maxillofac Surg 1993;51(7):762–7 [discussion: 767–8].

156. Leiser Y, Abu-El-Naaj I, Peled M. Odontogenic myxoma–a case series and review of the surgical management. J Craniomaxillofac Surg 2009;37(4):206–9.

157. Lamberg MA, Calonius BP, Makinen JE, et al. A case of malignant myxoma (myxosarcoma) of the maxilla. Scand J Dent Res 1984;92(4):352–7.

158. Pahl S, Henn W, Binger T, et al. Malignant odontogenic myxoma of the maxilla: case with cytogenetic confirmation. J Laryngol Otol 2000;114(7):533–5.

SELECT NEOPLASMS OF THE SINONASAL TRACT

Joaquín J. García, MD[a],*, Bruce M. Wenig, MD[b]

KEYWORDS

- Schneiderian papilloma • Lobular capillary hemangioma • Pyogenic granuloma
- Glomangiopericytoma • Sinonasal-type hemangiopericytoma
- Sinonasal undifferentiated carcinoma • Rhabdomyosarcoma • Olfactory neuroblastoma
- Mucosal malignant melanoma

ABSTRACT

The sinonasal tract (SNT) includes the nasal cavity and paranasal sinuses (maxillary, ethmoid, frontal, and sphenoid) and may give rise to a variety of nonneoplastic and neoplastic proliferations, including benign and malignant neoplasms. The benign neoplasms of the SNT include epithelial neoplasms of surface epithelial origin, minor salivary gland origin, and mesenchymal origin. The spectrum of malignant neoplasms of the SNT includes epithelial malignancies, sinonasal undifferentiated carcinoma, malignant salivary gland neoplasms, neuroectodermal neoplasms, neuroendocrine neoplasms, melanocytic neoplasm, and sarcomas. This article concentrates on some of the more common types of benign and malignant neoplasms.

SCHNEIDERIAN PAPILLOMAS

The mucosa that lines the nasal cavity and paranasal sinuses is ectodermal in origin, arising from the nasal placodes and invaginating to ultimately form the sinonasal cavities and lacrimal apparatus.[1] Before 1971, myriad designations were applied to papillomas of the sinonasal mucosa. In 1971, Hyams[2] reported on the clinical and pathologic features of 315 papillomas, introducing a unifying classification system. The clinical and histopathologic features of papillomas in this study gave rise to a triad of sinonasal papilloma subtypes: inverted, fungiform, and oncocytic schneiderian papillomas. These tumors represent between 0.4% and 4.7% of all sinonasal tumors.[3] Representation of each subtype ranges dramatically between studies and institutions. Nevertheless, inverted papillomas are commonly thought to be the most frequent (62%), followed by the fungiform (32%) and oncocytic types (6%).[2,4–8] Similar to other sinonasal neoplasms, schneiderian papillomas typically present with unilateral obstruction and/or epistaxis. They are most commonly observed in young adults and involve the maxillary and ethmoid sinuses. Exclusive involvement of the sphenoid and frontal sinuses is rare and extension from another sinus should be considered more likely.[9–11]

SCHNEIDERIAN PAPILLOMAS, INVERTED-TYPE

OVERVIEW

Inverted (endophytic) schneiderian papillomas are the most common subtype of sinonasal papilloma; unfortunately, the diagnostic and therapeutic challenges they present wreak havoc in the medical community because of their propensity for local destruction and recurrence. Additionally, most investigators have reported an association with

[a] Department of Laboratory Medicine and Pathology, Mayo Clinic College of Medicine, 200 First Street Southwest, Rochester, MN 55905, USA
[b] Department of Diagnostic Pathology and Laboratory Medicine, Beth Israel Medical Center, St. Luke's-Roosevelt Hospitals, Room 34, Silver Building 11th Floor, First Avenue at 16th Street, New York, NY 10003, USA
* Corresponding author.
E-mail address: garcia.joaquin@mayo.edu

Surgical Pathology 4 (2011) 1093–1125
doi:10.1016/j.path.2011.08.015

malignancy. Similar to their fungiform counterpart, inverted papillomas are largely considered associated with human papillomavirus (HPV).[6,7,12–27] One source of confusion is that HPV genome discovery in these lesions has spanned between 0 and 100% of cases.[28] Although inverted papillomas have been discovered in both young and old patients, they are most common in patients between ages 40 and 70 years and are up to 5 times more likely in men.[2,11,29–39] These tumors are only rarely seen in children.[31] Similar to their oncocytic counterpart, inverted papillomas most frequently arise from the lateral nasal wall and commonly extend into the sinuses (maxillary and ethmoid sinuses more often than sphenoid and frontal).[34,35,37,38] Less than 10% of inverted papillomas originate from the nasal septum.[40] Rarely, inverted papillomas are described in peculiar anatomic sites: middle ear–mastoid, nasopharynx, and lacrimal sac, for example.[41–44] Also uncommon is the presence of veritable bilateral disease. Several case series describe bilateral inverted papillomas in 0 to 10% of cases.[2,4,29,32,37,45] Given the destructive biologic potential of inverted papillomas, the possibility of septal perforation and extension into the contralateral compartment should first be considered. Addressing the impact of residual microscopic disease and tumor implantation at the time of initial surgery is essentially futile.

There is considerable debate regarding the role of HPV in the etiopathogenesis of inverted papillomas. A deluge of conflicting results has been reported in this most common subtype.[17,32] Using immunoperoxidase stains, polymerase chain reaction, and in situ hybridization, HPV has been declared present in 0 to 100% of inverted papillomas.[6,7,13–27,46,47] Generally speaking, most pathologists consider at least a remote relationship between HPV and inverted papillomas; the ubiquity and impact of this infection remains controversial. Reports that EBV is a role player in the neoplastic pathway have also been challenged by conflicting data.[28,46,48]

Imaging findings serve as a major centerpiece to the diagnosis and management of inverted schneiderian papillomas. Because their presentation varies with respect to location and extent of disease, accurate radiologic assessment is paramount to correct surgical approach and, in some cases, radiotherapy. Although inverted schneiderian papillomas classically present as a unilateral polypoid nasal mass that expands the nasal fossa and displaces the septum, these radiologic features are not pathognomonic.[49] Bone erosion and invasion are not uncommon findings[11,29]; however, such a discovery should alert clinicians to the possibility of malignancy.

GROSS FEATURES

Inverted schneiderian papillomas are usually pale pink or gray, firm, and polypoid fragments of soft tissue. They tend to be more vascular than what is seen in the typically translucent sinonasal inflammatory polyps.

MICROSCOPIC FEATURES

Inverted schneiderian papillomas are primarily distinguished from their fungiform counterpart (discussed later) by their growth pattern. Inverted papillomas exhibit a pushing border into the underlying stroma (**Fig. 1**). This growth pattern is typical and should not be mistaken for malignancy (eg, nonkeratinizing carcinoma) although such a possibility should be considered. The surface is composed of varying degrees (5–30 cells thick) of hyperplastic epithelium.[28] These cells are classically squamous, columnar, or ciliated in nature. Interspersed mucous cells are a nearly universal finding (see **Fig. 1**). So-called transmigrating neutrophils are commonly seen within the epithelium, sometimes forming microabscesses. Other inflammatory cells, including eosinophils and lymphocytes, can be seen sprinkled in both the surface epithelium and underlying stroma. Mitotic activity is occasionally noted in a basal and parabasal distribution. The basement membrane of inverted papillomas tends to be attenuated and sometimes imperceptible.

The stroma of inverted papillomas can be loose and myxoid or densely fibrous. Overt desmoplasia should inspire serious consideration for well-differentiated squamous cell carcinoma, either de novo or arising within an inverted papilloma. Up to 20% of cases may exhibit dysplasia.[2,26,50,51] Furthermore, the presence of foci of keratinizing squamous epithelium may be an indicator of the possible presence of carcinoma. Such findings warrant sampling of the entire surgical specimen

Key Features
SCHNEIDERIAN PAPILLOMAS, INVERTED-TYPE

1. Most frequently arise from lateral nasal wall and paranasal sinuses (maxillary and ethmoid)

2. Considered to have at least a remote relationship to HPV

3. Has been seen in association with conventional squamous cell carcinoma and other epithelial malignancies

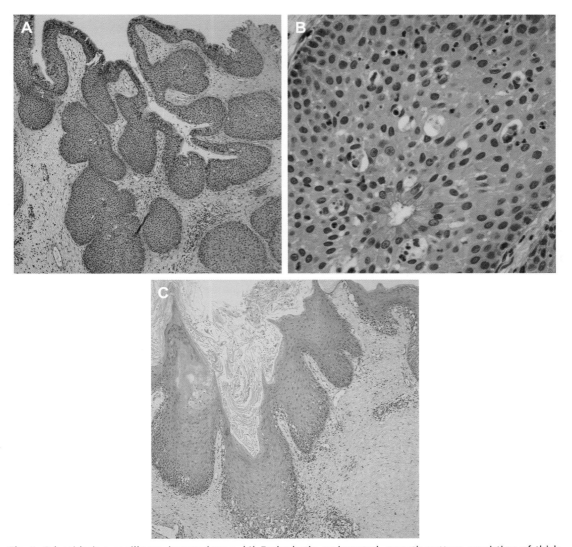

Fig. 1. Schneiderian papilloma, inverted-type. (*A*) Endophytic, or inverted, growth pattern consisting of thickened epithelial nests arising from the surface and growing down into the stroma; the surface epithelium has undergone squamous metaplasia. (*B*) The epithelial proliferation is noteworthy for uniformity of nuclei maintaining consistency in polarity, absence of cytologic atypia, scattered cysts, and identifiable intraepithelial mucocytes. (*C*) The presence of keratinizing squamous epithelium is considered an atypical feature in schneiderian papillomas and, when present, raises concern for the possibility of a coexisting squamous cell carcinoma or the development into a squamous cell carcinoma. In this setting all of the resected tissue should be processed for histologic evaluation.

and thorough histopathologic examination, using level sections when appropriate.

DIFFERENTIAL DIAGNOSIS

Inverted schneiderian papilloma has notoriously been confused with sinonasal inflammatory polyps, respiratory epithelial adenomatoid hamartoma (REAH), inverted ductal papilloma, squamous cell carcinoma, and verrucous carcinoma. Although sinonasal inflammatory polyps may possess areas of squamous metaplasia, the general lack of a downward growth pattern, dramatic epithelial hyperplasia, and transmigrating neutrophils should be a dissuasion from making this mistake. Moreover, sinonasal inflammatory polyps commonly have an edematous stroma, thickened or hyalinized basement membrane, an uncommon attribute of

△△ **Differential Diagnosis**
SCHNEIDERIAN PAPILLOMAS,
INVERTED-TYPE

- Sinonasal inflammatory polyp
- REAH
- Inverted ductal papillomas
- Squamous cell carcinoma
- Verrucous carcinoma

 Pitfalls
SCHNEIDERIAN PAPILLOMAS,
INVERTED-TYPE

! The growth pattern of inverted papillomas should not be mistaken for malignancy (eg, nonkeratinizing squamous cell carcinoma).

! Concern about the presence of dysplasia or carcinoma should be followed by histopathologic evaluation of the entire surgical specimen because up to 20% of cases may exhibit dysplasia and less than 10% harbor invasive squamous cell carcinoma.

inverted papilloma. Not infrequently, however, schneiderian papillomas may be seen coexisting with changes of inflammatory polyps. REAH is classically composed of many glandular islands invested by a thick basement membrane. REAH also lacks a significant degree of epithelial proliferation or neutrophilic infiltrate. Inverted ductal papilloma arises from within the lumen of a minor salivary gland excretory duct; this intraluminal growth pattern is unlike the inward growth observed in inverted papillomas. Ruling out the presence of invasive squamous cell carcinoma requires diligently ensuring the absence of cytologic pleomorphism, elevated mitotic activity (superficial layer), atypical mitotic figures, stromal invasion, and, in some cases, desmoplasia. Nonkeratinizing carcinoma typically shows interconnecting/ramifying cords of tumor characterized by malignant cytomorphology.

DIAGNOSIS

The diagnosis of inverted schneiderian papillomas is based exclusively on histologic criteria.

TREATMENT AND PROGNOSIS

The primary treatment modality of all schneiderian papillomas is complete surgical removal when feasible. Complete en bloc excision via lateral rhinotomy and medial maxillectomy and excision of the mucosa of the ipsilateral paranasal sinuses are often the goals of surgical management.[28,33] Even extensive resections can be fraught with recurrences, which range from 0 to 30%.[11] Smaller lesions may be removed by way of endoscopic sinonasal surgery.[32,52] Radiation therapy has generally been invoked in the setting of unresectable lesions, rapid recurrences, or squamous cell carcinoma arising from an inverted papilloma[33,38,53]; however, this practice has been met with concerns for the possibility of inducing malignant transformation.[29,53–55] Inverted papillomas have an approximately 10% risk

of being associated with epithelial malignancies—although the reported incidence has ranged dramatically.[2,4,6,11,25,26,29,30,33–37,45,47,51,55–59] These cases most frequently feature conventional squamous cell carcinoma; nevertheless, verrucous carcinoma, spindle cell carcinoma, adenocarcinoma, clear cell carcinoma, and mucoepidermoid carcinoma have also been reported.[28] Malignancies have been described as both synchronous and metachronous. In such cases, a surgical pathology report should contain at least the following items: (1) the type of malignancy associated with the papilloma, (2) the histologic grade of the malignant component, and (3) the approximate percentage of the malignant component. Some investigators have suggested that the development of squamous cell carcinoma in these cases is related to high-risk HPV types 16 and 18.[23,26,47]

SCHNEIDERIAN PAPILLOMAS, FUNGIFORM-TYPE

OVERVIEW

Fungiform (exophytic/septal/squamous papillomas) schneiderian papilloma represents the second most common type of sinonasal papilloma. It is typically seen in patients in the third to sixth decade of life and discovered in men more frequently than women by approximately 2 to 10 ratio.[2,56] Unlike its inverted and oncocytic counterparts, the vast majority of fungiform papillomas arise from the nasal septum—most often the anterior septum.[32,60] Although fungiform papilloma has been observed on the lateral walls, this is only thought to represent between 4% and 21% of cases.[2,30,32] Even though multifocality has been reported,[7] bilateral disease is most frequently a consequence of septal perforation and subsequent direct extension rather than bona fide multifocal disease.[61]

The etiopathogenesis of fungiform schneiderian papillomas is an area of significant debate because study results have been conflicting at best. Several studies have discovered a high incidence of HPV infection (50%–100%) in fungiform papillomas, particularly in types 6 and 11, with rare involvement by types 16 and 57b.[6,8,28,32,46] Although most pathologists do not contest the ability to identify HPV genomes incorporated into neoplastic cells, their role in pathogenesis—if any—remains a subject of debate.

GROSS FEATURES

Fungiform schneiderian papilloma is composed of pale pink or gray, soft to semifirm masses, occasionally with a prominent papillary or cauliflower-like architecture grossly. Much like inverted schneiderian papilloma, it usually appears more vascular than sinonasal inflammatory polyps.

MICROSCOPIC FEATURES

Histologically, fungiform schneiderian papilloma shows an exophytic pattern of growth composed of papillary fronds with fibrovascular cores lined by a thickened, nonkeratinizing epithelium (**Fig. 2**). When surface keratinization is exhibited, it is typically focal and likely subtle. The stratified epithelium (5–20 cells thick) is a constellation of squamous, ciliated, pseudostratified columnar respiratory, transitional (intermediate), and mucous cells.[28] The basement membrane of fungiform schneiderian papilloma is usually thin or attenuated. Scattered mitotic figures are not uncommon. A certain degree of cytologic atypia is to be expected because these are papillary lesions with intraluminal growth that are subjected to repeated trauma and coarse "living conditions." To this end, caution should be used when applying the terms, *dysplastic* or *squamous cell carcinoma in situ*, to fungiform schneiderian papillomas. Although squamous cell carcinoma has reportedly arisen in fungiform schneiderian papillomas,[56] this is considered a rare event.[28]

Key Features
SCHNEIDERIAN PAPILLOMAS, FUNGIFORM-TYPE

1. Most frequently arise from the nasal septum

2. Likely related to HPV

3. An association with squamous cell carcinoma has been described but is largely considered a rare event

Differential Diagnosis
SCHNEIDERIAN PAPILLOMAS, FUNGIFORM-TYPE

- Cutaneous papillomas (nasal vestibule)
- Exophytic/papillary squamous cell carcinoma

DIFFERENTIAL DIAGNOSIS

Consideration must be given to cutaneous papillomas, such as verruca vulgaris, that arise from the nasal vestibule. This diagnostic pitfall may be avoided by recognizing the presence of subcutaneous hair follicles and/or extensive lesional keratinization. Minor salivary gland tissue and septal cartilage, as would be suspected, suggest disease of sinonasal origin. Moreover, the presence of mucous, ciliated respiratory, or transitional (intermediate) cells should dissuade suggesting cutaneous origin.

DIAGNOSIS

The diagnosis of fungiform schneiderian papilloma is primarily based on histologic features. Challenging cases in which it cannot be determined if sufficient inward growth is present to meet criteria for inverted schneiderian papilloma can occur. In these scenarios, reevaluate the clinical and radiologic findings should be evaluated, primarily the origin of the lesion (ie, septal versus lateral wall).

TREATMENT AND PROGNOSIS

The primary treatment modality of schneiderian papillomas is complete surgical removal. Unfortunately, recurrences occur frequently. In most cases, recurrence is thought to be a consequence of incomplete removal rather than a function of bona fide multifocality.

Pitfalls
SCHNEIDERIAN PAPILLOMAS, FUNGIFORM-TYPE

! Cutaneous papillomas, such as verruca vulgaris, arising from the nasal vestibule can be distinguished by the presence of subcutaneous hair follicles and/or extensive lesional keratinization and the absence of intraepithelial mucocytes, minor salivary gland tissue, and septal cartilage.

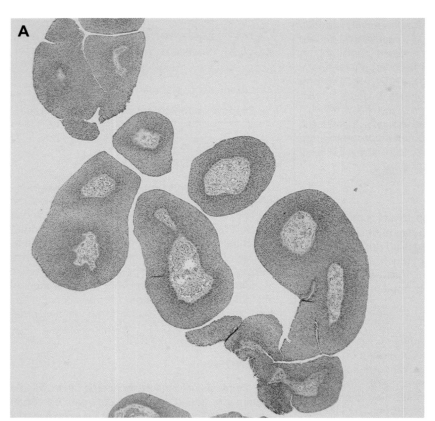

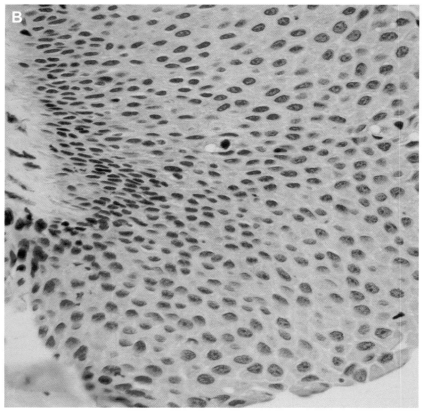

Fig. 2. Schneiderian papilloma, exophytic (septal)-type. (*A*) The tumor has a papillary or exophytic growth. (*B*) The epithelium is similar to that seen in inverted papillomas, including cytomorphologic uniformity and identification of intraepithelial mucocytes.

SCHNEIDERIAN PAPILLOMAS, ONCOCYTIC-TYPE

OVERVIEW

Oncocytic (cylindrical cell/columnar cell papillomas) schneiderian papillomas represent the least common subtype of sinonasal papilloma observed.[2,5,6,62–64] Like the inverted and fungiform papilloma, oncocytic schneiderian papilloma arises from the schneiderian membrane of the nose and paranasal sinuses. This variant shares clinical features with the inverted schneiderian papilloma but remains distinct in its histomorphology and relationship to HPV. These patients are typically older than 50 years of age and show no gender preference.[28] Similar to inverted papilloma, this lesion typically arises from the lateral nasal wall or sinuses and most commonly affects the maxillary and ethmoid sinuses.[32,60] Unlike its inverted counterpart, the pathogenesis of oncocytic papillomas is considered unrelated to HPV infection.[6–8,14]

GROSS FEATURES

Oncocytic schneiderian papilloma shares the gross features illustrated by other subtypes.

MICROSCOPIC FEATURES

Oncocytic schneiderian papilloma may demonstrate a mix of architectural appearances due to its alternating exophytic and endophytic growth patterns. Tumor cells display a range in epithelial stratification but are typically multilayered (2–8 cells thick) and pseudostratified. Tall columnar and cuboidal cells with well-defined borders enveloping modest amounts of eosinophilic and fine granular cytoplasm can be seen lining papillae and forming solid nests (**Fig. 3**). Ultrastructural studies have revealed a significant concentration of mitochondria within these cells.[62] Tumor cell nuclei are typically round to oval with vesicular chromatin and contain inconspicuous nucleoli. Occasionally, prominent surface cilia and intracytoplasmic mucin are exhibited. Common to all three papillomas are microcysts containing transmigrating neutrophils (microabscesses). In most cases, scattered mucous cells are also appreciated. Epidermoid cytomorphologic features are minimal if not absent and mitotic activity is low. Oncocytic schneiderian papillomas with a prominent inward growth pattern often display a fibrous stroma.

These papillomas should be sampled generously and examined thoroughly because the incidence of synchronous or metachronous invasive carcinoma, between 4% and 17% of cases, rivals that what is observed in inverted papillomas.[2,62–64] For this reason, cases with even focal cytomorphologic atypia should be scrutinized for the presence of dysplasia or carcinoma.

DIFFERENTIAL DIAGNOSIS

Oncocytic schneiderian papillomas bring up a challenging differential. Consideration must be given to rhinosporidiosis and adenocarcinoma. The microcystic spaces colonized by mucous cells within oncocytic schneiderian papillomas may be mistaken for rhinosporidiosis; more specifically, the sporangia of rhinosporidiosis. This diagnostic error may be avoided by identifying sporangia in the submucosa—often accompanied by a foreign body giant cell reaction—as well as the epithelium. Another microscopic finding that aids in circumventing this dilemma is the recognition of oncocytic cells, a finding not observed in rhinosporidiosis. Adenocarcinoma can be a diagnostic consideration. In contrast to oncocytic schneiderian papillomas, adenocarcinomas show complex glandular growth with back-to-back glands lacking intervening stroma and are characterized by a single cell type. Such features are not identified in oncocytic schneiderian papillomas.

Key Features
SCHNEIDERIAN PAPILLOMAS, ONCOCYTIC-TYPE

1. Most frequently arise from lateral nasal wall and paranasal sinuses (maxillary, ethmoid)

2. Likely unrelated to HPV

3. Has been seen in association with conventional squamous cell carcinoma and other epithelial malignancies

---

△△ **Differential Diagnosis**
SCHNEIDERIAN PAPILLOMAS, ONCOCYTIC-TYPE

- Rhinosporidiosis
- Adenocarcinoma of salivary gland origin
- Adenocarcinoma of non-salivary gland origin

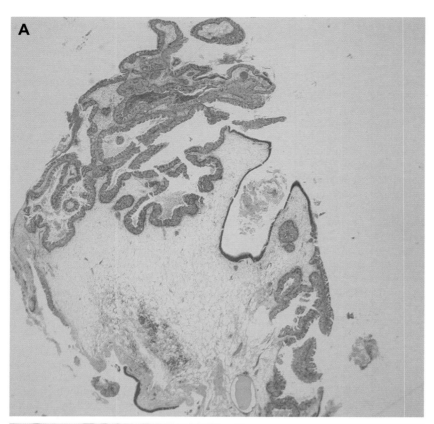

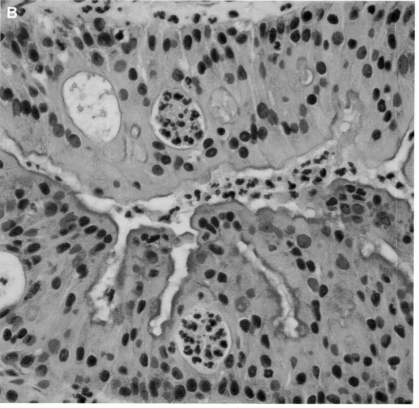

Fig. 3. Schneiderian papilloma, oncocytic-type. (*A*) Exophytic and endophytic epithelial cell proliferation occurring in a background of edematous stroma. (*B*) The cells consist of cells an eosinophilic to granular cytoplasm (oncocytes) with uniform, round nuclei and intraepithelial mucin cysts containing amorphous pink material and/or neutrophils; cilia can be seen at the outer surface of the epithelial proliferation.

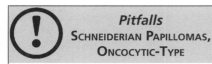

Pitfalls
SCHNEIDERIAN PAPILLOMAS,
ONCOCYTIC-TYPE

! Absence of complex glandular growth and presence of cilated cells with oncocytic cytoplasm allows for differentiation from adenocarcinoma.

DIAGNOSIS

The diagnosis of oncocytic schneiderian papillomas is almost exclusively based on histologic appearance.

TREATMENT AND PROGNOSIS

The primary treatment modality of schneiderian papillomas is surgical removal. This often means a lateral rhinotomy and medial maxillectomy. Recurrence rates may exceed 25% and are predominantly due to incomplete removal. Malignant transformation in these neoplasms has been documented and is thought to parallel the incidence found in inverted schneiderian papillomas.[2,30,62,63] The prognosis of patients with coexisting invasive malignancy is a function of type, grade, and extent of invasive disease. As discussed previously, when invasive disease is encountered within schneiderian papillomas, a surgical pathology report should contain at least the following items:

1. Type of malignancy associated with the papilloma
2. Histologic grade of the malignant component
3. Approximate percentage of the malignant component.

LOBULAR CAPILLARY HEMANGIOMA (PYOGENIC GRANULOMA)

OVERVIEW

Hartzell used the term, granuloma pyogenicum, in 1904 to describe the vascular proliferation currently referred to as lobular capillary hemangioma (LCH).[65] This designation was rooted in the perception that it represented a response to a pyogenic agent. LCH primarily occurs on skin and mucous membranes and is common in the head and neck and frequently observed on the lip, nose, oral mucosa/gingiva, and tongue.[65] Nasal lesions are most likely to originate from the anterior nasal septum, or Little's area. Similar to other lesions of the SNT, the most common

presentation is a painless, bleeding mass. The duration of symptoms lasts from weeks to months. There is a slight male predilection and patients are usually in the fourth to fifth decades of life. Although several investigators have proposed that LCH represents a vascular reaction to repeated trauma or injury,[66–69] others think it is a spontaneous benign endothelial proliferation in the vast majority of cases.[65] One peculiar feature of LCH is its presentation in the setting of pregnancy or oral contraceptive use. Pregnancy-associated LCH development and regression have been linked to the interplay between vascular endothelial growth factor, basic fibroblast growth factor, tumor necrosis factor α, and other molecules.[70–73]

GROSS FEATURES

LCHs are usually brown-gray, smooth, and polypoid or nodular masses. A common feature is focal surface ulceration.

MICROSCOPIC FEATURES

The microscopic features of LCH are distinct, characterized by a submucosal vascular proliferation arranged in lobules or clusters composed of central capillaries and smaller ramifying tributaries surrounded by and intimately associated with the granulation tissue and a mixed chronic inflammatory cell infiltrate) (**Fig. 4**). The central capillaries vary in caliber as well as in shape and in more mature lesions may show a staghorn appearance. The endothelial cell lining may be prominent and may display endothelial tufting as well as mitoses, but atypical mitoses are not identified. There is absence of intercommunication of vascular spaces as seen in angiosarcomas and an absence of cytologic atypia or atypical mitoses. The designation of active LCH can be used in conjunction with those lesions showing an increase in mitotic activity; however, these active lesions carry no additional

Key Features
LOBULAR CAPILLARY HEMANGIOMA
(PYOGENIC GRANULOMA)

1. Most frequently arise from the anterior nasal septum (Little area)

2. Uncertain etiology (history of trauma in select cases)

3. Occasionally presents in the setting of pregnancy or oral contraceptive use

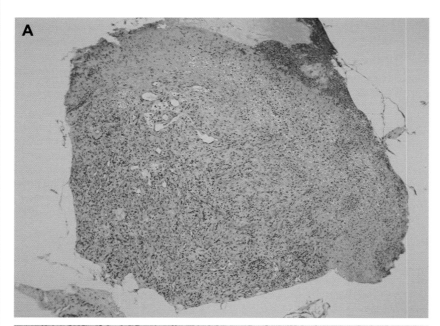

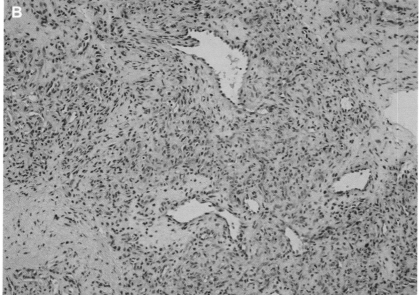

Fig. 4. Intranasal LCH. (*A*) Polypoid lesion with surface ulceration and associated fibrinoid necrosis and the presence of a submucosal proliferation, including dilated, irregularly shaped vascular spaces surrounded by a cellular proliferation. (*B*) The blood vessels may ramify with a staghorn appearance but there is no intercommunicating of the vascular channels; the vessels are lined by flattened endothelial cells and are surrounded by granulation tissue with a chronic inflammatory cell infiltrate.

risk of aggressive behavior or of transformation to an angiosarcoma. The surface ciliated respiratory epithelium may be intact with or without squamous metaplasia but is often ulcerated with associated fibrinoid necrosis.

Immunoreactivity is almost invariable to CD31, CD34, factor VIII–related antigen, and *Ulex europaeus I* lectin. Glucose transporter 1 staining is negative.

DIFFERENTIAL DIAGNOSIS

Diagnostic consideration must be given to glomangiopericytoma (sinonasal-type hemangiopericytoma), angiosarcoma, and Kaposi sarcoma. LCH, unlike glomangiopericytoma, is composed of several cell types (fibroblasts, inflammatory, and endothelial cells) rather than a single cell type and lacks perivascular hyalinization, the latter a common

Fig. 4. (*C, D*) The blood vessels may ramify with a staghorn appearance but there is no inter-communicating of the vascular channels; the vessels are lined by flattened endothelial cells and are surrounded by granulation tissue with a chronic inflammatory cell infiltrate.

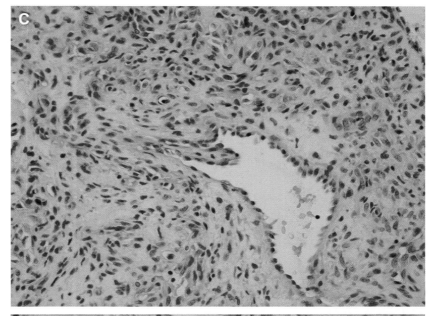

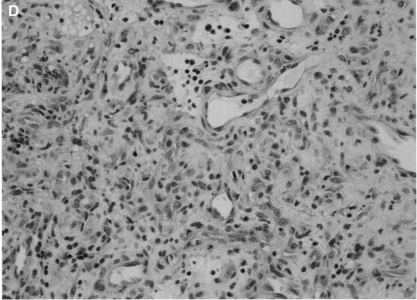

feature in glomangiopericytoma. Angiosarcoma may be duly ruled out by the absence of interconnecting/ramifying vascular channels, vascular endothelial cell tufting, absence of overt nuclear pleomorphism, increased mitotic activity, and the presence of atypical mitotic figures. The spindle cell proliferation, slit-like vascular spaces, extracellular hyaline globules, and absence of human herpesvirus 8 staining by immunohistochemistry seen in Kaposi sarcoma is not observed in LCH.

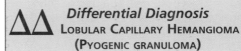

Differential Diagnosis
LOBULAR CAPILLARY HEMANGIOMA
(PYOGENIC GRANULOMA)

- Glomangiopericytoma (sinonasal-type hemangiopericytoma)
- Angiosarcoma
- Kaposi sarcoma

Pitfalls
LOBULAR CAPILLARY HEMANGIOMA (PYOGENIC GRANULOMA)

! Combination of cell types and absence of interconnecting (ramifying) vascular spaces should preclude a diagnosis of sinonasal-type hemangiopericytoma and angiosarcoma, respectively.

Juvenile hemangiomas are typically glucose transporter 1 immunoreactive.

DIAGNOSIS

The diagnosis of LCH includes the thorough evaluation of submitted material and the exclusion of other benign and malignant neoplasms.

TREATMENT AND PROGNOSIS

LCHs are treated with complete surgical excision. Recurrences are infrequent and should invoke consideration of a vascular proliferation with a more resilient biologic behavior.

GLOMANGIOPERICYTOMA (SINONASAL-TYPE HEMANGIOPERICYTOMA)

OVERVIEW

Stout and Murray offered the original description of hemangiopericytoma in 1942.[74] In terms of its histogenesis, pericytes are largely considered the cell of origin, but this opinion has been challenged.[75,76] Although this tumor is more common in the lower extremities and retroperitoneum, approximately 20% of all cases occur in the head and neck (nasal cavity, paranasal sinuses, orbit, scalp, face, and neck).[74,77–80] Hemangiopericytoma of the sinonasal cavity (glomangiopericytoma) has not exhibited the range of biologic behavior clinicians are accustomed to in other anatomic sites and for this reason were termed, *sinonasal-type hemangiopericytoma*.[81–83] The overall light microscopic and immunohistochemical staining shares more features with glomus tumors, hence the consideration that these tumors be called *glomangiopericytomas*.[84] Just as glomangiopericytomas tend to show more banal histologic features, they are also remarkable for lower rates of recurrence and metastasis. Conventional histopathologic parameters for predicting aggressive behavior show little value when applied to glomangiopericytomas.[77,85]

Most glomangiopericytomas originate from the nasal cavity but frequently involve the paranasal sinuses by way of direct extension. Exclusive involvement of the paranasal sinuses is a less frequent phenomenon.[84,86] Glomangiopericytomas are most common in the fifth to seventh decades of life and show an approximately equal gender distribution.[76,77,80,84] Nasal obstruction and epistaxis are typical complaints at presentation. Symptoms show an average duration of 10 months.[84] Imaging studies frequently exhibit bone erosion and sclerosis. These neoplasms are rare, but their morphologic and immunophenotypic profiles pose diagnostic challenges to surgical pathologists.

GROSS FEATURES

Glomangiopericytomas are usually received as fragments of pale pink to dark red soft, edematous, or friable tissue. Surface ulceration may or may not be present.

MICROSCOPIC FEATURES

The vast majority of glomangiopericytomas shows a distinct histologic appearance. They are typically polypoid and submucosal, often showing a thin rim of stroma between sinonasal mucosa and unencapsulated tumor (grenz zone). Connection with the overlying mucosa, squamous metaplasia, and surface ulceration are not uncommon findings.[86] The growth pattern may be sheet-like, nodular, fascicular, whorled, or mixed and its borders with adjacent stroma are often well delineated (**Fig. 5**). Native submucosal structures can be either displaced or enveloped by the neoplastic population. Monotonous oval to fusiform tumor cell nuclei with vesicular or hyperchromatic chromatin and occasional nucleoli exhibit equal spacing, sometimes within short to medium length

Key Features
GLOMANGIOPERICYTOMA (SINONASAL-TYPE HEMANGIOPERICYTOMA)

1. May originate from pericytes based on morphologic, immunohistochemical, and electron microscopic features (also bears resemblance to glomus tumors)

2. Shows less aggressive behavior than hemangiopericytoma of other anatomic sites (lower rates of recurrence and metastasis)

3. Typically immunoreactive for vimentin, smooth muscle actin, muscle-specific actin, and factor XIIIa

Fig. 5. Sinonasal-type hemangiopericytoma. (*A*) The tumor is submucosal without involvement of the surface epithelium and is characterized by its diffuse growth. (*B*) The vascular spaces vary in size and shape and often are characterized by the presence of perivascular (peritheliomatous) hyalinization. (*C*) The neoplastic cells are uniform in size and shape and have round to oval nuclei with fine nuclear chromatin and an indistinct cytoplasm situated in and around endothelial-lined vascular spaces, the latter including perivascular (peritheliomatous) hyalinization.

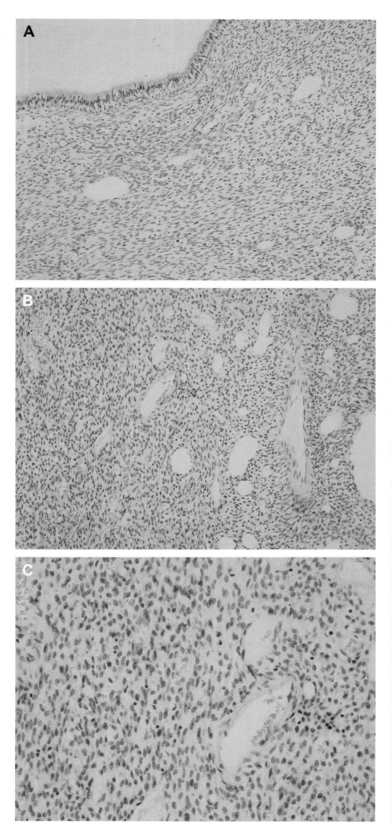

fascicles (see **Fig. 5**). Tumor cells with clear, amphophilic or eosinophilic cytoplasm bound by indistinct cell borders are set within a peculiar hemangiopericytoma-like vascular background. More specifically, the vascular network is composed of several branching staghorn thin-walled vessels with luminal diameters ranging from slit-like to gaping and ectatic. Electron microscopy has revealed tumor cells are set apart from blood vessels by basal lamina or a basal lamina-like substance.[86–88] The volume of this material is variable both within and between cases. Perivascular hyalinization, myxoid change, interstitial collagen deposition, and inflammation are common. Mitotic activity is low and necrosis is rarely encountered. Bone invasion and destruction are seldom events but may forecast an increased probability of recurrence and death from disease.[84]

In a comprehensive study from the files of the Armed Forces Institute of Pathology, Thompson and colleagues[84] reported on the immunophenotype of 104 cases of glomangiopericytoma: vimentin (98%), smooth muscle actin (92%), muscle-specific actin (77%), factor XIIIa (78%), and laminin (52%). Immunoreactivity is usually not displayed for CD31, CD34, factor VIII–related antigen, Bcl-2, S-100, glial fibrillary acidic protein (GFAP), neuron-specific enolase (NSE), CD117, desmin, keratins, and CD68.[84]

DIFFERENTIAL DIAGNOSIS

The architectural and vascular patterns of glomangiopericytoma are manifested in several other mesenchymal neoplasms. Common histologic mimics include LCH, nasopharyngeal angiofibroma, schwannoma (neurilemmoma), fibrosarcoma, leiomyosarcoma, and solitary fibrous tumor. LCH is a richly vascular proliferation with a lobular growth pattern that lacks the perivascular hyalinization of glomangiopericytoma. The diversity of cell types in LCH (fibroblasts, inflammatory, and endothelial cells) also assists in making this distinction. Angiofibroma occurs almost exclusively in young adolescent boys whereas glomangiopericytoma occurs in the fifth to seventh decades of life in both men and women. Schwannoma may show histomorphologic overlap with glomangiopericytoma but are strongly and diffusely immunoreactive for S-100, an attribute foreign to the latter. Fibrosarcoma and leiomyosarcoma are more likely to show nuclear pleomorphism and elevated mitotic rates when compared with glomangiopericytoma. Solitary fibrous tumor notoriously resembles hemangiopericytoma; its occurrence is extremely rare in the SNT. The

---

> ⚠️ **Differential Diagnosis**
> **GLOMANGIOPERICYTOMA**
> (SINONASAL-TYPE HEMANGIOPERICYTOMA)
>
> - LCH (pyogenic granuloma)
> - Angiofibroma
> - Schwannoma (neurilemmoma)
> - Fibrosarcoma
> - Leiomyosarcoma
> - Solitary fibrous tumor

presence of ropey keloidal collagen bundles and thin-walled blood vessels found in solitary fibrous tumor should dissuade making a diagnosis of glomangiopericytoma. Moreover, solitary fibrous tumor is classically diffusely positive for CD34 and Bcl-2 but negative for desmin, smooth muscle actin, and muscle-specific actin, findings inconsistent with glomangiopericytoma. More current classification schemes include solitary fibrous tumor with hemangiopericytoma.

DIAGNOSIS

The diagnosis of glomangiopericytoma is based on morphologic and immunophenotypic grounds.

TREATMENT AND PROGNOSIS

Patients are treated by local surgical excision with adequate margins.[80,89–91] Few studies have examined the efficacy of chemotherapy and radiation in hemangiopericytoma of the head and neck; application of these modalities is not recommended as primary treatment and tends to be used in the context of unresectable and/or metastatic disease, if at all.[75,80,89,92–94] Enzinger and Smith[77] reviewed cases of hemangiopericytoma from a variety of anatomic sites and reported worse clinical outcomes when hypercellularity, nuclear atypia, necrosis, increased mitotic activity (four or more mitotic figures per 10 high-power fields) and large tumors (≥6.5 cm in greatest dimension were encountered). Nuclear pleomorphism, significant mitotic activity, and necrosis are rare findings in glomangiopericytomas.[84,95] Kowalski and Paulino[96] have suggested that tumor cell immunoreactivity for MIB-1, a monoclonal antibody to a recombinant peptide that corresponds to the Ki-67 complementary DNA fragment present in the nuclei of proliferating cells, may correlate with biologic behavior and carry prognostic value in cases of glomangiopericytoma. Flow cytometric

> ### ⚠ Pitfalls
> ### GLOMANGIOPERICYTOMA (SINONASAL-TYPE HEMANGIOPERICYTOMA)
>
> ! Glomangiopericytoma exhibits submucosal diffuse growth composed of a single cell type and associated prominent vascularity, including foci of perivascular hyalinization, whereas LCH is a vascular proliferation with or without lobular pattern of growth composed of an admixture of cell types.

studies have disclosed a diploid DNA pattern and low S-phase in most tumor cells.[97] Moreover, tumors within the SNT often present earlier than peripheral sites—namely, before they reach 6.5 cm in size. To this end, it should come as no surprise that most cases constitute low-grade neoplasms with infrequent recurrences (approximately 15% of cases) and only rare metastases.[78,79,82,84,95,98] Thompson and colleagues[84] discovered an 88% 5-year survival in their cohort of 104 patients.

MALIGNANT NEOPLASMS OF THE SINONASAL TRACT

OVERVIEW

Malignant neoplasms of the nasal cavity and paranasal sinuses are rare, accounting for only 3% of head and neck tumors.[99] The maxillary sinus is involved in 70% to 80% of cases, followed by the ethmoid sinus (10%–20%).[100] Primary disease of the sphenoid and frontal sinuses is uncommon.[101] Understanding of nasal and paranasal sinus malignancies has been hampered by the heterogeneity of anatomic origin, tissue origin, histopathology, extent (stage), patient characteristics, and management strategies. The proximity of these tumors to critical anatomic structures, such as the orbit, dura, brain, cranial nerves, and cranial arteries, poses significant challenge in management. The 5-year survival for paranasal sinus cancer is approximately 30% to 40%.[102–105] Patients who present with malignant neck adenopathy carry a 5-year survival of less than 10%.[103,106–108] To this end, local control of advanced disease is a significant problem, even with the advent of improved imaging and surgical technology.

The most common tumors include squamous cell carcinoma (50%–80%), salivary gland type malignancies (eg, adenoid cystic carcinoma), sinonasal nonsalivary gland adenocarcinomas, SNUC, and ONB (esthesioneuroblastoma).[100] Nonepithelial malignancies, such as sarcomas, are typically managed with multiple modalities (surgery, radiotherapy, and chemotherapy).[100]

When tumors involve both the nasal cavity and paranasal sinuses, they have often been classified as sinonasal. Making this distinction should be attempted because tumors confined to the nasal vault have a more favorable outcome.[109–111] Similarly, tumors that originate from the palate and extend superiorly have a more favorable outcome than those from the maxillary sinus that involve the palate.[112] Several staging systems have been proposed and used in the medical literature.[113–116] This has led to a stage migration phenomenon, where the most aggressive lower stage cases are reclassified as more advanced cases. This is largely related to the advancement of computed tomography (CT) and positron emission tomography (PET).[109,117] Malignancies involving the frontal and sphenoid sinuses are typically considered a result of direct extension rather than primary disease. No formal staging systems have been designed for malignancies arising from these sites. The ability, or lack thereof, for local control determines the clinical course of disease.[104] Tumors that extend from the sinus to the dura, orbit, or cranium exhibit a poor outcome.[106,118,119]

Malignant sinonasal tumors are usually treated with a combination of radical surgical resection and postoperative radiotherapy, particularly in advanced stage disease.[103,104,109] In the absence of metastatic disease, surgery remains the cornerstone of management and should strive to achieve negative margins because it most likely portends better overall survival.[118,120–122] In patients who are not ideal surgical candidates, radiation alone is often suggested. Radiation in the absence of surgical intervention of paranasal cancers shows a 5-year survival of 30% to 40%.[108,110,123,124] Nevertheless, an ideal treatment strategy has not been agreed on for these patients. Patients with advanced disease show an overall poor outcome regardless of therapy. Although malignant adenopathy is likely best managed with combined surgery and radiotherapy, less is known about how to manage clinically node negative patients. This latter patient cohort ultimately shows nodal disease in 10% to 15% of cases.[110,125] The role of chemotherapy remains uncertain.

SINONASAL UNDIFFERENTIATED CARCINOMA

OVERVIEW

SNUC was first described in 1986 by Frierson and colleagues.[126] They invoked the use of this designation for a clinically aggressive sinonasal epithelial malignancy of uncertain histogenesis with or without neuroendocrine differentiation that lacks squamous or glandular differentiation.[126] Frierson emphasized the importance of recognizing SNUC as a distinct clinicopathologic entity because it appeared more aggressive than most, if not all, sinonasal malignancies. There are no known etiologic agents that incite pathogenesis, viral pathogens included.[127,128] Although SNUC represents a rare malignancy of the SNT, its recognition is of supreme importance to surgeons and medical oncologists because it presents distinct clinical and biologic features. SNUC typically presents as a rapidly enlarging mass that devastates tissue planes and bone within the nasal vault and paranasal sinuses with ease.[126,129] Penetration of orbital bones and the cranial cavity is not uncommon. Metastases to distant anatomic sites (cervical lymph nodes, bone, brain, and liver) have also been documented.[127]

SNUC has been observed in virtually every age group with the sixth decade of life the median age at presentation.[127,128,130,131] There is a 2:1 to 3:1 predilection for men.[131] The local extent of disease at the time of presentation may explain the presenting symptoms of nasal obstruction, epistaxis, proptosis, visual disturbances, and facial pain.[126] The acute onset—usually weeks to months—of these symptoms is considered characteristic for SNUC. Imaging studies often show extensive destruction of vital anatomic structures, including the cranial and orbital bones and cranial nerves.[131]

GROSS FEATURES

SNUCs are usually large (>4 cm in greatest dimension), are pale white or gray, and show areas that range from soft to friable. Large resection specimens show invasion into several anatomic compartments and structures. The margins of involvement can be difficult to delineate grossly.

MICROSCOPIC FEATURES

SNUC is almost invariably hypercellular and tumor cells are arranged in a variety of architectural patterns, including solid, sheet-like, organoid, lobular, trabecular, and ribbons (**Fig. 6**). The neoplasm is typically submucosal in location without involvement of the surface epithelium, which is often ulcerated; occasionally, direct continuity to the surface epithelial may be seen and, rarely, severe dysplasia/carcinoma in situ may be present. The neoplastic infiltrate lacks evidence of cellular differentiation (squamous cell, glandular, etc) and tumor cells are polygonal, are of considerable size, and often have ill-defined cell membranes. Nuclei range from medium to large in size and are classically pleomorphic. The chromatin is hyperchromatic or vesicular and shows inconspicuous to prominent nucleoli. Nuclear-to-cytoplasmic ratios are typically high and tumor cell cytoplasm is most often eosinophilic. Mitotic activity is brisk and atypical mitotic figures are commonplace, as is apoptosis. Confluent or microscopic foci of tumor cell necrosis are frequently encountered. Angiolymphatic and perineural invasion are frequently noted. A neurofibrillary background and rosettes (eg, Flexner-Wintersteiner and Homer Wright) are distinctly absent.[132]

The original description of SNUC discouraged the inclusion of cases that showed any semblance of squamous differentiation (keratinization and intercellular bridges). More recently, Ejaz and Wenig proposed that cases with limited degree of squamous differentiation (<5%) meeting other clinical (rapidly enlarging mass involving SNT), histologic, and immunophenotypic (discussed later) parameters of SNUC should still be classified as SNUC.[133] The rationale for this is based on the fact that such cases model the lethal biologic course seen in cases of SNUC. With the identification of the NUT midline carcinoma, it is conceivable that cases with abrupt squamous differentiation may better be classified in this newer diagnostic category if NUT translocation is identified.

The immunophenotype for SNUC is consistent and useful when attempting to discriminate it from other sinonasal malignancies. Immunohistochemical stains using antibodies directed against epithelial antigens are consistently positive. Although immunoreactivity for pankeratins is usually strong and diffuse, CK4, CK5/6, and CK14 are negative.[127,133,134] The staining patterns of p63 and epithelial membrane antige are more variable but typically at least focally present.[127,133] In situ hybridization for Epstein-Barr–encoded RNA is negative. NSE, CD99 (O13; Ewing marker), and neuroendocrine markers (eg, synaptophysin, chromogranin, and CD56) can be present and typically are focal when identified. Diffuse and intense staining for neuroendocrine markers should prompt consideration for a possible diagnosis of a poorly differentiated neuroendocrine carcinoma.[135,136] Although focal S-100 staining can be encountered, melanocytic markers (HMB-45, Melan-A, and tyrosinase) are negative. Furthermore, S-100 protein staining lacks the peripheral (sustentacular cell-like) pattern seen in ONB.

Fig. 6. SNUC. (*A*) Invasive cellular tumor showing lobular growth, a frequent feature of this tumor; in addition to a lobular pattern, trabecular growth may be identified. (*B*) Confluent foci of necrosis are a common feature.

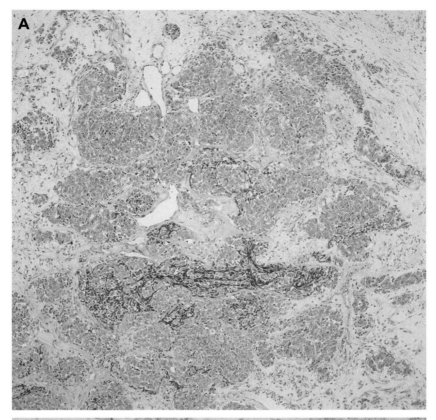

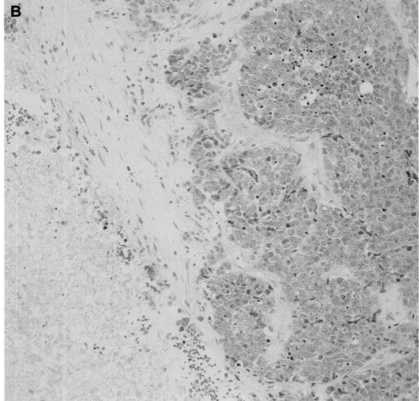

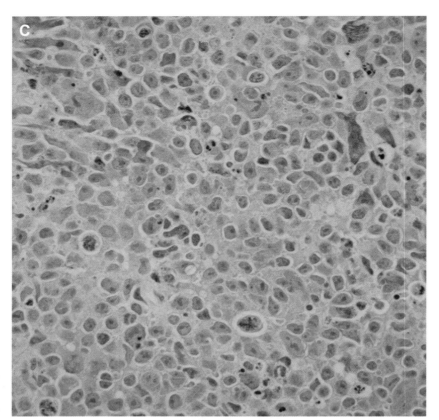

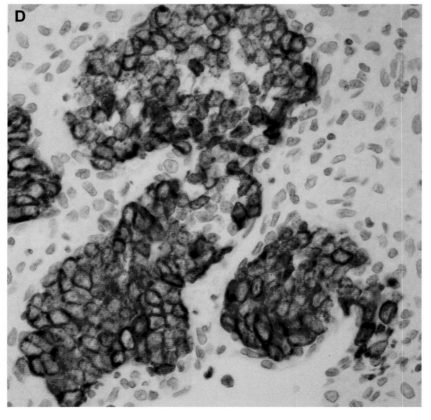

Fig. 6. (*C*) The neoplastic cells are polygonal to oval, composed of medium to large-sized, round to oval, hyperchromatic to vesicular nuclei, inconspicuous to prominent nucleoli, and a varying amount of eosinophilic-appearing cytoplasm with poorly defined cell membranes lacking evidence of cellular differentiation (squamous cell, glandular, etc); increased mitotic activity, including atypical mitoses and individual cell necrosis are present. (*D*) Diffuse cytokeratin immunoreactivity is present.

Key Features
SINONASAL UNDIFFERENTIATED CARCINOMA

1. Distinct clinicopathologic entity, including aggressive behavior, typically with signs and symptoms rapidly developing over a short period of time (weeks to months), representing important clinical parameters distinguish SNUC from other sinonasal malignancies

2. Morphologic features include submucosal lobular growth composed of a high-grade undifferentiated malignant neoplasm lacking evidence of cellular differentiation but with immunoreactivity for epithelial markers and absence of immunomarkers that might be indicative of an alternative diagnosis

Differential Diagnosis
SINONASAL UNDIFFERENTIATED CARCINOMA

- Poorly differentiated squamous cell carcinoma
- Small cell undifferentiated neuroendocrine carcinoma
- Nasopharyngeal nonkeratinizing carcinoma, undifferentiated-type
- MMM
- Rhabdomyosarcoma
- High-grade ONB
- Hematolymphoid malignancies (ie, NK/T-cell lymphoma)

Hematolymphoid markers (leukocyte common antigen, CD3, CD20, etc) and muscle markers (desmin, myogenin, myoglobin, and actins) are also negative.

DIFFERENTIAL DIAGNOSIS

SNUC must be distinguished from other high-grade epithelial and nonepithelial sinonasal malignancies using adjunct studies, such as immunohistochemistry and molecular studies. This has become increasingly important because targeted therapies in this anatomic region become more common and improve survival and quality of life. More specifically, SNUC must be separated from poorly differentiated squamous cell carcinoma, small cell undifferentiated neuroendocrine carcinoma, nasopharyngeal nonkeratinizing carcinoma undifferentiated-type, MMM, rhabdomyosarcoma, high-grade ONB, and hematolymphoid malignancies, such as natural killer (NK)/T-cell lymphoma.

SNUC can be discriminated from small cell undifferentiated neuroendocrine carcinoma because it lacks a diffuse and strong staining pattern for neuroendocrine markers (NSE, CD56, chromogranin, and synaptophysin). High-grade ONB can be separated from SNUC based on its absence of epithelial markers and the presence of diffuse staining with neuroendocrine markers (NSE, chromogranin, and synaptophysin) and S-100 positivity in a sustentacular pattern.[137] Confusion with the similarly named undifferentiated carcinoma of the nasopharynx may occur. In contrast to SNUC, nasopharyngeal undifferentiated carcinoma is invariably associated with Epstein-Barr virus, and in situ hybridization for

Epstein-Barr–encoded RNA is positive in the nasopharyngeal undifferentiated carcinoma but negative in SNUC. Melanoma, rhabdomyosarcoma, and hematolymphoid malignancies can be excluded with immunohistochemical profiling. Hematolymphoid malignancies may be p63 positive so the presence of p63 alone may not correlate to an epithelial neoplasm (eg, squamous cell or myoepithelial).

DIAGNOSIS

The diagnosis of SNUC is based on histologic, immunophenotypic, and, in some cases, molecular analysis.

TREATMENT AND PROGNOSIS

The prognosis of patients afflicted by SNUC is grim, despite aggressive therapy, and median survival is less than 18 months.[127,128] Patients are usually managed with surgical resection and adjuvant therapies, such as radiation and chemotherapy. The rapid growth and extent of local destruction renders it difficult to obtain negative surgical margins. Moreover, SNUC is notoriously nonresponsive to radiotherapy.[138,139]

Pitfalls
SINONASAL UNDIFFERENTIATED CARCINOMA

! Inappropriate histologic and immunohistochemical evaluation of high-grade sinonasal malignancies may result erroneous diagnosis and possible mismanagement of patients.

RHABDOMYOSARCOMA

OVERVIEW

Rhabdomyosarcoma (RMS) is a malignant neoplasm that originates from primitive skeletal muscle cells called rhabdomyoblasts. RMS only represents approximately 5% to 8% of adult and pediatric sarcomas, respectively; however, it is the most common sarcoma observed in the head and neck region.[131] Although parameningeal and orbital involvement is the most common, RMS can also be observed in the sinonasal cavity and nasopharynx. Men and women are equally affected and patients typically present in the first or second decade of life. Clinical manifestations of sinonasal RMS, much like other sinonasal malignancies, are nonspecific (nasal obstruction, epistaxis, proptosis, visual disturbances, and facial pain). The etiopathogenesis of RMS is unknown.

GROSS FEATURES

Gross examination of RMS is often unimpressive as the lesions are typically small—sometimes nothing more than a polyp. The term, *sarcoma botryoides*, designates a gross appearance of RMS rather than a histologic variant; namely, it describes polypoid or grape-like features. Sarcoma botryoides is occasionally glistening and myxoid as well. Approximately 25% of RMSs originating from the sinonasal cavity demonstrate a sarcoma botryoides appearance.

MICROSCOPIC FEATURES

The most common histologic variant of RMS in the head and neck is the embryonal type (71%).[140] Alveolar RMS is observed less frequently (13%) and pleomorphic RMS is rare.[140] Regardless of the morphologic variant, the rhabdomyoblast, the proposed cell of origin of RMS, can exhibit cells that are small and round, ribbon or strap-shaped, or enlarged and pleomorphic. The presence of cross-striations is not always identified; to this end, their absence should not dissuade one from making the diagnosis of RMS if other morphologic, immunophenotypic, and molecular criteria are met. An innocuous-appearing inflammatory infiltrate can potentially conceal neoplastic cells, possibly posing significant diagnostic challenge.

Embryonal RMS is characterized by tumor cells arranged in alternating areas of hypocellularity and hypercellularity. Neoplastic cells may arrange themselves densely in a subepithelial location; this is often referred to as a *cambium layer*. The background stroma can be edematous, myxoid, or fibrillary. Tumor cells can display both round and/or spindled morphology. Round or oval tumor cells possess hyperchromatic nuclei surrounded by cytoplasm that can demonstrate a variety of tinctorial appearances (basophilic, acidophilic, or amphophilic). Spindled tumor cells appear elongated or fusiform with central and hyperchromatic nuclei and eosinophilic to clear-appearing cytoplasm. Mitotic activity and tumor cell necrosis is not uncommon with either histologic appearance.

Alveolar RMS, which is more common in adults, is composed of noncohesive tumor cells arranged loosely around central hypocellular or empty spaces (alveoli) (**Fig. 7**). Some cases may display predominantly solid or trabecular growth patterns, with alveolar architecture only a focal feature. Whether alveolar, trabecular, or solid, the masses of tumor cells are separated from one another by fibrous septa that can be noticeably vascular. Neoplastic cells are round, oval, or spindle-shaped and possess hyperchromatic nuclei with occasional inconspicuous nucleoli. A

Key Features
RHABDOMYOSARCOMA

1. It is the most common sarcoma observed in the head and neck region

2. Sarcoma botryoides designates a gross appearance of RMS rather than a histologic variant

3. Alveolar subtype of RMS is characterized by t(2;13)q36;q14)

△△ *Differential Diagnosis*
RHABDOMYOSARCOMA

- Poorly differentiated squamous cell carcinoma
- Small cell undifferentiated neuroendocrine carcinoma
- MMM
- SNUC
- High-grade ONB
- Hematolymphoid malignancies (ie, NK/T-cell lymphoma)

Fig. 7. Alveolar rhabdo-myosarcoma. (*A*) Diffuse/solid growth with round to oval hyperchromatic nuclei, clear-appearing cytoplasm, and increased mitotic activity. (*B*) Loss of cellular cohesion, resulting in alveolar spaces.

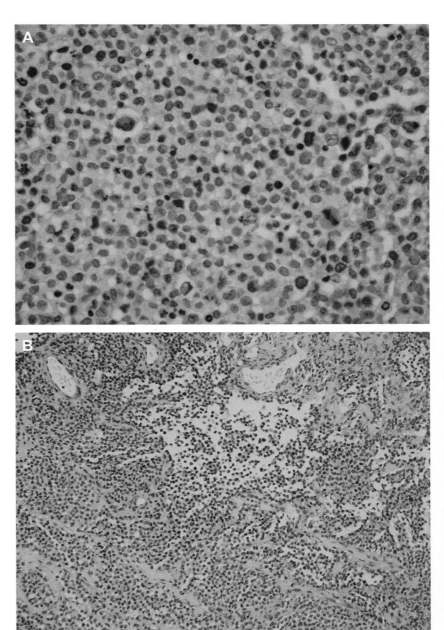

common feature of alveolar RMS is multinucleated giant cells with peripherally placed nuclei. Similar to embryonal RMS, increased mitotic activity, atypical mitotic figures, and necrosis are not infrequent.

Histochemical staining can be of benefit when considering the possibility of RMS as the cytoplasm of neoplastic cells contains glycogen (diastase-sensitive, periodic acid–Schiff positive). Masson trichrome and phosphotungstic acid–

hematoxylin stains can be used to accentuate intracytoplasmic myofibrils. As expected, mucicarmine is negative in tumor cells. Given the mesenchymal cell of origin for RMS, immunohistochemical stains for desmin, myoglobin, Myf4, muscle-specific actin, and vimentin are positive (see **Fig. 7**). Epithelial, hematolymphoid, neuroendocrine, and melanocytic markers are negative. The alveolar subtype of RMS is characterized by the t(2;13)q36;q14) translocation. This can be

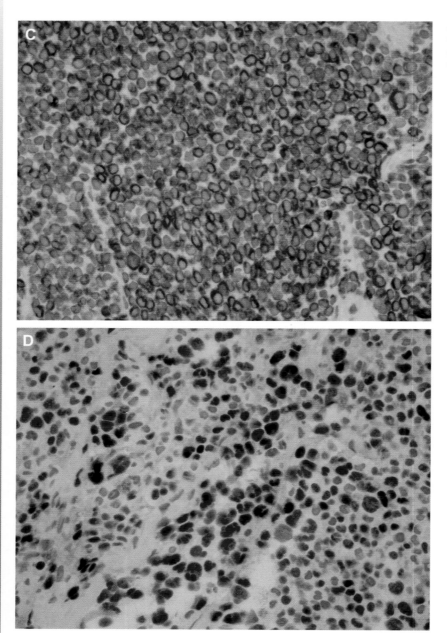

Fig. 7. (C) Desmin and (D) myogenin immunoreactivity confirm the diagnosis.

elicited in most cases of alveolar RMS using fluorescence in situ hybridization or reverse transcription–polymerase chain reaction.

DIFFERENTIAL DIAGNOSIS

Although uncommon in older patients, RMS should be a diagnostic consideration for a high-grade sinonasal malignancy in any age group. Furthermore, RMS must be separated from entities, such as poorly differentiated squamous cell carcinoma, small cell undifferentiated neuroendocrine carcinoma, lymphoepithelial carcinoma of the SNT, MMM, high-grade ONB, and hematolymphoid malignancies, such as NK/T-cell lymphoma.

DIAGNOSIS

The diagnosis of RMS is based on histologic, immunophenotypic, and, in some cases, molecular findings.

Pitfalls
RHABDOMYOSARCOMA

! Although more common in the first or second decade of life, adults can also be affected; alveolar RMS is the most common histologic subtype in adults.

! Inappropriate histologic, immunohistochemical, and molecular evaluation of high-grade sinonasal malignancies may result in mismanagement of patients.

TREATMENT AND PROGNOSIS

Unlike many other high-grade sinonasal malignancies, surgical resection of RMS is not always the primary therapeutic goal. The role of surgery is often limited to resection of small lesions or tissue diagnosis in unresectable or metastatic cases (regional lymph nodes, lungs, bone marrow, meninges, brain, liver, pancreas, kidney, and heart). On making a tissue diagnosis of RMS, therapeutic algorithms take age, anatomic site, and disease stage into account. Because RMS has a proclivity for bone marrow involvement, bone marrow aspiration/biopsy is central to clinical staging. The 5-year survival of RMS in the head and neck is approximately 80%.[131]

OLFACTORY NEUROBLASTOMA

OVERVIEW

ONB, also known as esthesioneuroblastoma, has long been considered to originate from the olfactory membrane of the SNT. More specifically, evidence acquired from light and electron microscopic studies suggests that ONB arises from bipolar neurons of the olfactory membrane.[141] ONB shows a subtle female predominance and bimodal age peak in the second and sixth decades of life; the median age is approximately 50 years.[141] Clinical manifestations commonly include epistaxis and nasal obstruction. Less frequently, facial pain, anosmia, excessive lacrimation, and visual disturbances are reported.

GROSS FEATURES

ONB is most commonly a small (<1 cm), soft, polypoid, mass covered by sinonasal mucosa.

MICROSCOPIC FEATURES

The pioneer of the current grading system used for ONB, Hyams, suggested a four-tier (grade) system. Grade I, the most differentiated, is characterized by monotonous tumor cells arranged in a predominantly lobular architecture. Neoplastic cells have round nuclei with vesicular or powdery chromatin with or without inconspicuous nucleoli. Tumor cell nests are set within neurofibrillary material and separated by a highly vascularized stroma. Homer Wright pseudorosettes are common. Calcification is variably identified. Mitotic activity and necrosis are virtually nonexistent in grade I lesions. Grade II lesions are discriminated from their lower-grade counterpart by their increased nuclear pleomorphism and indefinite neurofibrillary background. The designation of grade III ONB is reserved for tumors with limited lobular architecture, poorly defined or focal neurofibrillary background, hyperplastic cells nests with even more anaplasia, elevated mitotic activity, and atypical mitoses. Although Flexner-Wintersteiner rosettes are observed in a minority of cases, calcifications are absent. Lastly, grade IV ONB shows marked anaplasia, including pleomorphic nuclei and noticeable eosinophilic nucleoli (**Fig. 8**). Mitotic figures—some of which are atypical—and necrosis are not uncommon. As expected, grade IV lesions generally lack a distinct neurofibrillary network and calcifications.

Understanding the immunoprofile of ONB is instrumental to distinguishing it from other SNT neoplasms. Typically, it is a combination of markers and not any one alone that assists in the diagnosis of ONB. NSE remains the most sensitive marker for ONB, although it is nonspecific and can be seen in a wide array of tumor types.[137,142,143] Immunohistochemical staining for S-100 protein likely provides the most usefulness in differentiating ONB from other entities. Although staining can be variable, S-100 protein typically highlights sustentacular cells lining the tumor lobules in a peripheral pattern, a unique feature when

Key Features
OLFACTORY NEUROBLASTOMA

1. Originates from the olfactory membrane of the SNT

2. Submucosal lobular growth that in lower-grade ONBs include identifiable neurofibrillary material separated by a highly vascularized stroma

3. S-100 protein highlights peripherally situated sustentacular cells but may only be focally present in higher-grade tumors

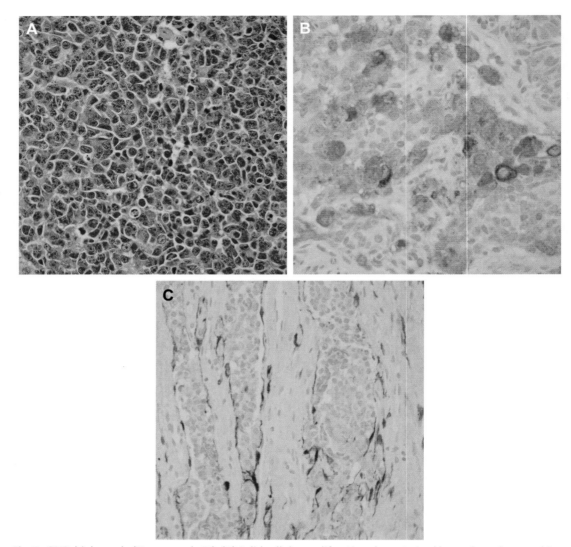

Fig. 8. ONB, high-grade (Hyams grade IV). (*A*) Solid cellular proliferation characterized by nuclear pleomorphism, dispersed nuclear chromatin, inconspicuous to identifiable nucleoli, and increased mitotic activity; in this grade tumor, there is an absence of cellular differentiation (eg, neurofibrillary component), making identification of this neoplasm as an ONB difficult. Immunohistochemical staining assists in the diagnosis, including (*B*) diffuse NSE and (*C*) peripheral (sustentacular cell-like) S-100 protein staining with absence of epithelial markers, melanocytic markers, and hematolymphoid markers.

compared with other SNT neoplasms (see **Fig. 8**). Typically ONBs lack staining with epithelial markers (eg, cytokeratins, epithelial membrane antigen, and p63) although in any given case such staining may focally be seen. Diffuse immunoreactivity for keratin should prompt consideration of alternative diagnoses including epithelial and neuroendocrine neoplasms. GFAP, chromogranin, synaptophysin, CD56, and Leu-7 (CD57) expression are also inconsistent. Finally, electron

microscopy has shown the neoplastic cells of ONB to harbor dense-core neurosecretory granules that range from 80 nm to 25 nm in greatest dimension.[137]

DIFFERENTIAL DIAGNOSIS

The differential diagnosis for ONB is similar to that of other sinonasal malignancies, namely, MMM,

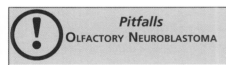

Differential Diagnosis
OLFACTORY NEUROBLASTOMA

- Poorly differentiated squamous cell carcinoma
- Small cell undifferentiated neuroendocrine carcinoma
- MMM
- Rhabdomyosarcoma
- SNUC
- Hematolymphoid malignancies (ie, NK/T-cell lymphoma)

rhabdomyosarcoma, neuroendocrine carcinoma, and, in higher-grade lesions, SNUC.

DIAGNOSIS

The diagnosis of ONB is rooted in light microscopic and immunophenotypic features, although low-grade ONB can often be strongly suspected with light microscopic evaluation alone.

TREATMENT AND PROGNOSIS

The primary treatment of ONB is surgical and complete resection imparts greater prognostic significance than clinical stage.[141] Full-course radiotherapy is often used on an adjuvant basis. Chemotherapy has been used in cases where complete resection is not possible and/or metastatic disease. The overall survival of ONB is favorable: 78% at 5 years, 71% at 10 years, and 68% at 15 years.[144] Approximately one-third of patients experience cervical lymph node metastasis.[131]

Pitfalls
OLFACTORY NEUROBLASTOMA

! Failure to evaluate high-grade sinonasal malignancies with NSE and S-100 protein immunostaining can result in overlooking the diagnosis.

! In the presence of diffuse cytokeratin staining, a diagnosis of ONB should be questioned.

MUCOSAL MALIGNANT MELANOMA

OVERVIEW

Malignant melanoma of the head and neck represents 15% to 25% of all cases of malignant melanoma.[133] Although MMM represents only a minority of these cases (approximately 6%–8%)—the majority is of ocular origin—it maintains extreme importance from a diagnostic and therapeutic standpoint.[133] There is a male predilection and wide age range of affected individuals. Most commonly, patients are between the sixth and eighth decades of life.[131] Presenting symptoms include epistaxis, facial pain, hoarseness, and dysphagia. MMM originates more commonly in the nasal vault than it does the paranasal sinuses; however, involvement of both compartments is not uncommon, either as a consequence of direct extension or multicentricity. With respect to the nasal vault, MMM can declare itself in the septum, lateral wall, middle turbinate, and inferior turbinate.[131] Paranasal involvement classically originates from the maxillary (antrum) or ethmoid sinuses.[131]

GROSS FEATURES

MMM may show a range of gross appearances: flat or polypoid, pink-white, or brown-black. The margins of the tumor may be difficult, if not impossible, to demarcate without microscopic evaluation.

MICROSCOPIC FEATURES

Ulceration of the surface mucosa is not an uncommon finding. Similar to malignant melanoma in other anatomic sites, MMM can showcase spindled, epithelioid, or mixed cytomorphology. Architecturally, the spindle cell variant of MMM shows tumor cells arranged in storiform and/or fascicular patterns composed of elongated to oval-appearing pleomorphic nuclei with vesicular to hyperchromatic chromatin (Fig. 9). The presence of nucleoli is variable, inconspicuous in some cases and prominent in others. The architectural patterns of epithelioid MMM include alveolar, nested,

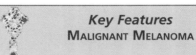

Key Features
MALIGNANT MELANOMA

1. Peak incidence is sixth to eighth decades of life
2. Tumor cells may exhibit spindled, epithelioid, or mixed cytomorphology

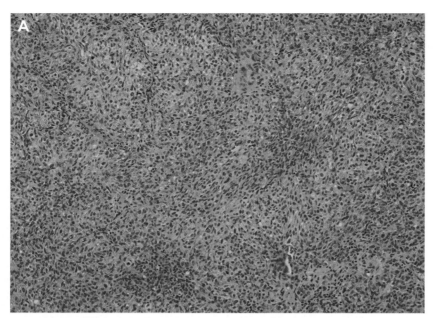

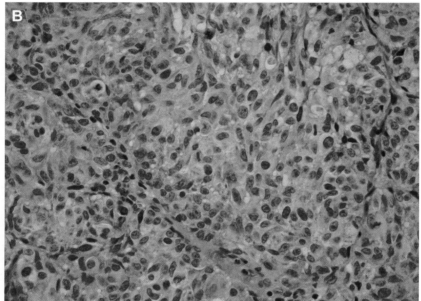

Fig. 9. Sinonasal MMM. (*A*) The neoplastic infiltrate includes solid, lobular, and fascicular growth patterns. (*B*) The neoplastic cells composed of round to oval to spindle-shaped, pleomorphic nuclei with vesicular to hyperchromatic nuclei, nuclear molding, prominent eosinophilic nucleoli, and eosinophilic cytoplasm; in most cases of mucosal melanomas, there is an absence of readily identifiable intracytoplasmic melanin pigment.

organoid, trabecular, or solid. Tumor cells are usually markedly atypical with enlarged nuclei (high nuclear-to-cytoplasmic ratios), prominent eosinophilic nucleoli, and nuclear grooves. Nuclear molding and pseudoinclusions are occasionally identified. Tumor cell cytoplasm may be clear, pink, or eosinophilic. In some cases, the nuclei are eccentrically placed imparting a plasmacytoid appearance. As discussed previously, in any given case there may be an admixture of spindled and epithelioid cell populations. Mitotic activity, atypical mitoses, and necrosis are commonly seen. Less common features include tumor giant cells and, rarely, glandular or squamous differentiation.

Surface involvement in the form of junctional or pagetoid changes is not commonly identified and is not required in the diagnosis because these neoplasms may originate in the submucosa. Pigmentation (melanin) is frequently encountered; however, as much as one-third of MMM cases exhibit no pigmentation.[133]

MMMs are typically immunoreactive for vimentin, S-100 protein, HMB-45, tyrosinase, and Melan-A (**Fig. 10**).[145,146] Immunostains for epithelial markers (cytokeratin and epithelial membrane antigen), carcinoembryonic antigen, neuroendocrine markers, hematolymphoid markers, and mesenchymal markers (eg, desmin and actins) are negative.

DIFFERENTIAL DIAGNOSIS

Much like other high-grade malignancies of the SNT, MMM must be distinguished from poorly

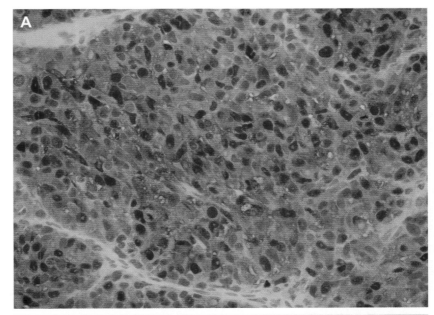

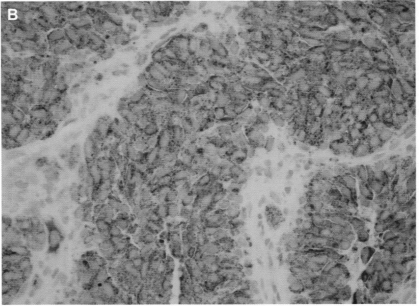

Fig. 10. Sinonasal MMM. (*A*) S-100 protein and (*B*) HMB-45 staining. Melan A, tyrosinase, and vimentin reactivity was also present (not shown).

Differential Diagnosis
MALIGNANT MELANOMA

- Poorly differentiated squamous cell carcinoma
- Small cell undifferentiated neuroendocrine carcinoma
- SNUC
- Rhabdomyosarcoma
- High-grade ONB
- Hematolymphoid malignancies (ie, NK/T-cell lymphoma)

differentiated squamous cell carcinoma, small cell undifferentiated neuroendocrine carcinoma, lymphoepithelial carcinoma of the SNT, MMM, rhabdomyosarcoma, high-grade ONB, and hematolymphoid malignancies such as NK/T-cell lymphoma.

DIAGNOSIS

The diagnosis of MMM is based on the immunophenotypic profile of tumor cells.

TREATMENT AND PROGNOSIS

The prognosis for patients with MMM is grave, with less than 30% surviving beyond 5 years.[131] Unlike its cutaneous counterpart, the prognosis of MMM cannot be stratified based on tumor depth—this is largely due to microanatomic differences between these sites. Complete surgical resection is the primary goal of treatment; the usefulness of radiotherapy and chemotherapy is uncertain. Metastatic disease is not infrequent, often spreading to lymph nodes, lungs, and brain.

Pitfalls
MALIGNANT MELANOMA

! A small percentage of cases is S-100 protein negative (approximately 10%–15%); all cases where a diagnosis of MMM I suspected should include staining for melanocytic markers, including HMB-45, tyrosinase, and Melan-A.

REFERENCES

1. Batsakis JG. Pathology consultation. Nasal (Schneiderian) papillomas. Ann Otol Rhinol Laryngol 1981; 90(2 Pt 1):190–1.
2. Hyams VJ. Papillomas of the nasal cavity and paranasal sinuses. A clinicopathological study of 315 cases. Ann Otol Rhinol Laryngol 1971;80(2): 192–206.
3. Lampertico P, Russell WO, Maccomb WS. Squamous papilloma of upper respiratory epithelium. Arch Pathol 1963;75:293–302.
4. Weissler MC, Montgomery WW, Turner PA, et al. Inverted papilloma. Ann Otol Rhinol Laryngol 1986; 95(3 Pt 1):215–21.
5. Michaels L, Young M. Histogenesis of papillomas of the nose and paranasal sinuses. Arch Pathol Lab Med 1995;119(9):821–6.
6. Buchwald C, Franzmann MB, Jacobsen GK, et al. Human papillomavirus (HPV) in sinonasal papillomas: a study of 78 cases using in situ hybridization and polymerase chain reaction. Laryngoscope 1995;105(1):66–71.
7. Sarkar FH, Visscher DW, Kintanar EB, et al. Sinonasal Schneiderian papillomas: human papillomavirus typing by polymerase chain reaction. Mod Pathol 1992;5(3):329–32.
8. Weiner JS, Sherris D, Kasperbauer J, et al. Relationship of human papillomavirus to Schneiderian papillomas. Laryngoscope 1999;109(1):21–6.
9. Batsakis JG, Suarez P. Schneiderian papillomas and carcinomas: a review. Adv Anat Pathol 2001; 8(2):53–64.
10. Peters BW, O'Reilly RC, Willcox TO Jr, et al. Inverted papilloma isolated to the sphenoid sinus. Otolaryngol Head Neck Surg 1995;113(6):771–7.
11. Lawson W, Ho BT, Shaari CM, et al. Inverted papilloma: a report of 112 cases. Laryngoscope 1995; 105(3 Pt 1):282–8.
12. Harris MO, Beck JC, Terrell JE, et al. Expression of human papillomavirus 6 in inverted papilloma arising in a renal transplant recipient. Laryngoscope 1998;108(1 Pt 1):115–9.
13. Fu YS, Hoover L, Franklin M, et al. Human papillomavirus identified by nucleic acid hybridization in concomitant nasal and genital papillomas. Laryngoscope 1992;102(9):1014–9.
14. Judd R, Zaki SR, Coffield LM, et al. Sinonasal papillomas and human papillomavirus: human papillomavirus 11 detected in fungiform Schneiderian papillomas by in situ hybridization and the polymerase chain reaction. Hum Pathol 1991;22(6):550–6.
15. Kashima HK, Kessis T, Hruban RH, et al. Human papillomavirus in sinonasal papillomas and squamous cell carcinoma. Laryngoscope 1992;102(9): 973–6.

16. McLachlin CM, Kandel RA, Colgan TJ, et al. Prevalence of human papillomavirus in sinonasal papillomas: a study using polymerase chain reaction and in situ hybridization. Mod Pathol 1992;5(4):406–9.

17. Wu TC, Trujillo JM, Kashima HK, et al. Association of human papillomavirus with nasal neoplasia. Lancet 1993;341(8844):522–4.

18. Respler DS, Jahn A, Pater A, et al. Isolation and characterization of papillomavirus DNA from nasal inverting (schneiderian) papillomas. Ann Otol Rhinol Laryngol 1987;96(2 Pt 1):170–3.

19. Syrjänen S, Happonen RP, Virolainen E, et al. Detection of human papillomavirus (HPV) structural antigens and DNA types in inverted papillomas and squamous cell carcinomas of the nasal cavities and paranasal sinuses. Acta Otolaryngol 1987;104(3–4):334–41.

20. Weber RS, Shillitoe EJ, Robbins KT, et al. Prevalence of human papillomavirus in inverted nasal papillomas. Arch Otolaryngol Head Neck Surg 1988;114(1):23–6.

21. Brandwein M, Steinberg B, Thung S, et al. Human papillomavirus 6/11 and 16/18 in Schneiderian inverted papillomas. In situ hybridization with human papillomavirus RNA probes. Cancer 1989;63(9):1708–13.

22. Bryan RL, Bevan IS, Crocker J, et al. Detection of HPV 6 and 11 in tumours of the upper respiratory tract using the polymerase chain reaction. Clin Otolaryngol Allied Sci 1990;15(2):177–80.

23. Siivonen L, Virolainen E. Transitional papilloma of the nasal cavity and paranasal sinuses. Clinical course, viral etiology and malignant transformation. ORL J Otorhinolaryngol Relat Spec 1989;51(5):262–7.

24. Ishibashi T, Tsunokawa Y, Matsushima S, et al. Presence of human papillomavirus type-6-related sequences in inverted nasal papillomas. Eur Arch Otorhinolaryngol 1990;247(5):296–9.

25. Furuta Y, Shinohara T, Sano K, et al. Molecular pathologic study of human papillomavirus infection in inverted papilloma and squamous cell carcinoma of the nasal cavities and paranasal sinuses. Laryngoscope 1991;101(1 Pt 1):79–85.

26. Beck JC, McClatchey KD, Lesperance MM, et al. Presence of human papillomavirus predicts recurrence of inverted papilloma. Otolaryngol Head Neck Surg 1995;113(1):49–55.

27. Ogura H, Fujiwara T, Hamaya K, et al. Detection of human papillomavirus type 57 in a case of inverted nasal papillomatosis in Japan. Eur Arch Otorhinolaryngol 1995;252(8):513–5.

28. Barnes L. Schneiderian papillomas and nonsalivary glandular neoplasms of the head and neck. Mod Pathol 2002;15(3):279–97.

29. Snyder RN, Perzin KH. Papillomatosis of nasal cavity and paranasal sinuses (inverted papilloma, squamous papilloma). A clinicopathologic study. Cancer 1972;30(3):668–90.

30. Christensen WN, Smith RR. Schneiderian papillomas: a clinicopathologic study of 67 cases. Hum Pathol 1986;17(4):393–400.

31. Eavey RD. Inverted papilloma of the nose and paranasal sinuses in childhood and adolescence. Laryngoscope 1985;95(1):17–23.

32. Buchwald C, Franzmann MB, Tos M. Sinonasal papillomas: a report of 82 cases in Copenhagen County, including a longitudinal epidemiological and clinical study. Laryngoscope 1995;105(1):72–9.

33. Myers EN, Fernau JL, Johnson JT, et al. Management of inverted papilloma. Laryngoscope 1990;100(5):481–90.

34. Phillips PP, Gustafson RO, Facer GW. The clinical behavior of inverting papilloma of the nose and paranasal sinuses: report of 112 cases and review of the literature. Laryngoscope 1990;100(5):463–9.

35. Outzen KE, Grøntved A, Jørgensen K, et al. Inverted papilloma of the nose and paranasal sinuses: a study of 67 patients. Clin Otolaryngol Allied Sci 1991;16(3):309–12.

36. Dolgin SR, Zaveri VD, Casiano RR, et al. Different options for treatment of inverting papilloma of the nose and paranasal sinuses: a report of 41 cases. Laryngoscope 1992;102(3):231–6.

37. Bielamowicz S, Calcaterra TC, Watson D. Inverting papilloma of the head and neck: the UCLA update. Otolaryngol Head Neck Surg 1993;109(1):71–6.

38. Lawson W, Le Benger J, Som P, et al. Inverted papilloma: an analysis of 87 cases. Laryngoscope 1989;99(11):1117–24.

39. Pelausa EO, Fortier MA. Schneiderian papilloma of the nose and paranasal sinuses: the University of Ottawa experience. J Otolaryngol 1992;21(1):9–15.

40. Kelly JH, Joseph M, Carroll E, et al. Inverted papilloma of the nasal septum. Arch Otolaryngol 1980;106(12):767–71.

41. Wenig BM. Schneiderian-type mucosal papillomas of the middle ear and mastoid. Ann Otol Rhinol Laryngol 1996;105(3):226–33.

42. Astor FC, Donegan JO, Gluckman JL. Unusual anatomic presentations of inverting papilloma. Head Neck Surg 1985;7(3):243–5.

43. Sulica RL, Wenig BM, Debo RF, et al. Schneiderian papillomas of the pharynx. Ann Otol Rhinol Laryngol 1999;108(4):392–7.

44. Hampal S, Hawthorne M. Hypopharyngeal inverted papilloma. J Laryngol Otol 1990;104(5):432–4.

45. Osborn DA. Transitional cell growths of the upper respiratory tract. J Laryngol Otol 1956;70(10):574–88.

46. Gaffey MJ, Frierson HF, Weiss LM, et al. Human papillomavirus and Epstein-Barr virus in sinonasal Schneiderian papillomas. An in situ hybridization

and polymerase chain reaction study. Am J Clin Pathol 1996;106(4):475–82.

47. Klemi PJ, Joensuu H, Siivonen L, et al. Association of DNA aneuploidy with human papillomavirus-induced malignant transformation of sinonasal transitional papillomas. Otolaryngol Head Neck Surg 1989;100(6):563–7.

48. Macdonald MR, Le KT, Freeman J, et al. A majority of inverted sinonasal papillomas carries Epstein-Barr virus genomes. Cancer 1995;75(9):2307–12.

49. Som PM, Dillon WP, Sze G, et al. Benign and malignant sinonasal lesions with intracranial extension: differentiation with MR imaging. Radiology 1989;172(3):763–6.

50. Norris HJ. Papillary lesions of the nasal cavity and paranasal sinuses. II. Inverting papillomas. A study of 29 cases. Laryngoscope 1963;73:1–17.

51. Abildgaard-Jensen J, Greisen O. Inverted papillomas of the nose and the paranasal sinuses. Clin Otolaryngol Allied Sci 1985;10(3):135–43.

52. Stankiewicz JA, Girgis SJ. Endoscopic surgical treatment of nasal and paranasal sinus inverted papilloma. Otolaryngol Head Neck Surg 1993;109(6):988–95.

53. Suh KW, Facer GW, Devine KD, et al. Inverting papilloma of the nose and paranasal sinuses. Laryngoscope 1977;87(1):35–46.

54. Mabery TE, Devine KD, Harrison EG Jr. The problem of malignant transformation in a nasal papilloma: report of a case. Arch Otolaryngol 1965;82:296–300.

55. Woodson GE, Robbins KT, Michaels L. Inverted papilloma. Considerations in treatment. Arch Otolaryngol 1985;111(12):806–11.

56. Norris HJ. Papillary lesions of the nasal cavity and paranasal sinuses: part i exophytic (squamous) papillomas. A study of 28 cases. Laryngoscope 1962;72(12):1784–98.

57. Skolnik EM, Loewy A, Friedman JE. Inverted papilloma of the nasal cavity. Arch Otolaryngol 1966;84(1):61–7.

58. Segal K, Atar E, Mor C, et al. Inverting papilloma of the nose and paranasal sinuses. Laryngoscope 1986;96(4):394–8.

59. Lesperance MM, Esclamado RM. Squamous cell carcinoma arising in inverted papilloma. Laryngoscope 1995;105(2):178–83.

60. Ferlito A. The World Health Organization's revised classification of tumours of the larynx, hypopharynx, and trachea. Ann Otol Rhinol Laryngol 1993;102(9):666–9.

61. Batsakis JG. The pathology of head and neck tumors: nasal cavity and paranasal sinuses, part 5. Head Neck Surg 1980;2(5):410–9.

62. Barnes L, Bedetti C. Oncocytic Schneiderian papilloma: a reappraisal of cylindrical cell papilloma of the sinonasal tract. Hum Pathol 1984;15(4):344–51.

63. Ward BE, Fechner RE, Mills SE. Carcinoma arising in oncocytic Schneiderian papilloma. Am J Surg Pathol 1990;14(4):364–9.

64. Kapadia SB, Barnes L, Pelzman K, et al. Carcinoma ex oncocytic Schneiderian (cylindrical cell) papilloma. Am J Otolaryngol 1993;14(5):332–8.

65. Mills SE, Cooper PH, Fechner RE. Lobular capillary hemangioma: the underlying lesion of pyogenic granuloma. A study of 73 cases from the oral and nasal mucous membranes. Am J Surg Pathol 1980;4(5):470–9.

66. Anderson CF. Granuloma pyogenicum of the oral cavity; report of a case. Oral Surg Oral Med Oral Pathol 1953;6(11):1325–32.

67. Bhaskar SN, Jacoway JR. Pyogenic granuloma—clinical features, incidence, histology, and result of treatment: report of 242 cases. J Oral Surg 1966;24(5):391–8.

68. Kerr DA. Granuloma pyogenicum. Oral Surg Oral Med Oral Pathol 1951;4(2):158–76.

69. Leyden JJ, Master GH. Oral cavity pyogenic granuloma. Arch Dermatol 1973;108(2):226–8.

70. Yuan K, Wing LY, Lin MT. Pathogenetic roles of angiogenic factors in pyogenic granulomas in pregnancy are modulated by female sex hormones. J Periodontol 2002;73(7):701–8.

71. Pacifici R, Brown C, Puscheck E, et al. Effect of surgical menopause and estrogen replacement on cytokine release from human blood mononuclear cells. Proc Natl Acad Sci U S A 1991;88(12):5134–8.

72. Tabibzadeh S, Satyaswaroop PG, von Wolff M, et al. Regulation of TNF-alpha mRNA expression in endometrial cells by TNF-alpha and by oestrogen withdrawal. Mol Hum Reprod 1999;5(12):1141–9.

73. Yuan K, Lin MT. The roles of vascular endothelial growth factor and angiopoietin-2 in the regression of pregnancy pyogenic granuloma. Oral Dis 2004;10(3):179–85.

74. Stout AP. Hemangiopericytoma; a study of 25 cases. Cancer 1949;2(6):1027–54, illust.

75. Kuo FY, Lin HC, Eng HL, et al. Sinonasal hemangiopericytoma-like tumor with true pericytic myoid differentiation: a clinicopathologic and immunohistochemical study of five cases. Head Neck 2005;27(2):124–9.

76. McMaster MJ, Soule EH, Ivins JC. Hemangiopericytoma. A clinicopathologic study and long-term followup of 60 patients. Cancer 1975;36(6):2232–44.

77. Enzinger FM, Smith BH. Hemangiopericytoma. An analysis of 106 cases. Hum Pathol 1976;7(1):61–82.

78. Batsakis JG, Rice DH. The pathology of head and neck tumors: vasoformative tumors, part 9B. Head Neck Surg 1981;3(4):326–39.

79. Walike JW, Bailey BJ. Head and neck hemangiopericytoma. Arch Otolaryngol 1971;93(4):345–53.

80. Billings KR, Fu YS, Calcaterra TC, et al. Hemangio-pericytoma of the head and neck. Am J Otolaryngol 2000;21(4):238–43.

81. Compagno J. Hemangiopericytoma-like tumors of the nasal cavity: a comparison with hemangiopericytoma of soft tissues. Laryngoscope 1978;88(3):460–9.

82. Compagno J, Hyams VJ. Hemangiopericytoma-like intranasal tumors. A clinicopathologic study of 23 cases. Am J Clin Pathol 1976;66(4):672–83.

83. Gorenstein A, Facer GW, Weiland LH. Hemangio-pericytoma of the nasal cavity. Otolaryngology 1978;86(3 Pt 1):ORL405–15.

84. Thompson LD, Miettinen M, Wenig BM. Sinonasal-type hemangiopericytoma: a clinicopathologic and immunophenotypic analysis of 104 cases showing perivascular myoid differentiation. Am J Surg Pathol 2003;27(6):737–49.

85. Díaz-Flores L, Gutiérrez R, Varela H, et al. Micro-vascular pericytes: a review of their morphological and functional characteristics. Histol Histopathol 1991;6(2):269–86.

86. Eichhorn JH, Dickersin GR, Bhan AK, et al. Sino-nasal hemangiopericytoma. A reassessment with electron microscopy, immunohistochemistry, and long-term follow-up. Am J Surg Pathol 1990;14(9):856–66.

87. Dardick I, Hammar SP, Scheithauer BW. Ultrastruc-tural spectrum of hemangiopericytoma: a compara-tive study of fetal, adult, and neoplastic pericytes. Ultrastruct Pathol 1989;13(2–3):111–54.

88. Nunnery EW, Kahn LB, Reddick RL, et al. Heman-giopericytoma: a light microscopic and ultrastruc-tural study. Cancer 1981;47(5):906–14.

89. Carew JF, Singh B, Kraus DH. Hemangiopericyto-ma of the head and neck. Laryngoscope 1999;109(9):1409–11.

90. Catalano PJ, Brandwein M, Shah DK, et al. Sino-nasal hemangiopericytomas: a clinicopathologic and immunohistochemical study of seven cases. Head Neck 1996;18(1):42–53.

91. Hervé S, Abd Alsamad I, Beautru R, et al. Manage-ment of sinonasal hemangiopericytomas. Rhinol-ogy 1999;37(4):153–8.

92. Delsupehe KG, Jorissen M, Sciot R, et al. Heman-giopericytoma of the head and neck: a report of four cases and a literature review. Acta Otorhinolar-yngol Belg 1992;46(4):421–7.

93. Backwinkel KD, Diddams JA. Hemangiopericyto-ma. Report of a case and comprehensive review of the literature. Cancer 1970;25(4):896–901.

94. Mira JG, Chu FC, Fortner JG. The role of radio-therapy in the management of malignant heman-giopericytoma: report of eleven new cases and review of the literature. Cancer 1977;39(3):1254–9.

95. Yasui R, Minatogawa T, Kanoh N, et al. Nasal septal hemangiopericytoma-like tumor: a case report with an immunohistochemical study. Am J Rhinol 2001;15(4):267–70.

96. Kowalski PJ, Paulino AF. Proliferation index as a prognostic marker in hemangiopericytoma of the head and neck. Head Neck 2001;23(6):492–6.

97. el-Naggar AK, Batsakis JG, Garcia GM, et al. Sino-nasal hemangiopericytomas. A clinicopathologic and DNA content study. Arch Otolaryngol Head Neck Surg 1992;118(2):134–7.

98. Marianowski R, Wassef M, Herman P, et al. Nasal haemangiopericytoma: report of two cases with literature review. J Laryngol Otol 1999;113(3):199–206.

99. Carrau RL, Myers EM, Johnson JT. Paranasal sinus carcinoma—diagnosis, treatment, and prognosis. Oncology (Williston Park) 1992;6(1):43–50 [discus-sion: 55–6].

100. Day TA, Beas RA, Schlosser RJ, et al. Management of paranasal sinus malignancy. Curr Treat Options Oncol 2005;6(1):3–18.

101. Bhattacharyya N. Factors predicting survival for cancer of the ethmoid sinus. Am J Rhinol 2002;16(5):281–6.

102. Kondo M, Ogawa K, Inuyama Y, et al. Prognostic factors influencing relapse of squamous cell carci-noma of the maxillary sinus. Cancer 1985;55(1):190–6.

103. Giri SP, Reddy EK, Gemer LS, et al. Management of advanced squamous cell carcinomas of the maxillary sinus. Cancer 1992;69(3):657–61.

104. Alvarez I, Suárez C, Rodrigo JP, et al. Prognostic factors in paranasal sinus cancer. Am J Otolaryng-ol 1995;16(2):109–14.

105. Kaplan I, Anavi Y, Manor R, et al. The use of molec-ular markers as an aid in the diagnosis of glandular odontogenic cyst. Oral Oncol 2005;41(9):895–902.

106. Gullane PJ, Conley J. Carcinoma of the maxillary sinus. A correlation of the clinical course with orbital involvement, pterygoid erosion or pterygo-palatine invasion and cervical metastases. J Otolaryngol 1983;12(3):141–5.

107. Robin PE, Powell DJ. Regional node involvement and distant metastases in carcinoma of the nasal cavity and paranasal sinuses. J Laryngol Otol 1980;94(3):301–9.

108. Neal AJ, Habib F, Hope-Stone HF. Carcinoma of the maxillary antrum treated by pre-operative radio-therapy or radical radiotherapy alone. J Laryngol Otol 1992;106(12):1063–6.

109. Harbo G, Grau C, Bundgaard T, et al. Cancer of the nasal cavity and paranasal sinuses. A clinico-pathological study of 277 patients. Acta Oncol 1997;36(1):45–50.

110. Logue JP, Slevin NJ. Carcinoma of the nasal cavity and paranasal sinuses: an analysis of radical radiotherapy. Clin Oncol (R Coll Radiol) 1991;3(2):84–9.

111. Parsons JT, Kimsey FC, Mendenhall WM, et al. Radiation therapy for sinus malignancies. Otolaryngol Clin North Am 1995;28(6):1259–68.

112. Truitt TO, Gleich LL, Huntress GP, et al. Surgical management of hard palate malignancies. Otolaryngol Head Neck Surg 1999;121(5):548–52.

113. Lederman M. Tumours of the upper jaw: natural history and treatment. J Laryngol Otol 1970;84(4):369–401.

114. Sakai S, Hamasaki Y. Proposal for the classification of carcinoma of the paranasal sinuses. Acta Otolaryngol 1967;63(1):42–8.

115. Carinci F, Farina A, Padula E, et al. Primary malignancies of the nasal fossa and paranasal sinuses: comparison between UICC classification and a new staging system. J Craniofac Surg 1997; 8(5):405–12.

116. Cantú G, Solero CL, Mariani L, et al. A new classification for malignant tumors involving the anterior skull base. Arch Otolaryngol Head Neck Surg 1999;125(11):1252–7.

117. Slevin NJ, Collins CD, Hastings DL, et al. The diagnostic value of positron emission tomography (PET) with radiolabelled fluorodeoxyglucose (18F-FDG) in head and neck cancer. J Laryngol Otol 1999; 113(6):548–54.

118. Rutter MJ, Furneaux CE, Morton RP. Craniofacial resection of anterior skull base tumours: factors contributing to success. Aust N Z J Surg 1998; 68(5):350–3.

119. Bilsky MH, Kraus DH, Strong EW, et al. Extended anterior craniofacial resection for intracranial extension of malignant tumors. Am J Surg 1997;174(5):565–8.

120. Janecka IP, Sen C, Sekhar L, et al. Treatment of paranasal sinus cancer with cranial base surgery: results. Laryngoscope 1994;104(5 Pt 1):553–5.

121. McCutcheon IE, Blacklock JB, Weber RS, et al. Anterior transcranial (craniofacial) resection of tumors of the paranasal sinuses: surgical technique and results. Neurosurgery 1996;38(3):471–9 [discussion: 479–80].

122. Mouriaux F, Martinot V, Pellerin P, et al. Survival after malignant tumors of the orbit and periorbit treated by exenteration. Acta Ophthalmol Scand 1999;77(3):326–30.

123. Waldron JN, O'Sullivan B, Warde P, et al. Ethmoid sinus cancer: twenty-nine cases managed with primary radiation therapy. Int J Radiat Oncol Biol Phys 1998;41(2):361–9.

124. Haylock BJ, John DG, Paterson IC. The treatment of squamous cell carcinoma of the paranasal sinuses. Clin Oncol (R Coll Radiol) 1991;3(1):17–21.

125. Sisson GA Sr, Toriumi DM, Atiyah RA. Paranasal sinus malignancy: a comprehensive update. Laryngoscope 1989;99(2):143–50.

126. Frierson HF Jr, Mills SE, Fechner RE, et al. Sinonasal undifferentiated carcinoma. An aggressive neoplasm derived from schneiderian epithelium and distinct from olfactory neuroblastoma. Am J Surg Pathol 1986;10(11):771–9.

127. Cerilli LA, Holst VA, Brandwein MS, et al. Sinonasal undifferentiated carcinoma: immunohistochemical profile and lack of EBV association. Am J Surg Pathol 2001;25(2):156–63.

128. Jeng YM, Sung MT, Fang CL, et al. Sinonasal undifferentiated carcinoma and nasopharyngeal-type undifferentiated carcinoma: two clinically, biologically, and histopathologically distinct entities. Am J Surg Pathol 2002;26(3):371–6.

129. Bashir AA, Robinson RA, Benda JA, et al. Sinonasal adenocarcinoma: immunohistochemical marking and expression of oncoproteins. Head Neck 2003; 25(9):763–71.

130. Gallo O, Graziani P, Fini-Storchi O. Undifferentiated carcinoma of the nose and paranasal sinuses. An immunohistochemical and clinical study. Ear Nose Throat J 1993;72(9):588–90.

131. Wenig BM. Undifferentiated malignant neoplasms of the sinonasal tract. Arch Pathol Lab Med 2009; 133(5):699–712.

132. Smith SR, Som P, Fahmy A, et al. A clinicopathological study of sinonasal neuroendocrine carcinoma and sinonasal undifferentiated carcinoma. Laryngoscope 2000;110(10 Pt 1):1617–22.

133. Ejaz A, Wenig BM. Sinonasal undifferentiated carcinoma: clinical and pathologic features and a discussion on classification, cellular differentiation, and differential diagnosis. Adv Anat Pathol 2005;12(3):134–43.

134. Franchi A, Moroni M, Massi D, et al. Sinonasal undifferentiated carcinoma, nasopharyngeal-type undifferentiated carcinoma, and keratinizing and nonkeratinizing squamous cell carcinoma express different cytokeratin patterns. Am J Surg Pathol 2002;26(12):1597–604.

135. Mills SE. Neuroectodermal neoplasms of the head and neck with emphasis on neuroendocrine carcinomas. Mod Pathol 2002;15(3):264–78.

136. Rosenthal DI, Barker JL Jr, El-Naggar AK, et al. Sinonasal malignancies with neuroendocrine differentiation: patterns of failure according to histologic phenotype. Cancer 2004;101(11):2567–73.

137. Hirose T, Scheithauer BW, Lopes MB, et al. Olfactory neuroblastoma. An immunohistochemical, ultrastructural, and flow cytometric study. Cancer 1995;76(1):4–19.

138. Kramer D, Durham JS, Sheehan F, et al. Sinonasal undifferentiated carcinoma: case series and systematic review of the literature. J Otolaryngol 2004;33(1):32–6.

139. Kim BS, Vongtama R, Juillard G. Sinonasal undifferentiated carcinoma: case series and

literature review. Am J Otolaryngol 2004;25(3): 162–6.

140. Newton WA Jr, Soule EH, Hamoudi AB, et al. Histopathology of childhood sarcomas, Intergroup Rhabdomyosarcoma Studies I and II: clinicopathologic correlation. J Clin Oncol 1988;6(1):67–75.

141. Mills SE, Frierson HF Jr. Olfactory neuroblastoma. A clinicopathologic study of 21 cases. Am J Surg Pathol 1985;9(5):317–27.

142. Choi HS, Anderson PJ. Olfactory neuroblastoma: an immuno-electron microscopic study of S-100 protein-positive cells. J Neuropathol Exp Neurol 1986;45(5):576–87.

143. Frierson HF Jr, Ross GW, Mills SE, et al. Olfactory neuroblastoma. Additional immunohistochemical characterization [see comment]. Am J Clin Pathol 1990;94(5):547–53.

144. Eden BV, Debo RF, Larner JM, et al. Esthesioneuroblastoma. Long-term outcome and patterns of failure—the University of Virginia experience. Cancer 1994;73(10):2556–62.

145. Franquemont DW, Mills SE. Sinonasal malignant melanoma. A clinicopathologic and immunohistochemical study of 14 cases. Am J Clin Pathol 1991;96(6):689–97.

146. Prasad ML, Jungbluth AA, Iversen K, et al. Expression of melanocytic differentiation markers in malignant melanomas of the oral and sinonasal mucosa. Am J Surg Pathol 2001;25(6): 782–7.

SQUAMOUS CELL CARCINOMA OF THE ORAL CAVITY AND OROPHARYNX

Justin A. Bishop, MD[a], James J. Sciubba, DMD, PhD[b],
William H. Westra, MD[c],*

KEYWORDS

- Head and neck squamous cell carcinoma • Human papillomavirus
- Basaloid squamous cell carcinoma • Spindle cell type: sarcomatoid carcinoma
- Papillary squamous cell carcinoma • Verrucous carcinoma • Pseudoepitheliomatous hyperplasia
- Necrotizing sialometaplasia

ABSTRACT

The most common malignancy to involve the oral cavity and oropharynx is squamous cell carcinoma (SCC). Because these oral cancers share an origin from the squamous epithelium, the pathology of oral SCC might be expected to be uniform and its diagnosis repetitive. In reality, the morphologic diversity in SCC, along with the propensity for reactive processes of the oral cavity to mimic SCC histologically, renders its diagnosis one of the more challenging in surgical pathology. This article discusses variants of oral and oropharyngeal SCC and highlights those features that help distinguish human papillomavirus–related from human papillomavirus–unrelated SCC.

CONVENTIONAL SQUAMOUS CELL CARCINOMA

OVERVIEW

The oral cavity is comprised of two anatomically distinct compartments—the oral cavity proper and the oropharynx—and carcinomas arising from these distinct compartments deserve separate consideration. The oral cavity proper encompasses the oral tongue (anterior two-thirds of tongue in front of the V-shaped sulcus terminalis), gingiva, buccal mucosal, floor of mouth, and hard palate. Most squamous cell carcinomas (SCCs) arising in the oral cavity proper are tobacco related. The oropharynx is comprised of the soft palate, base of tongue, and palatine tonsils. This anatomic region is more frequently targeted by oncogenic human papillomavirus, and these human papillomavirus (HPV)-related SCCs are discussed later. Conventional oral SCCs tend to occur in patients older than 50 years, and they predominate in men (male-to-female ratio 3:1).[1,2] Carcinogen exposure, diet, and pre-existing medical conditions may all play a role, individually or in combination, in the development of oral cancer. The synergistic effect of tobacco smoking and alcohol use represents the dominant risk factor,[1,2] although smokeless tobacco is a major cause of oral SCC in those parts of the world where the practice of chewing betel quid is common.[3] Other factors, including immunosuppression, nutritional deficiencies, and poor oral hygiene, may further contribute to the development of oral SCC.[1]

[a] Johns Hopkins Medical Institutions, 600 North Wolfe Street, Pathology 401, Baltimore, MD 21287, USA
[b] Milton J. Dance, Jr. Head and Neck Center, Greater Baltimore Medical Center, 6569 North Charles Street, Suite 401, Baltimore, MD 21204, USA
[c] Johns Hopkins Medical Institutions, 401 North Broadway, Weinberg 2242, Baltimore, MD 21231, USA
* Corresponding author.
E-mail address: wwestra@jhmi.edu

Surgical Pathology 4 (2011) 1127–1151
doi:10.1016/j.path.2011.07.002

GROSS/CLINICAL FEATURES OF SCC

Invasive oral SCCs are generally preceded by clinically visible but asymptomatic premalignant alterations of the oral mucosa known as leukoplakia and erythroplakia (**Fig. 1**). *Leukoplakia* is a clinical term that refers to a white patch in the oral cavity. Leukoplakia varies in thickness, and its surface features range from granular to nodular to fissured. *Erythroplakia* is a clinical term that refers to a red patch of the oral mucosa. It tends to have a soft and velvety appearance. These white and red lesions are sometimes, but not always, associated with histologic evidence of premalignant or malignant changes. Erythroplakia is much likely than leukoplakia to be associated with dysplasia or carcinoma.

The gross appearance of invasive SCC is highly variable depending on the extent of local tumor spread. Early invasion (ie, microinvasion) within an area of leukoplakia or erythroplakia is not apparent on visual inspection alone. With more advanced tumor growth, the macroscopic appearance may range from subtle thickening of the mucosa to flat ulcers to fungating masses. On cut section, invasive oral SCCs are firm and grayish white, typically with ulceration of the overlying epithelium.

MICROSCOPIC FEATURES OF SCC

Squamous dysplasia refers to neoplastic alterations of the surface epithelium before invasion into the subepithelial tissues. These changes include architectural disturbances (eg, irregular epithelial stratification, loss of polarity of the basal cells, drop-shaped rete ridges, increased mitotic activity, premature keratinization of individual cells, and keratin pearls within rete pegs) and cytologic abnormalities (eg, atypical mitotic forms, nuclear enlargement with hyperchromasia, and cellular pleomorphism). The World Health Organization currently recommends that these changes be graded on a scale of 1 to 4 based on the severity of the atypia and extent of epithelial involvement.[1] Although terminology varies, atypia limited to the lower one-third of the epithelium is generally referred to as *mild dysplasia*, atypia limited to the lower two-thirds of the epithelium as *moderate dysplasia*, and atypia extending upward into the upper one-third as *severe dysplasia* (**Fig. 2**). A diagnosis of squamous carcinoma in situ is reserved for lesions where the architectural atypia is full thickness and the degree of cytologic atypia is pronounced.

Invasion usually occurs in a background of surface dysplasia and is seen microscopically as extension of atypical squamous cells beyond the basement membrane into the underlying subepithelial tissues. The term, *microinvasion*, refers to stromal invasion that is limited to the most superficial aspect of the lamina propria (generally within 1 to 2 mm below the basement membrane of the adjacent non-neoplastic epithelium).[4] The invasive nests of squamous cells tend to be irregular and infiltrative, and they elicit a desmoplastic stromal reaction that includes fibrosis, edema, chronic inflammation, and sometimes a foreign body giant cell reaction to keratin debris.

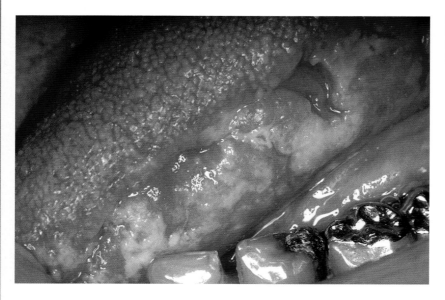

Fig. 1. Mixed erythroleukoplakia with areas of erosion, atrophy, and ulceration.

Fig. 2. Progressive stages of squamous dysplasia. When the cellular and architecture disturbances are mild and limited to the lower third of the epithelium, the dysplasia is graded as mild (*A*). With progression, the atypia becomes more fully developed and extends into the middle third (*B*)—moderate dysplasia—and then upper third (*C*)—severe dysplasia of the epithelium.

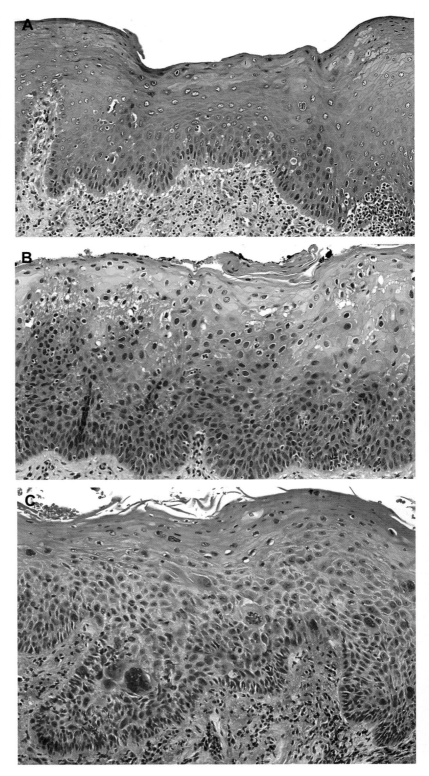

With advancing invasion, SCC infiltrates the musculature of the tongue and may extend into adjacent structures (eg, mandible). Conventional oral SCC tends to infiltrate as cohesive rounded nests, irregular cords, individual cells, or some combination of these patterns (**Fig. 3**). The invasive component may be either keratinized or nonkeratinized, and its histologic grade varies from well-differentiated carcinomas resembling non-neoplastic squamous epithelium (eg, abundant glassy eosinophilic cytoplasm, mild nuclear atypia, and well-developed intercellular bridges) to poorly differentiated carcinomas comprised of immature cells with marked nuclear atypia, numerous mitoses, and atypical mitotic forms. For poorly differentiated carcinoma, evidence of keratin production in the form of keratin pearls or single cells with cytoplasmic keratinization may be crucial in establishing its squamous nature. For poorly differentiated tumors where there is no evidence of keratinization on routine histology, immunohistochemistry may be needed to confirm its epithelial nature and eliminate the possibility of a lymphoma or a mucosal melanoma. A basic immunohistochemical panel includes epithelial markers (eg, cytokeratins), lymphoid markers (eg, common leukocyte antigen, CD3, and CD20), and melanocytic markers (eg, S-100, melanin-A, and HMB-45).

DIFFERENTIAL DIAGNOSIS OF SCC

Atypia of the surface epithelium can be encountered in a spectrum of reactive, regenerative, and

Differential Diagnosis
ATYPIA OF SURFACE SQUAMOUS EPITHELIUM

- Squamous dysplasia
- Radiation-induced epithelial atypia
- Re-epithelialization of ulcer bed
- Local irritation/trauma
- Candida mucositis
- Herpetic ulcer with viral cytopathic changes
- Nutritional deficiencies (eg, iron, folate, and vitamin B_{12})

reparative processes that are not neoplastic in nature and have no potential to progress toward malignancy. The distinction between a true squamous dysplasia and some non-neoplastic process may be straightforward in cases of severe dysplasia/carcinoma in situ where the cytologic and architectural atypia is highly developed but less reliable in milder forms of dysplasia where the atypia is less profound and may overlap with a reactive/reparative process. The alterations noted in the surface epithelium must be carefully interpreted in light of the entire histologic picture. Squamous atypia in association with ulceration, intense acute inflammation, viral cytopathic changes,

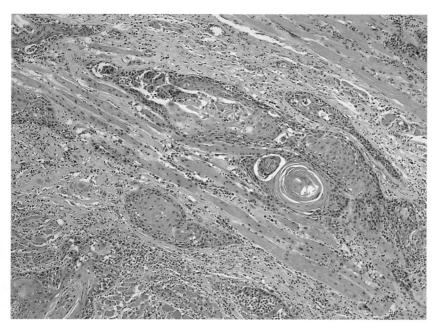

Fig. 3. Conventional squamous cell carcinoma of the oral tongue. Squamous nests infiltrate between skeletal muscle fibers. Some of the nests exhibit keratin pearl formations. The invasive nests incite fibrosis and inflammation in the surrounding stroma.

infestation by fungal hyphae, or radiation-induced stromal alterations should prompt consideration of a reactive/reparative process.

Invasion beyond the basement membrane is an important finding that signals the onset of malignancy such that its diagnosis should not be rendered lightly. Extension of dysplastic squamous epithelium within the ducts and acini of seromucinous glands is still limited by a basement membrane and thus should not be interpreted as microinvasion. Pseudoepitheliomatous hyperplasia is a non-neoplastic proliferation of the squamous epithelium with irregular downward extension of the squamous rete into the submucosa. Pseudoepitheliomatous hyperplasia can be encountered in various chronic inflammatory conditions, but it is most fully developed when it arises in association with a granular cell tumor. In this context, pseudoepitheliomatous hyperplasia exhibits deep downward extension into the stroma by irregular and angulated tongues of squamous epithelium (**Fig. 4**). The presence of deep keratin pearls, mild cellular atypia, and mitotic figures may further blur its distinction from well-differentiated conventional SCC. Unlike SCC, pseudoepitheliomatous hyperplasia related to granular cell tumor is not associated with surface dysplasia or with a desmoplastic stromal reaction. Instead, the stroma between the tongues of squamous epithelium is packed by nests and sheets of granular cells characterized by abundant eosinophilic, granular cytoplasm (see **Fig. 4**). The granular cell is strongly S-100 positive.

Pitfalls
PSEUDOEPITHELIOMATOUS HYPERPLASIA

! Irregular tongues of squamous epithelium with downward into subepithelial tissues

! Absence of surface dysplasia

! Minimal cytologic atypia

! May be associated with a granular cell tumor in its most fully developed form

! An S-100 immunostain can be useful in confirming the presence of an associated granular cell tumor

Histologically, the repopulation of infarcted ducts and acini by a proliferation of metaplastic squamous epithelium can mimic invasive SCC (**Fig. 5**). Microscopic features that are helpful in distinguishing necrotizing sialometaplasia from invasive SCC include the presence of ischemic necrosis of the minor salivary gland lobules, the common background changes of ulceration and inflammation, the absence of overt cytologic features of malignancy, and confinement of the proliferative process to the framework of the pre-existing minor salivary gland lobules. The latter finding is seen as rounded squamous nests that maintain the lobular architecture of a minor salivary gland unit—a pattern that contrasts with the jagged irregularity of invasive SCC. Some

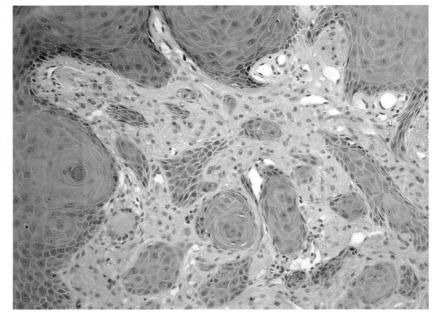

Fig. 4. Granular cell tumor with associated pseudoepitheliomatous hyperplasia. Angulated nests of squamous epithelium bud off the surface epithelium and extend downward into the subepithelial tissues mimicking well-differentiated squamous cell carcinoma. The stroma between the squamous nests is packed with cells characterized by eosinophilic to amphopuilic granular cytoplasm.

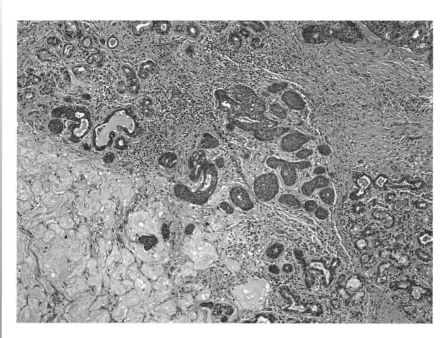

Fig. 5. Necrotizing sialometaplasia. Metaplastic squamous epithelium grows within the preserved frame work of an infarcted minor salivary gland lobule. An ischemic lobule, seen as pools of mucin, is present on the left side of the figure.

investigators have used immunohistochemical markers for myoepithelial cells (eg, actin, p63, and calponin) in an effort to highlight the intact myoepithelial layer around the metaplastic squamous nests in necrotizing squamous metaplasia.[5]

PROGNOSIS OF SCC

Prognosis of oral SCC is most strongly influenced by the extent of tumor spread (ie, tumor stage).

Oral SCC is notorious for its ability to infiltrate local structures and metastasize by way of lymphatics to regional lymph nodes along the jugular chain. Hematogenous spread to distant sites (eg, lungs) is less common. Histologic grading is much less important than tumor staging in predicting clinical outcomes.[6] Histopathologic parameters that do portend a worse prognosis include angiolymphatic invasion, perineural invasion, depth of invasion, and the presence of extracapsular spread for those SCCs that have metastasized to regional lymph nodes.[7] The pattern of invasion

---

(!) **Pitfalls**
NECROTIZING SIALOMETAPLASIA

! Classically occurs on the hard palate but can be encountered in other head and neck sites

! Ischemic injury of minor salivary glands during early stages of lesional evolution (often not present during advanced stages of lesional progression)

! Often arises in a background of ulceration and inflammation

! Overtly malignant cytologic features are not developed

! Rounded squamous nests that maintain the lobular architecture of the minor salivary gland

---

 Differential Diagnosis
ATYPICAL SQUAMOUS PROLIFERATIONS EXTENDING INTO STROMA

• Invasive squamous cell carcinoma

• Extension of dysplastic squamous epithelium within the ducts and acini of seromucinous glands

• Radiated minor salivary gland ducts and lobules

• Pseudoepitheliomatous hyperplasia

• Necrotizing sialometaplasia

along the advancing tumor front also carries some prognostic weight. Expansive growth characterized by large cohesive nests with a well-defined pushing margin is associated with a better prognosis; whereas a more infiltrative pattern of irregular strands of tumor cells is associated with a poorer prognosis.[8,9] Oral SCCs often arise from a field of molecular genetic alterations that are distributed throughout large tracts of the respiratory system (field cancerization).[10,11] As a result, patients who develop an oral SCC are at an elevated risk of developing a second synchronous or metachronous SCC in their oral cavity or elsewhere in the respiratory tract.

PAPILLARY VARIANT OF SQUAMOUS CELL CARCINOMA

OVERVIEW

The hallmark feature of the papillary variant of squamous cell carcinoma is its exophytic growth with finger-like papillary projections. This outward projection stands in sharp contrast to the infiltrative character of most conventional oral SCCs. Although oncogenic types of the HPV have been identified in some papillary SCCs,[12–14] the vast majority of papillary SCCs generally do not arise from a pre-existing HPV-associated squamous papillomas (ie, carcinomatous transformation of a squamous papilloma).

GROSS/CLINICAL FEATURES OF PAPILLARY SCC

Papillary SCC appears grossly as a friable, exophytic, cauliflower-like mass. It may have a broad-based attachment to the oral mucosa, or it may project from the oral mucosa along a thin stalk. This exophytic growth tends to overshadow any endophytic (ie, infiltrative) component.

MICROSCOPIC FEATURES OF PAPILLARY SCC

The trademark feature of papillary SCC, namely its papillary extensions, is histologically characterized by a multilayered squamous epithelium supported by a central fibrovascular core (**Fig. 6**A). Architecturally it is structured like a squamous papilloma but, unlike a benign papilloma, its fronds are lined by cytologically malignant squamous cells (see **Fig. 6**B). In the papillary variant of SCC, the presence of invasion may be elusive and difficult to identify in small biopsy specimens. In large part this reflects shortcoming of the diagnostic biopsy: When dealing with large exophytic masses, a limited biopsy is often too superficial to evaluate the base of the tumor for invasive growth. Some investigators advocate that all papillary SCCs should be regarded as malignant even when invasion cannot be established on histologic grounds.[4]

DIFFERENTIAL DIAGNOSIS OF PAPILLARY SCC

Papillary SCCs are primarily distinguished from benign squamous papillomas on cytologic grounds. In papillary SCCs, the papillary fronds are lined by dyspolarized layers of pleomorphic cells exhibiting overtly malignant cytologic features. Although squamous papillomas frequently demonstrate viral-related cellular atypia and basal cell hyperplasia, the degree of this atypia is not as severe as encountered in papillary SCC. Squamous papillomas are benign proliferations driven by nononcogenic (ie, low-risk) types of human papilloma virus (primarily types 6 and 11), whereas papillary SCCs are malignant neoplasms that, in some instances, are caused by oncogenic types of HPV.[12–14] Type specific HPV in situ hybridization can sometimes inform the differential diagnosis. In effect, the detection of low-risk but not high-risk HPV in a squamous papillary lesion supports the diagnosis of squamous papilloma.

PROGNOSIS OF PAPILLARY SCC

Some studies have suggested that patients with papillary SCCs have a better prognosis than patients with conventional SCCs.[15] This improved prognosis may in part reflect its limited invasiveness. Even for large papillary SCCs, the bulk of tumor growth is outward rather than inwardly invasive.

Key Features
PAPILLARY VARIANT OF SQUAMOUS CELL CARCINOMA

- Frond-like projects of squamous epithelium supported by delicate fibrovascular cores (ie, papillary architecture)

- Cellular pleomorphism, increased mitotic activity, and abnormal maturation (ie, cytologically malignant)

- Frank stromal invasion may be an elusive finding, particularly in superficial biopsies of exuberantly exophytic masses

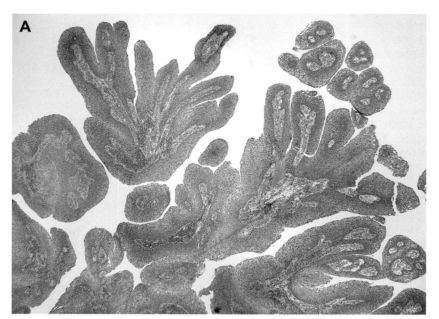

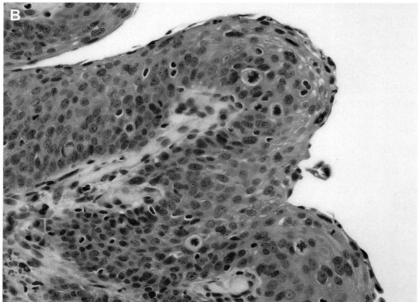

Fig. 6. Papillary variant of squamous cell carcinoma. The defining feature of papillary squamous cell carcinoma is architectural growth characterized by exophytic finger-like projections (*A*). Unlike a benign squamous papilloma, the fibrovascular cores are lined by cytologically malignant cells (*B*).

VERRUCOUS CARCINOMA

OVERVIEW

Verrucous carcinoma is a singular type of well-differentiated squamous cell carcinoma that is set apart on the basis of its warty exophytic appearance, broad pushing pattern of invasion, slow growth, and inability to metastasize.[16] In the oral cavity, chronic smokeless tobacco is the primary etiologic factor.[1,17]

GROSS/CLINICAL FEATURES OF VERRUCOUS CARCINOMA

Verrucous carcinoma grossly appears as a broad-based plaque that is sharply demarcated from the

> ### Key Features
> #### VERRUCOUS CARCINOMA
>
> - Warty corrugated surface comprised of spires of acanthosis with hyperkeratosis
> - Invasive front is broad and pushing rather than irregular and infiltrative
> - Minimal cellular atypia
> - May be locally destructive but harbors no potential for metastatic spread
> - Complete excision is curative

surrounding mucosa. Its surface is irregularly thickened and exhibits grayish white warty projections (**Fig. 7**). In contrast to conventional SCC, surface ulceration is not seen in verrucous carcinoma.

MICROSCOPIC FEATURES OF VERRUCOUS CARCINOMA

Verrucous carcinoma is characterized by marked epithelial thickening. The pattern of this epithelial thickening is distinctive with respect to both its superficial and deep components. The surface of the epithelium is highly corrugated owing to the presence of spires of acanthosis (**Fig. 8**). These spires are separated by crypts packed with keratin, and they are capped by layers of parakeratin. The deeper zone at its interface with

the underlying stroma is broad and club-shaped. Verrucous carcinoma differs from conventional SCC in that it infiltrates the stroma not as irregular nests and cords but as expansive rete pegs with a pushing border (**Fig. 9**). The cellular features of verrucous carcinoma are nonthreatening. The pleomorphism, disorderly maturation, atypical mitoses, and other atypical cytologic features that characterize most forms of malignancy are not well developed in verrucous carcinoma.

Although verrucous carcinoma is usually encountered as a localized lesion arising in men who have chronically used smokeless tobacco, it also occurs in association with a rare intraoral process known as proliferative verrucous leukoplakia—a multifocal squamous proliferation involving the oral cavity of mainly women, characterized by a strong propensity toward recurrence and progression toward invasive SCC.[1,18] The histopathological features vary over time, ranging from simple squamous hyperplasia to verrucous hyperplasia to verrucous carcinoma to papillary SCC to conventional SCC.

DIFFERENTIAL DIAGNOSIS OF VERRUCOUS CARCINOMA

Verrucous carcinoma lacks the cytologic atypia and pattern of irregular infiltration that characterize other forms of SCC. Consequently, verrucous carcinoma can be difficult to recognize as a variant of SCC. The main differential diagnosis is between verrucous carcinoma and verrucous hyperplasia. The distinction rests on the finding of pushing growth beyond the basement membrane and

Fig. 7. Verrucous carcinoma. The surface of the tongue is carpeted by broad-based thickened warty lesion with white keratotic projections.

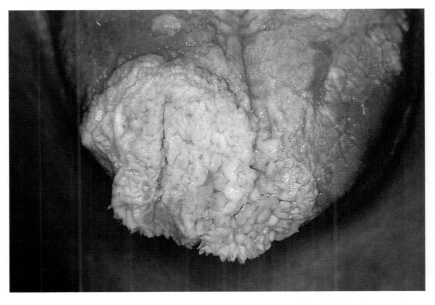

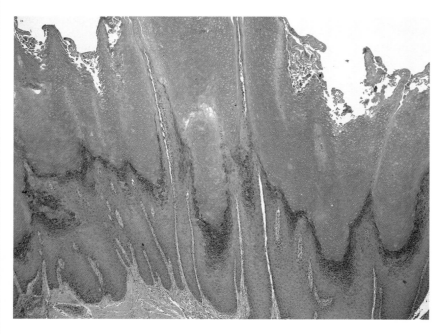

Fig. 8. Verrucous carcinoma. The surface of a verrucous carcinoma is thick and corrugated owing to broad irregular zone of keratin and parakeratin. Its base is broad and pushing. Verrucous carcinoma lacks the overtly malignant cytologic features of conventional squamous cell carcinoma.

into the subepithelial tissues (see **Fig. 9**). Recognition of invasive growth is seldom easy and may not even be possible in superficial biopsies where the base of the lesion is not well represented for histologic evaluation of its relationship to the underlying stroma and adjacent mucosa. Surgeons are encouraged to obtain biopsies that are sufficient in depth to capture the base of the lesion and sufficient in breadth to display the relationship of the verrucous proliferation with an adjacent zone of uninvolved mucosa.

PROGNOSIS OF VERRUCOUS CARCINOMA

Although verrucous carcinomas are invasive neoplasms that can be locally destructive, they have no potential to metastasize.[19,20] Accordingly,

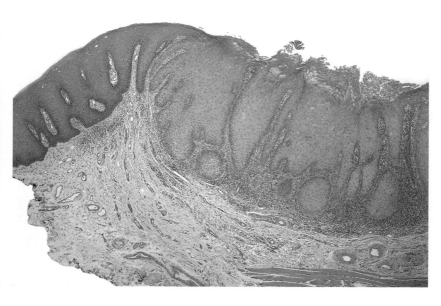

Fig. 9. Verrucous carcinoma. Verrucous carcinoma invades in a burrowing fashion. This downward growth is often best appreciated at the interface of the verrucous carcinoma with the adjacent epithelium.

complete resection is curative, and there is no need for treatment of the neck for regional lymph node metastases. Conventional squamous carcinomas can sometimes arise in association with a verrucous carcinoma. Because the presence of a conventional SCC may alter both prognosis and therapy, complete submission of a verrucous carcinoma for histologic evaluation of an associated conventional component is mandatory. Verrucous carcinomas have a high association with metachronous and synchronous SCCs of the head and neck, such that a diagnosis of verrucous carcinoma necessitates a thorough head and neck evaluation and close patient follow-up.[20,21]

SPINDLE CELL VARIANT OF SQUAMOUS CELL CARCINOMA (SARCOMATOID CARCINOMA)

OVERVIEW

The spindle cell variant of SCC is a biphasic tumor that, in addition to conventional SCC, also harbors a spindle cell element (**Figs. 10** and **11**). Although the spindle cells may take on a highly mesenchymal appearance, they are derived from the surface squamous epithelium.[22,23]

GROSS/CLINICAL FEATURES OF SARCOMATOID CARCINOMA

The spindle cell variant of SCCs classically presents as polypoid mass with an ulcerated surface.[22]

Key Features
SPINDLE CELL VARIANT OF SQUAMOUS CELL CARCINOMA

- A biphasic SCC with dual conventional and spindle cell components
- Typically presents as a polypoid mass with an ulcerated surface
- The conventional component is present as invasive nests of SCC and/or surface dysplasia
- The spindle cell component takes on a mesenchymal appearance and may even exhibit heterologous elements (eg, bone formation)
- Immunohistochemistry may or may not be helpful in confirming the epithelial origin of the malignant spindled cells
- Prognosis is more related to the degree of endophytic growth than the overall size of the polypoid mass

MICROSCOPIC FEATURES OF SARCOMATOID CARCINOMA

The epithelial nature of this variant is best appreciated and most fully expressed in the conventional component represented by nests of infiltrating squamous cell and/or dysplasia of the surface epithelium. The epithelial nature of the spindle cell component is less obvious. The spindled shape of the tumor cells along with their

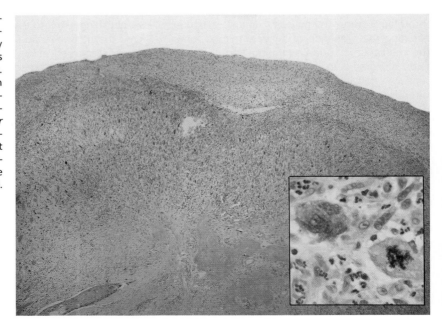

Fig. 10. Spindle cell variant of squamous carcinoma. This variant typically grows as a polypoid mass with an ulcerated surface. Its biphasic nature is seen here as a tongue of invasive conventional squamous carcinoma (*lower left*) and a zone of undifferentiated malignant mesenchymal-like cells (*inset*). Heterologous bone formation is present (*center*).

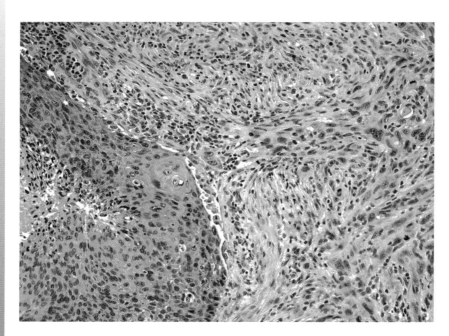

Fig. 11. Spindle cell variant of squamous cell carcinoma. An invasive nest of conventional squamous cell carcinoma is associated with fascicles of malignant spindle cells resembling a sarcoma.

discohesive growth is more reminiscent of a mesenchymal process. The spindle cell proliferation sometimes undergoes heterologous differentiation (eg, bone formation or cartilage formation), further heightening confusion with a true mesenchymal neoplasm (see **Fig. 10**). In most cases, the malignant nature of the spindle cell component is obvious. They are highly pleomorphic with numerous mitotic figures, including the presence of atypical mitotic forms. The cellularity is variable ranging from individual cells dispersed in an edematous stroma to densely cellular proliferations in fascicular formations.

DIFFERENTIAL DIAGNOSIS OF SARCOMATOID CARCINOMA

Distinguishing the spindle cell variant of SCC from a sarcoma largely rests on the demonstration of epithelial differentiation. Any association with a conventional SCC component, either in the form of an invasive SCC or dysplasia of the surface epithelial, is regarded as sufficient confirmation of the epithelial nature of the spindle cell component. The value of this finding, however, is limited in those cases where the conventional component has been completely overrun by the spindled component and the dysplastic surface epithelium

has been totally ulcerated. In these instances, evidence for epithelial differentiation may require an immunohistochemical approach that includes immunostains for a wide spectrum of cytokeratins. Not all spindle cell variants of SCC are cytokeratin positive. For those carcinomas that are not, the strategic use of other immunohistochemical markers, such as p63 and p53, may be useful in establishing a link to their epithelial origin.[23,24]

At the other extreme, the spindle cells may be singly dispersed in an edematous and inflamed background, causing confusion with a florid reactive granulation tissue (**Fig. 12**). Careful inspection of the cellular features is necessary because the spindled cells of SCC exhibit greater degrees of pleomorphism. Although mitotic activity may be elevated in reactive and neoplastic conditions alike, atypical mitoses are more restricted to the spindle cell variant of SCC. The use of immunohistochemical stains for cytokeratin and p63 may sometimes be helpful in establishing a diagnosis, keeping in mind that the absence of staining does not necessarily exclude the diagnosis of sarcomatoid carcinoma.

PROGNOSIS OF SARCOMATOID CARCINOMA

The prognosis of the spindle cell SCC is more directly related to the degree of endophytic growth than it is to overall tumor size.[22] Paradoxically,

Fig. 12. Spindle cell variant of squamous cell carcinoma. The malignant cells are present in a background of ulceration, edema, and inflammation, causing confusion with inflamed granulation tissue.

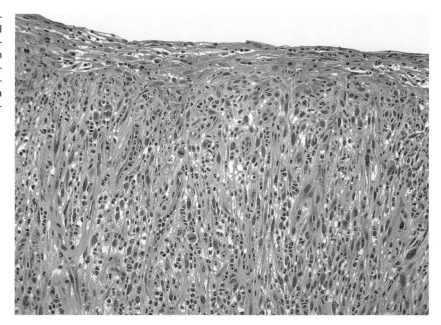

even a large bulky polypoid tumor may have a favorable outcome as long as the invasive portion is shallow.

ACANTHOLYTIC VARIANT OF SCC

OVERVIEW

The acantholytic variant of SCC is marked by dyskeratosis with disruptions of intercellular connections within the nests of invasive SCC, a process

Key Features
ACANTHOLYTIC VARIANT OF SQUAMOUS CELL CARCINOMA

- Acantholysis refers to a pattern of dyskeratosis with dissolution of cellular connections resulting in the formation of pseudoluminal spaces

- Unlike true glandular formations, the pseudolumina contain dyskeratotic cells and cellular debris but not mucin

- The acantholytic component often demonstrates direct transition with conventional SCC and is associated with surface dysplasia

known as acantholysis. The consequent formation of gland-like spaces gives the false impression of a glandular neoplasm (hence, the term, *pseudoglandular SCC*), whereas the formation of anastamosing channel-like spaces gives the erroneous impression of a vascular neoplasm (hence, the term, *angiosarcoma-like SCC*). The acantholytic pattern is set apart as a variant of SCC mostly due to its penchant to morphologically mimic these other neoplasms, but it is similar to conventional SCC in other respects, including prognosis and therapy.

GROSS/CLINICAL FEATURES OF ACANTHOLYTIC VARIANT

Other than its predilection for the vermillion border of the lip,[25] there are no gross features that distinguish acantholytic from conventional SCC.

MICROSCOPIC FEATURES OF ACANTHOLYTIC VARIANT

Like conventional SCC, the acantholytic variant typically is seen as invasive nests of SCC arising from a dysplastic surface epithelium. Discohesion with dropout of dyskeratotic cells from the center of the nests results in the formation of pseudolumina. Careful inspection often reveals the presence of dyskeratotic cells and cellular debris within the center of some of these spaces.

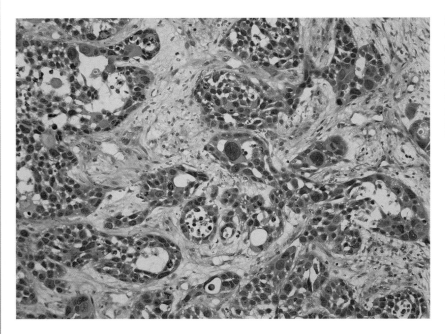

Fig. 13. Acantholytic variant of squamous cell carcinoma, pseudoglandular pattern. Discohesion with dropout of dyskeratotic cells results in the formation of pseudolumina. Cellular debris can be seen within some of the pseudolumina.

DIFFERENTIAL DIAGNOSIS OF ACANTHOLYTIC VARIANT

The presence of gland-like spaces may cause confusion with adenocarcinoma, adenosquamous carcinoma, and mucoepidermoid carcinoma (**Fig. 13**). The use of special stains for mucin production can be useful in confirming the absence of true glandular differentiation. When the pseudolumina form irregular anastamosing channels, acantholysis may be mistaken for a vasoformative process, such as angiosarcoma

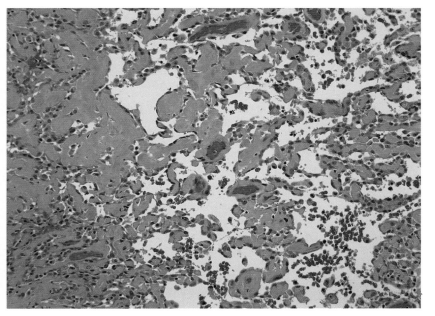

Fig. 14. Acantholytic variant of squamous cell carcinoma, angiosarcoma-like pattern. Acantholysis within the squamous nests results in the formation of irregular and anastamosing channels resembling an angiosarcoma.

(**Fig. 14**). A thorough histologic evaluation usually discloses areas of direct transition with more conventional SCC. If doubts persist, immunohistochemical stains for endothelial markers (eg, CD31 and CD34) can be helpful in confirming the absence of vascular differentiation. As a means of supporting squamous epithelial origin, a p63 stain is more helpful than general cytokeratin stains because epithelioid angiosarcomas are often cytokeratin positive.

BASALOID SQUAMOUS CELL CARCINOMA

OVERVIEW

Basaloid squamous cell carcinoma is a variant of SCC that is set apart by its prominent basaloid morphology and by its aggressive clinical behavior.[1]

Gross/Clinical Features of Basaloid Squamous Cell Carcinoma

Basaloid SCC appears as a firm indurated mass. Relative to the extent of visible surface alterations, the degree of submucosal growth may be disproportionately large prompting clinical consideration of a salivary gland carcinoma or a soft tissue sarcoma. On cut section, basaloid SCCs are typically tan-white, infiltrative, and necrotic.[4]

MICROSCOPIC FEATURES OF BASALOID SQUAMOUS CELL CARCINOMA

Basaloid SCCs take origin from the basilar portion of the surface epithelium, invading and filling the subepithelial tissues as expanding nests and lobules (**Fig. 15**). The presence of cellular

---

Key Features
BASALOID SQUAMOUS
CELL CARCINOMA

- Lobular growth of immature cells with a high nuclear to cytoplasmic ratio

- Aggressive clinical behavior

- The diagnosis requires the presence of a SCC component

  ○ Surface dysplasia

  ○ Invasive SCC

  and/or

  ○ Zones of abrupt keratinization

---

necrosis within the center of the tumor lobules is a common finding. The tumor cells often palisade at the periphery of the lobules. Dense eosinophilic stromal matrix is sometimes deposited between the tumor cells and within duct-like formations. The term, *basaloid*, refers to the immature appearance of the tumor cells. They exhibit a high nuclear to cytoplasmic ratio, lacking the abundant eosinophilic cytoplasm indicating more mature squamous differentiation. Some areas of the tumor must show unambiguous squamous differentiation, although these areas are, by definition, dominated by the basaloid component. This squamous element may take the form of surface dysplasia, an associated conventional invasive SCC, or abrupt zones of keratinization within the basaloid nests (see **Fig. 15**).

DIFFERENTIAL DIAGNOSIS OF BASALOID SQUAMOUS CELL CARCINOMA

Basaloid SCC may exhibit morphologic overlap with other tumors characterized by a prominent basaloid morphology, including the solid variant of adenoid cystic carcinoma, small cell carcinoma, and HPV-associated SCC. Unlike basaloid SCC, the solid variant of adenoid cystic carcinoma is not associated with a squamous component. It can be safely eliminated from the differential diagnosis when surface dysplasia, zones of keratinization, and/or an invasive keratinized SCC are identified. Conversely, the absence of a squamous component and the presence of a classic cribriform growth pattern support the diagnosis of adenoid cystic carcinoma. The distinction of basaloid SCC from small cell carcinoma generally requires the integration of histologic and immunohistochemical findings. Immunohistochemical evidence of neuroendocrine differentiation (eg, positivity for chromogranin, synaptophysin, and CD56) in a high-grade carcinoma characterized by nuclear hyperchromasia, nuclear molding, and extreme mitotic activity supports the diagnosis of small cell carcinoma over basaloid SCC. TTF-1 is variable expressed in small cell carcinomas, but it is not expressed in basaloid SCCs. High molecular weight cytokeratins (eg, CK 5/6 and CK903) are consistently expressed in basaloid SCCs, but they are not expressed in most small cell carcinomas.[26,27]

SCCs caused by HPV consistently demonstrate basaloid features, even to the point where they cannot be distinguished from basaloid SCC on histologic grounds. Morphologic similarities aside, these HPV-related SCCs do not share the same aggressive clinical behavior that characterizes the basaloid SCC.[28] Determination of HPV tumor

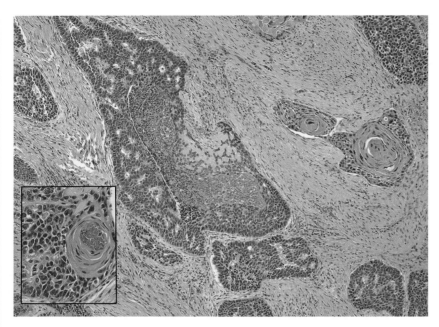

Fig. 15. Basaloid squamous cell carcinoma. The basaloid cells grow in a lobular pattern with central zones of necrosis. The conventional component may take the form of a separate discrete nests of squamous cell carcinoma (*right side*) or as zones of abrupt keratinization within the basaloid nests (*inset*).

status is currently the only reliable means of differentiating a highly aggressive basaloid SCC from a prognostically favorable HPV-related SCC.

PROGNOSIS OF BASALOID SQUAMOUS CELL CARCINOMA

Basaloid SCC is an aggressive tumor that is associated with poor clinical outcomes and increased rates of regional and distant metastases.[29,30] Even when matched stage for stage, some investigators believe that the basaloid SCC behaves more aggressively than conventional SCC.[31–33]

HPV-RELATED SQUAMOUS CELL CARCINOMA

OVERVIEW

Recent work suggests considerable differences between some SCCs of the oral cavity/oropharynx. One particularly relevant subgroup can be defined by the identification of HPV DNA. Although the incidence of tobacco-related SCC of the head and neck has stabilized, the incidence of HPV-related SCC has been increasing by 11% over the past two decades.[34] These HPV-related SCCs are distinct from tobacco-related oral SCCs in several important respects, and their growing dominance is changing the landscape of head and neck oncology and having an impact on pathology practices.

Patients with HPV-related cancer look different from prototypic patients with tobacco-related SCC of the oral cavity. They tend to be white men who are younger, of higher socioeconomic status, and more highly educated.[2,35,36] They are often nonsmokers who do not abuse alcohol.[37] Instead, the rising incidence of HPV-related SCC of the head and neck is being driven by nontraditional behavioral and environmental factors related to high-risk sexual practices. The major risk factors overlap with those associated with

Key Features
HPV-RELATED SQUAMOUS CELL CARCINOMA

- Incidence is increasing in the United States

- Patients tend to be white men in their 40s, 50s, or 60s

- Patients are often nonsmokers and nondrinkers

- Major risk factors include high-risk sexual practices

- Preferential targeting of the oropharynx, in particular the lingual and palatine tonsils

- Associated with improved prognosis

HPV-related SCC of the uterine cervix, including a high total number of lifetime sexual partners, early age of first sexual intercourse, increased oral-vaginal and/or oral-anal contact, and infrequent use of barriers during sexual contact.[38,39] Marijuana has recently been implicated as a cofactor primarily related to its immunosuppressive effects.[40] Cannabinoids bind to receptors expressed on B cells, T cells, natural killer cells, macrophages, and dendritic cells in human tonsillar tissue. Binding, in turn, can suppress immune responses, diminish host responses to viral pathogens, and attenuate antitumor activity.

HPV-related SCC has a strong predilection for the oropharyngeal compartment of the oral cavity, in particular the lingual and palatine tonsils.[41,42] In the United States, 60% to 80% of those SCCs arising in the oropharynx are caused by oncogenic HPV (in particular type 16), but they are less frequently encountered in other anatomic sites of the head and neck, including the oral cavity proper.[41–43] In large part this site specificity reflects the unique microenvironment of the tonsillar tissues. The ultrastructural makeup of the squamous epithelium lining the tonsillar crypts (ie, the reticulated epithelium) may leave this highly specialized epithelium vulnerable to HPV infection.[2]

The unique spectrum of molecular genetic alterations associated with HPV infection is of both biologic and diagnostic relevance. A key step in HPV-related carcinogenesis is the transcription of the viral oncoprotein E7. E7 is known to functionally inactive the retinoblastoma (Rb) gene product, causing a perturbation of other key components of the critical Rb pathway.[44] As an example, functional inactivation of Rb by E7 is known to induce up-regulation of the p16 tumor suppressor gene product, reaching levels that can be readily detected by routine immunohistochemistry. P16 immunohistochemistry is now commonly used as a diagnostic assay to differentiate those oral SCCs that are HPV-related from those that are not.[43,45,46]

GROSS/CLINICAL FEATURES OF HPV-RELATED SQUAMOUS CELL CARCINOMA

Due to the propensity of HPV to target the epithelium lining the deep tonsillar crypts rather than the tonsillar surface, the findings associated with the early stages of tumorigenesis (eg, squamous dysplasia and microinvasion) have eluded visual inspection and clinical characterization. Unlike SCC of the oral cavity proper, HPV-related SCC of the oropharynx is generally not preceded by clinically visible patches of erythroplakia or leukoplakia. Tumor origin from deep within the tonsillar crypts may also explain the phenomenon of

metastatic spread to regional lymph nodes in the absence of a clinically apparent primary. With progressive tumor growth at the primary site, HPV-related SCCs typically are seen as firm bulky masses. The extent of submucosal spread is often disproportionately large relative to the surface component. On cut section, the normal gross architecture of the tonsil is effaced by a tan fleshy mass (Fig. 16). Cystic change is a common finding in those metastatic HPV-related SCCs involving cervical lymph nodes.[47]

MICROSCOPIC APPEARANCE AND DIFFERENTIAL DIAGNOSIS OF HPV-RELATED SQUAMOUS CELL CARCINOMA

HPV-SCC has a characteristic histologic appearance that sets them apart from conventional oral SCCs (Table 1). They typically take origin from the tonsillar crypts of the lingual and palatine tonsils. The surface epithelium does not show progression through the histologic stages of dysplasia that characterizes most conventional oral SCCs. When the surface epithelium is involved, it is usually due to secondary extension from a subjacent crypt. The tumor infiltrates as expansive lobules (Fig. 17). The tumor lobules are often permeated by infiltrating lymphocytes. Overt keratinization is usually absent or only focally present. The cells have a high nuclear to cytoplasmic ratio that imparts a basaloid appearance—a feature commonly taken as evidence to support a poorly differentiated tumor grade. These HPV-related SCCs closely resemble the specialized reticulated from which they are derived and might be more appropriately regarded as highly differentiated SCCs.

A subset of HPV-related SCCs of the oropharynx deviates from this characteristic morphology causing confusion with some other form of head and neck cancer. When the basaloid morphology is highly developed, HPV-related SCC may be histologically indistinguishable from the basaloid squamous variant of SCC (Fig. 18).[28] Some HPV-related SCCs demonstrate lymphoepithelial features, including tumor cells with syncytial cytoplasm, vesicular nuclei, and large central nucleoli dispersed in an inflammatory background as cell clusters or single cells (Fig. 19).[48] When these lymphoepithelial features are highly developed, an HPV-related SCC may be mistaken for an Epstein-Barr virus (EBV)-induced undifferentiated carcinoma of the nasopharynx. HPV-related SCCs can rarely exhibit a papillary pattern of growth.[12] In effect, a subset of papillary SCCs is represented by HPV-related SCC. When encountered as a lymph node metastasis, HPV-related

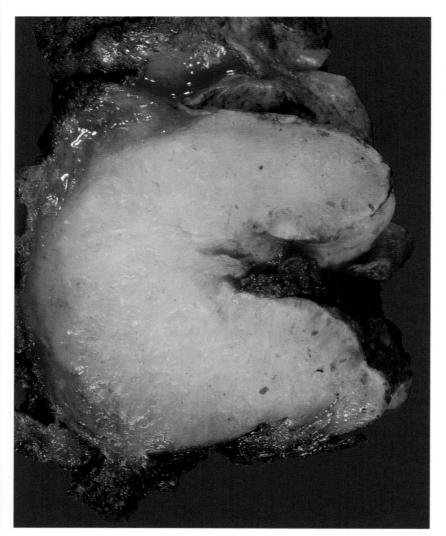

Fig. 16. HPV-related squamous cell carcinoma. On cut section, the normal architecture of the palatine tonsil has been effaced by an endophytic tan fleshy mass.

Table 1
Contrasting histologic features of conventional oral SCC and HPV-related oropharyngeal carcinoma

Histologic Features	Conventional Oral SCC	HPV-Related Oropharyngeal SCC
Origin	Surface epithelium	Reticulated epithelium lining the tonsillar crypts
Dysplasia of surface epithelium	Present	Absent
Architecture	Irregular cords and nests	Expanding lobules
Desmoplasia	Prominent	Often absent
Keratinization	Prominent	Minimal or absent
Differentiation	Moderately differentiated	Basaloid appearance often interpreted as poorly differentiated

Fig. 17. HPV-related squamous cell carcinoma. Lobules of nonkeratinized basaloid cells are surrounded by and permeated by infiltrating lymphocytes.

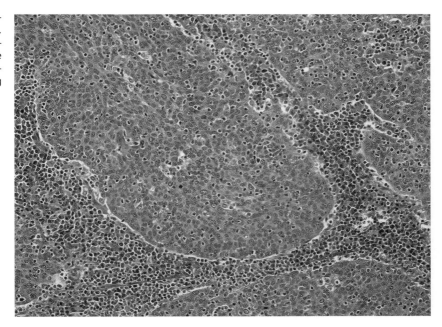

SCC often demonstrates cystic change—a pattern that recapitulates the tonsillar crypt (**Fig. 20**). These cystic metastases are commonly mistaken for branchial cleft cysts. In each of these instances, the differential diagnosis can be informed by HPV status. For basaloid carcinomas, HPV positivity is helpful in distinguishing the less-aggressive HPV-related SCC from the highly aggressive basaloid squamous cell carcinoma (see **Fig. 18**).[28] For lymphoepithelial carcinomas, HPV positivity points to oropharyngeal rather than nasopharyngeal origin (see **Fig. 19**).[48] For squamous-lined cysts of the lateral neck, HPV positivity confirms the metastatic nature of the lesion and points to the oropharynx as the most likely site of tumor origin (see **Fig. 20**).HPV testing has become a useful diagnostic tool in discerning site of tumor origin for those patients with clinically occult primary carcinomas who present with lymph node metastases.[45,49,50]

HPV TESTING OF CLINICAL SAMPLES

There is not yet a standard assay for HPV detection. Current methods included consensus and type-specific polymerase chain reaction (PCR) techniques, real-time PCR assays to quantify viral load, DNA in situ hybridization, and immunohistochemical detection of surrogate biomarkers (eg, p16 protein). Compared with PCR-based methods, in situ hybridization is a more practical tool for diagnostic pathologists.

1. The development of nonfluorescent chromogens now allows visualization of DNA hybridization using conventional light microscope allowing for histologic evaluation of viral distribution in tissue samples (see **Figs. 18–20**).
2. The introduction of various signal amplification steps has significantly improved the sensitivity of this technique, even to the point of viral detection down to one viral copy per cell.
3. Adaptation of in situ hybridization to formalin-fixed and paraffin-embedded tissues has made this technique compatible with standard tissue-processing procedures.

P16 immunohistochemistry is often advocated as a surrogate marker of HPV based on the findings that HPV integration with transcription of viral oncoproteins induces overexpression of p16 (see **Fig. 18**). As a surrogate marker, p16 overexpression is highly sensitive for the presence of HPV but not entirely specific.

PROGNOSIS OF HPV-RELATED SQUAMOUS CELL CARCINOMA

The presence of HPV is of considerable clinical relevance as these HPV-positive SCCs are associated with improved clinical outcomes relative to

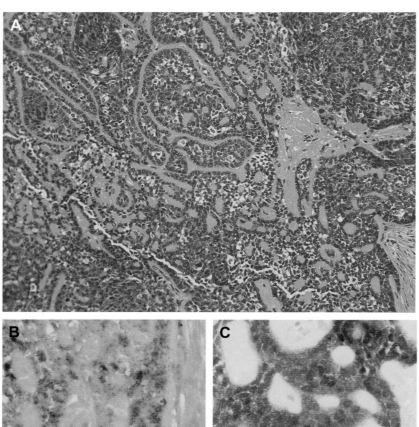

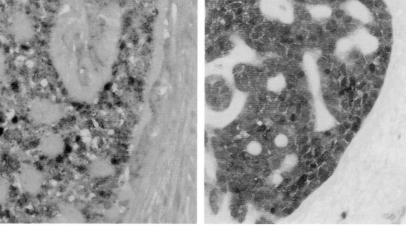

Fig. 18. HPV-related squamous cell carcinoma. This tumor has well-developed basaloid features, including the presence of intercellular stromal hyaline deposition (*A*). In these cases, HPV analysis using in situ hybridization (*B*) and/or p16 immunohistochemistry (*C*) may be the only reliable way to differentiate this HPV-related SCC from the aggressive basaloid variant of SCC.

their HPV-negative counterparts. HPV-positivity correlates with a lower risk of tumor progression and death.[41,51,52] The mechanisms underlying this favorable prognosis may involve the combined effects of immune surveillance to viral-specific tumor antigens, an intact apoptotic response to radiation, and the absence of widespread genetic alterations associated with smoking.[2] In the absence of field cancerization, patients may be less likely to develop second SCCs.

Fig. 19. HPV-related squamous cell carcinoma. (*A*) A germinal center is present on the left and a nest of tumor on the right. The tumor exhibits well-developed lymphoepithelial features, including syncitial cytoplasm, vesicular nuclei, prominent nucleoli, and a background of lymphocytes and plasma cells. (*B*) The detection of HPV-16 by in situ hybridization is helpful in distinguishing this HPV-related SCC from an EBV-related undifferentiated nasopharyngeal carcinoma.

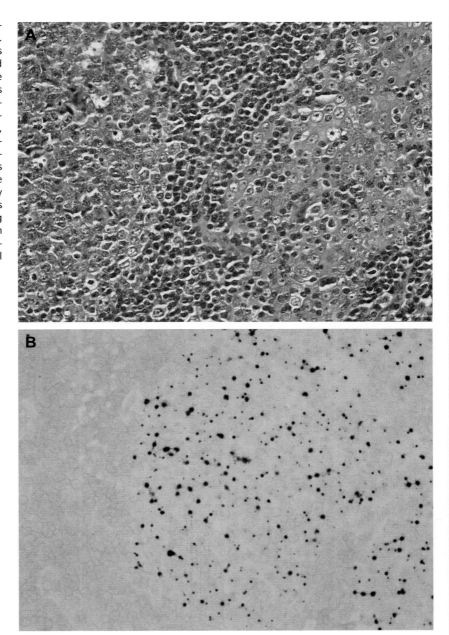

The development of therapeutic vaccine protocols to augment the host immune response to viral antigens holds promise as a strategy to further enhance tumor clearance. Although clinical studies have not yet documented the utility of preventive HPV vaccines, the vaccination of both boys and girls may potentially reduce the rate of HPV-associated oral SCC in future generations.

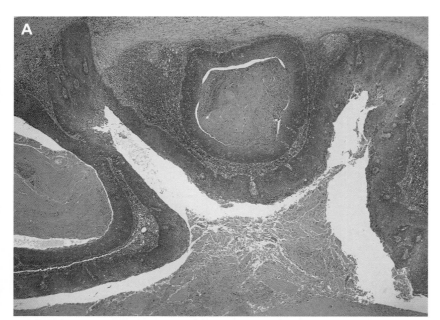

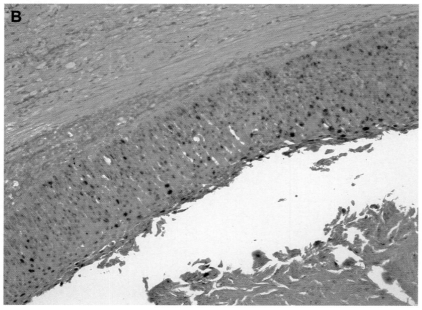

Fig. 20. Metastatic HPV-related squamous cell carcinoma. (*A*) When HPV-related SCCs of the oropharynx metastasize to regional lymph nodes, they often become cystic recapitulating the appearance of tonsillar crypts. (*B*) The presence of HPV in the squamous epithelium lining (high-risk HPV in situ hybridization) points to the oropharynx as the most likely site of tumor origin.

<table>
<tr><td>

Differential Diagnosis
ΔΔ VARIANTS OF SQUAMOUS
CELL CARCINOMA OF THE
ORAL CAVITY AND OROPHARYNX

Papillary variant

- Squamous papilloma with viral-related atypia

Verrucous carcinoma

- Verrucous hyperplasia

Spindle cell variant

- True sarcoma

- Florid granulation tissue

Acantholytic variant

- Gland-forming carcinomas (adenocarcinoma, adenosquamous cell carcinoma, and mucoepidermoid carcinoma)

- Angiosarcoma

Basaloid squamous cell carcinoma

- Solid variant of adenoid cystic carcinoma

- Small cell carcinoma

- HPV-related squamous cell carcinoma

HPV-related squamous cell carcinoma

- Basaloid squamous cell carcinoma

- EBV virus–related undifferentiated nasopharyngeal carcinoma

- Papillary variant of squamous cell carcinoma

- Branchial cleft cyst

</td></tr>
</table>

REFERENCES

1. Slootweg PJ, Eveson JW. Tumours of the oral cavity and oropharynx. In: Barnes L, Eveson JW, Reichart P, et al, editors. World Health Organization classification of tumours: pathology and genetics of head and neck tumours. Lyon (France): IARC Press; 2005. p. 163–208.

2. Pai SI, Westra WH. Molecular pathology of head and neck cancer: Implications for diagnosis, prognosis, and treatment. Annu Rev Pathol 2009;4:49–70.

3. Balaram P, Sridhar H, Rajkumar T, et al. Oral cancer in southern India: uhe influence of smoking, drinking, paan-chewing and oral hygiene. Int J Cancer 2002;98(3):440–5.

4. Wenig BM. Squamous cell carcinoma of the upper aerodigestive tract: precursors and problematic variants. Mod Pathol 2002;15(3):229–54.

5. Carlson DL. Necrotizing sialometaplasia: a practical approach to the diagnosis. Arch Pathol Lab Med 2009;133(5):692–8.

6. Roland NJ, Caslin AW, Nash J, et al. Value of grading squamous cell carcinoma of the head and neck. Head Neck 1992;14(3):224–9.

7. Greer RO. Pathology of malignant and premalignant oral epithelial lesions. Otolaryngol Clin North Am 2006;39(2):249–75, v.

8. Crissman JD, Liu WY, Gluckman JL, et al. Prognostic value of histopathologic parameters in squamous cell carcinoma of the oropharynx. Cancer 1984; 54(12):2995–3001.

9. Kirita T, Okabe S, Izumo T, et al. Risk factors for the postoperative local recurrence of tongue carcinoma. J Oral Maxillofac Surg 1994;52(2):149–54.

10. Califano J, van der Riet P, Westra W, et al. Genetic progression model for head and neck cancer: implications for field cancerization. Cancer Res 1996; 56(11):2488–92.

11. Slaughter DP, Southwick HW, Smejkal W. Field cancerization in oral stratified squamous epithelium; clinical implications of multicentric origin. Cancer 1953;6(5):963–8.

12. Jo VY, Mills SE, Stoler MH, et al. Papillary squamous cell carcinoma of the head and neck: frequent association with human papillomavirus infection and invasive carcinoma. Am J Surg Pathol 2009;33(11):1720–4.

13. Cobo F, Talavera P, Concha A. Review article: relationship of human papillomavirus with papillary squamous cell carcinoma of the upper aerodigestive tract: a review. Int J Surg Pathol 2008;16(2): 127–36.

14. Suarez PA, Adler-Storthz K, Luna MA, et al. Papillary squamous cell carcinomas of the upper aerodigestive tract: a clinicopathologic and molecular study. Head Neck 2000;22(4):360–8.

15. Thompson LD, Wenig BM, Heffner DK, et al. Exophytic and papillary squamous cell carcinomas of the larynx: a clinicopathologic series of 104 cases. Otolaryngol Head Neck Surg 1999;120(5):718–24.

16. Ackerman LV. Verrucous carcinoma of the oral cavity. Surgery 1948;23(4):670–8.

17. Walvekar RR, Chaukar DA, Deshpande MS, et al. Verrucous carcinoma of the oral cavity: a clinical and pathological study of 101 cases. Oral Oncol 2009;45(1):47–51.

18. Hansen LS, Olson JA, Silverman S Jr. Proliferative verrucous leukoplakia. A long-term study of thirty patients. Oral Surg Oral Med Oral Pathol 1985; 60(3):285–98.

19. Batsakis JG, Hybels R, Crissman JD, et al. The pathology of head and neck tumors: verrucous carcinoma, part 15. Head Neck Surg 1982;5(1): 29–38.

20. Medina JE, Dichtel W, Luna MA. Verrucous-squamous carcinomas of the oral cavity. A clinicopathologic

study of 104 cases. Arch Otolaryngol 1984;110(7):
437–40.

21. Slootweg PJ, Muller H. Verrucous hyperplasia or verrucous carcinoma. an analysis of 27 patients.
J Maxillofac Surg 1983;11(1):13–9.

22. Batsakis JG, Suarez P. Sarcomatoid carcinomas of
the upper aerodigestive tracts. Adv Anat Pathol
2000;7(5):282–93.

23. Ansari-Lari MA, Hoque MO, Califano J, et al. Immunohistochemical p53 expression patterns in sarcomatoid carcinomas of the upper respiratory tract.
Am J Surg Pathol 2002;26(8):1024–31.

24. Lewis JS, Ritter JH, El-Mofty S. Alternative epithelial
markers in sarcomatoid carcinomas of the head and
neck, lung, and bladder-p63, MOC-31, and TTF-1.
Mod Pathol 2005;18(11):1471–81.

25. Jones AC, Freedman PD, Kerpel SM. Oral adenoid
squamous cell carcinoma: a report of three cases
and review of the literature. J Oral Maxillofac Surg
1993;51(6):676–81.

26. Serrano MF, El-Mofty SK, Gnepp DR, et al. Utility of
high molecular weight cytokeratins, but not p63, in
the differential diagnosis of neuroendocrine and basaloid carcinomas of the head and neck. Hum Pathol
2008;39(4):591–8.

27. Morice WG, Ferreiro JA. Distinction of basaloid
squamous cell carcinoma from adenoid cystic and
small cell undifferentiated carcinoma by immunohistochemistry. Hum Pathol 1998;29(6):609–12.

28. Begum S, Westra WH. Basaloid squamous cell
carcinoma of the head and neck is a mixed variant
that can be further resolved by HPV status. Am J
Surg Pathol 2008;32(7):1044–50.

29. Wain SL, Kier R, Vollmer RT, et al. Basaloid-squa-
mous carcinoma of the tongue, hypopharynx, and
larynx: report of 10 cases. Hum Pathol 1986;
17(11):1158–66.

30. Raslan WF, Barnes L, Krause JR, et al. Basaloid
squamous cell carcinoma of the head and neck:
a clinicopathologic and flow cytometric study of 10
new cases with review of the english literature. Am
J Otolaryngol 1994;15(3):204–11.

31. Banks ER, Frierson HF Jr, Mills SE, et al. Basaloid
squamous cell carcinoma of the head and neck. A
clinicopathologic and immunohistochemical study
of 40 cases. Am J Surg Pathol 1992;16(10):939–46.

32. Klijanienko J, el-Naggar A, Ponzio-Prion A, et al. Basaloid squamous carcinoma of the head and neck.
immunohistochemical comparison with adenoid
cystic carcinoma and squamous cell carcinoma.
Arch Otolaryngol Head Neck Surg 1993;119(8):
887–90.

33. Winzenburg SM, Niehans GA, George E, et al. Basaloid squamous carcinoma: a clinical comparison of
two histologic types with poorly differentiated squamous cell carcinoma. Otolaryngol Head Neck Surg
1998;119(5):471–5.

34. Ernster JA, Sciotto CG, O'Brien MM, et al. Rising
incidence of oropharyngeal cancer and the role of
oncogenic human papilloma virus. Laryngoscope
2007;117(12):2115–28.

35. Sturgis EM, Cinciripini PM. Trends in head and neck
cancer incidence in relation to smoking prevalence: an emerging epidemic of human papillomavirus-associated cancers? Cancer 2007;
110(7):1429–35.

36. Shiboski CH, Schmidt BL, Jordan RC. Tongue and
tonsil carcinoma: Increasing trends in the U.S. population ages 20–44 years. Cancer 2005;103(9):
1843–9.

37. D'Souza G, Kreimer AR, Viscidi R, et al. Case-control
study of human papillomavirus and oropharyngeal
cancer. N Engl J Med 2007;356(19):1944–56.

38. Smith EM, Ritchie JM, Summersgill KF, et al. Age,
sexual behavior and human papillomavirus infection
in oral cavity and oropharyngeal cancers. Int J
Cancer 2004;108(5):766–72.

39. Heck JE, Berthiller J, Vaccarella S, et al. Sexual
behaviours and the risk of head and neck cancers:
a pooled analysis in the international head and
neck cancer epidemiology (INHANCE) consortium.
Int J Epidemiol 2010;39(1):166–81.

40. Gillison ML, D'Souza G, Westra W, et al. Distinct risk
factor profiles for human papillomavirus type 16-
positive and human papillomavirus type 16-negative
head and neck cancers. J Natl Cancer Inst 2008;
100(6):407–20.

41. Gillison ML, Koch WM, Capone RB, et al. Evidence
for a causal association between human papillomavirus and a subset of head and neck cancers. J Natl
Cancer Inst 2000;92(9):709–20.

42. Begum S, Cao D, Gillison M, et al. Tissue distribution
of human papillomavirus 16 DNA integration in
patients with tonsillar carcinoma. Clin Cancer Res
2005;11(16):5694–9.

43. Singhi AD, Westra WH. Comparison of human
papillomavirus in situ hybridization and p16 immunohistochemistry in the detection of human
papillomavirus-associated head and neck cancer
based on a prospective clinical experience. Cancer
2010;116(9):2166–73.

44. Hafkamp HC, Speel EJ, Haesevoets A, et al.
A subset of head and neck squamous cell carcinomas exhibits integration of HPV 16/18 DNA and
overexpression of p16INK4A and p53 in the
absence of mutations in p53 exons 5–8. Int J Cancer
2003;107(3):394–400.

45. Begum S, Gillison ML, Ansari-Lari MA, et al. Detection of human papillomavirus in cervical lymph nodes: a highly effective strategy for localizing site
of tumor origin. Clin Cancer Res 2003;9(17):
6469–75.

46. Klussmann JP, Gultekin E, Weissenborn SJ, et al.
Expression of p16 protein identifies a distinct entity

of tonsillar carcinomas associated with human papillomavirus. Am J Pathol 2003;162(3):747–53.

47. Goldenberg D, Begum S, Westra WH, et al. Cystic lymph node metastasis in patients with head and neck cancer: an HPV-associated phenomenon. Head Neck 2008;30(7):898–903.

48. Singhi AD, Stelow EB, Mills SE, et al. Lymphoepithelial-like carcinoma of the oropharynx: a morphologic variant of HPV-related head and neck carcinoma. Am J Surg Pathol 2010;34(6):800–5.

49. Cao D, Begum S, Ali SZ, et al. Expression of p16 in benign and malignant cystic squamous lesions of the neck. Hum Pathol 2010;41(4):535–9.

50. Begum S, Gillison ML, Nicol TL, et al. Detection of human papillomavirus-16 in fine-needle aspirates to determine tumor origin in patients with metastatic squamous cell carcinoma of the head and neck. Clin Cancer Res 2007;13(4):1186–91.

51. Ang KK, Harris J, Wheeler R, et al. Human papillomavirus and survival of patients with oropharyngeal cancer. N Engl J Med 2010;363(1):24–35.

52. Fakhry C, Westra WH, Li S, et al. Improved survival of patients with human papillomavirus-positive head and neck squamous cell carcinoma in a prospective clinical trial. J Natl Cancer Inst 2008;100(4):261–9.

COMMON LESIONS OF THE LARYNX AND HYPOPHARYNX

Joaquín J. García, MD[a], Mary S. Richardson, MD[b],*

KEYWORDS

- Laryngeal amyloidosis • Vocal cord polyp • Laryngeal cysts • Laryngeal papilloma
- Epithelial precursor lesions • Squamous cell carcinoma • Spindle cell carcinoma
- Basaloid squamous cell carcinoma • Papillary squamous cell carcinoma
- Neuroendocrine neoplasms

ABSTRACT

B enign and malignant lesions of the larynx and hypopharynx present an interesting and diverse spectrum of diagnostic entities, which may be infrequently encountered in routine surgical pathology practice. This article places emphasis on illustrating the classical pathologic characteristics, differential diagnosis, clinical significance, and presentation of common lesions unique to these sites. The initial diagnosis of these lesions is via small endoscopic biopsy. The nature of the biopsy requires careful assessment because many of the entities share subtle overlapping histologic features. The proper classification of these lesions, however, aids in the choice of appropriate treatment options.

observed in all age groups, and can be related to infection, smoking, or hypothyroidism. Common symptoms include breaking of the voice to hoarseness.

Location of polyps and nodules is usually at the vibratory middle third of the true vocal cord. The abuse of the voice incites injury within the space of Reinke, which may be limited to fluid collection (edematous/myxoid/fibrous nodule), fibrin leakage, and vascular dilation (fibrin, hyaline/vascular polyp).[1] The various histologic types of polyp and nodule are thought to represent a spectrum of tissue response to injury (edematous/myxoid/fibrinous) and/or healing (hyalinized/fibrous/vascular).[2]

LARYNGEAL (VOCAL CORD) NODULE OR POLYP

OVERVIEW

Laryngeal nodules or polyps, commonly referred to as *singer's nodules* or *vocal cord polyps*, are composed of vocal cord mucosa and stroma. Although pathologists may often use the terms nodule and polyp interchangeably in the larynx, clinicians make a distinction. Specifically, vocal cord nodules are usually bilateral, occur in young women, and are related to prolonged vocal cord abuse. Vocal cord polyps, however, are unilateral,

Key Features
VOCAL CORD NODULE/POLYP

- Usually located near vibratory midpoint of true vocal cord
- Classified according to dominant connective tissue component: edematous, myxoid, vascular, hyaline, or mixed type
- Surface epithelium may show extreme reactive changes, such as hyperplasia, metaplasia, or keratinization

[a] Department of Laboratory Medicine and Pathology, Mayo Clinic College of Medicine, 200 First Street Southwest, Rochester, MN 55905, USA
[b] Medical University of South Carolina, 171 Ashley Avenue, MSC 908, Charleston, SC 29425, USA
* Corresponding author.
E-mail address: richardm@musc.edu

Surgical Pathology 4 (2011) 1153–1175
doi:10.1016/j.path.2011.08.014
1875-9181/11/$ – see front matter © 2011 Published by Elsevier Inc.

GROSS

The macroscopic appearance of a vocal cord nodule is a smooth white surface, whereas the polyp is a sessile to pedunculated erythematous nodule. These lesions may be solitary (polyps) or bilateral and on opposing cord surfaces (nodules) of the vocal cord or on the cord adjacent to the ventricle (polyps).

MICROSCOPIC

From a histopathology standpoint, the vocal cord nodule and polyp represent a spectrum of similar findings (**Fig. 1**). The vocal cord nodule is a sube-pithelial collection of edematous and myxoid stroma and may have fibrinoid change. Polyps have been subdivided into four histologic types

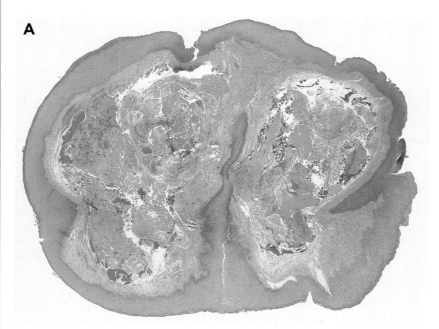

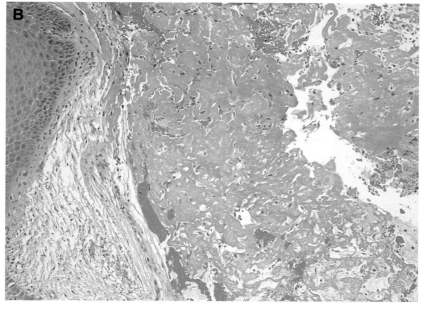

Fig. 1. Vocal cord polyp. (*A*) This polyp is composed of dilated vasculature with fibrin-like material. The fibrinoid material often resembles amyloid deposits. (*B*) However, note the delicate organizing capillaries within the fibrin and a Congo red stain would be negative.

based on the predominant features of the under-lying stroma:

1. Edematous or myxoid, myxoid, or loose stroma
2. Vascular, dilated vessels possibly showing granulation tissue and fibrin deposits
3. Fibrous, dense fibrous stroma with spindle cells
4. Hyalinized, composed of a collection of hyali-nized fibrin-like material adjacent to vessels.

The overlying mucosa may be keratinized, hyperplastic, or metaplastic in nature.

DIFFERENTIAL DIAGNOSIS

The differential diagnosis for vocal cord polyps includes amyloidosis, myxoma, neurofibroma con-tact ulcer, and spindle cell carcinoma (SpCC). The hyalinized or vascular type vocal cord polyp may be confused for amyloidosis; however, the Congo red stain is negative and adjacent tissue is unin-volved. Myxomas are exceedingly rare within the larynx and are an extensive lesion beyond the cord. Neurofibromas may be excluded because these lesions show appropriate S-100 immunore-activity. Contact ulcers are generally located on the vocal process of the arytenoids and composed of ulcerated granulation tissue.[3] Exuberant granu-lation tissue may be present within a vascular vocal cord polyp and the possibility of SpCC may be entertained. Surface dysplasia, marked cytologic atypia, and atypical mitoses, features of SpCC, however, are absent in vocal cord polyps.

PROGNOSIS

Simple excision of the polyp and modification of vocal habits may resolve the lesion and reduce the likelihood of recurrence. If the inciting cause is not altered, these lesions likely recur.

LARYNGEAL AMYLOIDOSIS

OVERVIEW

Amyloidosis refers to tissue accumulations of a heterogeneous family of extracellular insoluble fi-brillary protein. Within the head and neck, the most common sites for amyloid deposition are the larynx and tongue. Amyloid deposition in the tongue is usually associated with systemic AL amyloidosis (plasma cell dyscrasia or multiple myeloma).[4] In contrast, laryngeal amyloidosis is usually primary, the most common localized form of amyloidosis.[5] Laryngeal amyloidosis has been reported to precede systemic amyloidosis by several (8) years.[6] Laryngeal amyloid is a light chain type.

The reported age range is 18 to 65 years, with most series reporting means between 37 and 56 years without gender predilection. Although unusual, there are reported pediatric cases of laryngeal amyloidosis.[7] Laryngeal amyloidosis represents between 0.2% to 1.2% of benign tumors in the larynx.[7] The deposits often impair vocal function, which is commonly manifested as hoarseness, dyspnea, and dysphasia.

△△ Differential Diagnosis
VOCAL CORD NODULE/POLYP

- Amyloidosis—amyloid stains positive for Congo red by birefringence apple green
- Myxoma—exceedingly rare neoplasm within the larynx
- Contact ulcer—usually located on the aryte-noids, ulcerated granulation tissue
- Neurofibroma—S-100 positivity highlights this neoplasm
- SpCC—shows adjacent dysplastic mucosa, marked cytologic atypia, and abnormal mitotic figures

---

Key Features
LARYNGEAL AMYLOIDOSIS

- Lesions often polypoid and multiple
- Subepithelial, acellular, eosinophilic matrix
- Nodules of waxy deposits in a perivascular and periglandular arrangement
- Associated mixed inflammatory infiltrate and giant cell formation
- Congo red stain produces apple-green bire-fringence with polarized light

GROSS

On mucosal inspection, granular, bosselated, or polypoid submucosal nodules are noted. The average size of the deposits in one series was 1.6 cm.[7] The false cords are the most frequent sites affected, followed by the true cords and transglottic area. The deposits may be limited to just the larynx or may be multifocal disease within the upper respiratory tract.

MICROSCOPIC FINDINGS

Amyloid appears microscopically as a subepithelial, extracellular, acellular, homogeneous eosinophilic material in a sheeted or clefted nodular configuration. These extracellular deposits within stroma are readily identified, having a predilection for perivascular and periglandular distribution. A sparse lymphoblastic infiltrate is often identified adjacent to the deposits. Frequently, aggregates of multinucleated giant cells are seen surrounding amyloid deposits; however, the significance of these giant cells is not known.[4] Confirmation that a deposit is amyloid can be accomplished by performing the histochemical Congo red stain (**Fig. 2**). If positive for amyloid, the histochemical Congo red stain displays as apple green birefringence under polarized light.[5]

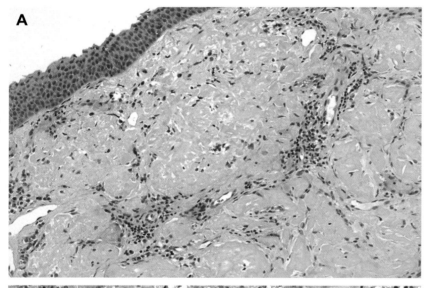

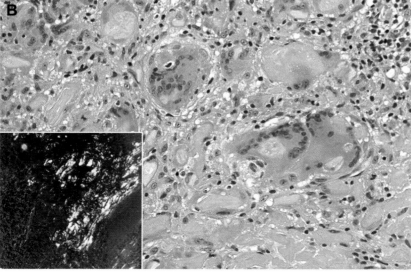

Fig. 2. Laryngeal amyloidosis. (*A*) Submucosal clefted nodules of a waxy eosinophilic matrix with scattered inflammatory cells (hematoxylin-eosin [H&E], original magnification ×10). (*B*) Numerous foreign body giant cells engulfing adjacent amyloid (H&E, original magnification ×40). Congo red stain displays a brick red staining pattern, which on exposure to polarized light, has apple-green birefringence (*inset*).

Differential Diagnosis
SUBEPITHELIAL EOSINOPHILIC
DEPOSITS

- Vocal cord polyp, hyaline vascular-type fibrinoid, and glassy
- Ligneous conjunctivitis—plaque-like deposits of acid mucopolysaccharides
- Lipoid proteinosis—deposits of hyaline lipoproteins, usually involving many sites beyond larynx
- Congo red stain negative in all of the above

DIFFERENTIAL DIAGNOSIS

The most common lesion of the vocal cord that can be confused with amyloid deposition is a vocal cord polyp of the hyaline vascular type. The hyaline is composed of fibrin deposits, which are negative with a Congo red evaluation. Other disorders included in the differential diagnosis have stromal deposits of mucopolysaccharides: ligneous conjunctivitis, a hereditary disease that may present with fibrous plaque deposits in the larynx or trachea, and lipoid proteinosis. The deposits in ligneous conjunctivitis and lipoid proteinosis are negative by Congo red stain.

TREATMENT AND PROGNOSIS

After a complete systemic work-up, conservative surgical excision of the deposits and long-term clinical follow-up is indicated. Conservative excision often helps restores vocal function; however, recurrent respiratory tract disease is not uncommon.

CYSTS

OVERVIEW

Cysts in the larynx are most commonly classified as ductal (75%, due to obstruction of mucous gland ducts) or saccular (25%, due to obstruction of orifice of laryngeal ventricle). Many of the cysts and cystic lesions (saccular cyst vs laryngocele) of this region cannot be separated on histologic criteria alone but additionally require clinical or

Fig. 3. Laryngeal cyst. (*A*) Ductal cyst. The collapse wall of the cyst is lined by an oncocytic epithelium. (*B*) Oncocytic cyst. The lining of this ductal cyst is a single cell thick lining without papillary enfoldings.

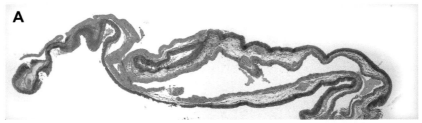

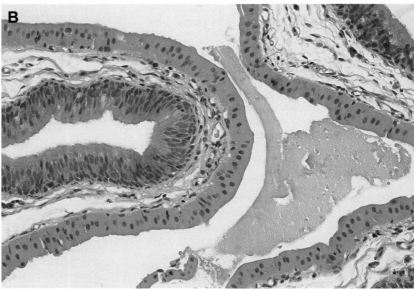

Key Features
LARYNGEAL CYSTS AND CYSTIC LESIONS

- Ductal cyst—small, arise from occluded ducts of seromucous glands, usually <1 cm

- Saccular cyst—mucus-filled cyst in appendix of ventricle range from 1 cm to 7 cm, may be long standing and suggested by a thickened basement membrane

- Oncocytic cyst—occurs in area of false cord and ventricle in patients older than 50 years, unilocular/cyst, lesions with papillary enfolding are designated as papillary cystadenomas, tendency to be multifocal and locally recur

- Laryngocele—distended ventricle filled with air, which communicates with the endolarynx, usually a radiologic diagnosis, may be associated with squamous cell carcinoma

radiologic input for exact location and etiology. These lesions can present at any age, although most occur in individuals after the fifth decade of life. The most common location for cysts is the supraglottis.[8–10]

Symptoms include hoarseness, coughing, sensation of a foreign body in the airway, and pain. Many cysts remain clinically silent and are merely an incidental finding at time of visualization of the endolarynx.

GROSS

Cysts of the larynx are raised submucosal distentions covered by a tense, often thin membrane (**Fig. 3**). Ductal cysts are usually small (<1 cm in diameter) whereas saccular cysts can become large (1–7 cm in diameter). The saccular cyst is a deeper submucosal mass filled with a watery or viscous mucous (see **Fig. 3**). Similarly, the laryngocele, a deep submucosal distention of the ventricle, is caused by entrapped air—this diagnosis is typically made on radiologic imaging.

MICROSCOPIC FINDINGS

Histologically, ductal and saccular cysts are lined by respiratory or squamous epithelium. Both of these cysts may be lined by an oncocytic epithelium, formerly classified as oncocytic cysts. Ductal cysts are commonly found in association with an adjacent seromucous gland. An oncocytic cyst lined by proliferating papillary oncocytic

structures may then be classified as an oncocytic cystadenoma.[9]

PROGNOSIS

Cysts are managed conservatively to avoid laryngeal scarring or stenosis. The cysts may be aspirated, deroofed, or excised. Cysts with oncocytic metaplastic epithelium are often multifocal and can recur becuase other adjacent mucosal glands may exhibit similar metaplastic change. These cysts are also removed by conservative surgical excision.

SQUAMOUS PAPILLOMA

OVERVIEW

The most common benign tumor of the larynx, squamous papilloma (SP), is causally related to the human papillomavirus (HPV). Clinically, SPs can be grouped according to the bimodal distribution of presentation (juvenile vs adult) and number of lesions (solitary or multiple). The juvenile form peaks usually before 5 years of age and is characterized by multiple lesions. The adult form is seen in the third to fifth decades, most often solitary lesions that infrequently recur and are more common in men. Recurrent respiratory papillomatosis (RRP) is the clinical term for the appearance of one or more viral-related (HPV genotypes, usually 6 or 11, rarely 16 or 18) SPs that have a tendency for recurrence and resistance to treatment. RRP can occur in juvenile (juvenile-onset) or

Key Features
SQUAMOUS PAPILLOMA

- Solitary lesion with papillary projections composed of delicate fibrovascular core covered by minimally keratinizing squamous epithelium with normal maturation, usually seen in adults

- Multiple or recurrent SPs are referred to as RRP

- RRP shows prominent basal and parabasal cell hyperplasia with often minimal cytopathic effect of HPV (koilocytosis)

- Detection of HPV DNA for subtype 6 and 11

- Predilection for sites of transition between with squamous and respiratory epithelium (squamociliary junction)

adult (adult-onset) patients. Reported estimated incidence of RRP in the United States is 4.3 per 100,000 children and 1.8 per 100,000 adults.[11,12] Two clinical forms of RRP are recognized based on severity of disease as determined by extent of papillomatosis at specific sites (aggressive vs nonaggressive). Aggressive clinical course is characterized by short durations between numerous recurrences. Aggressive RRP is most often seen within the juvenile-onset population, especially in those patients presenting before 3 years of age and infected with HPV 11.[11] RRP may extend into the trachea and bronchi (approximately 2%–15%); however, further involvement of the pulmonary parenchyma is a potentially ominous finding (15%–5%).[13,14] Malignant transformation of RRP to squamous cell carcinoma (SCC) is rare (1.6%).[11]

GROSS

SPs are exophytic, pedunculated, or broad-based sessile mucosal excrescences. They have white to pink lobulated or bosselated surfaces (**Fig. 4**). They can measure 1 cm or more in diameter but are usually removed as shards of tissue. The tumors are frequently located at natural and iatrogenic junctions of squamous and respiratory epithelium (squamociliary junction).[15]

MICROSCOPIC

The architectural arrangement of a papilloma is composed of a central fibrovascular core, which is surfaced with squamous epithelium (see **Fig. 4**A). The squamous epithelium may exhibit minimal keratinization, mild dysplastic changes, and even viral cytopathic effect (koilocytes). These lesions demonstrate positive staining for HPV by immunoperoxidase (45%) or by in situ hybridization.[11,16] SPs with atypia or mild dysplasia generally correlate with a more active clinical course. These papillomas display marked delay of maturation resulting in hyperplasia of the basal cell layers and persistence of nucleated cells in the superficial layers.[17] In a quiescent phase, the covering epithelium approximates normal squamous maturation. Malignant transformation is an unusual event and when SCC develops in SP it tends to be extremely well differentiated. In the reported cases of SP with malignant transformation where the HPV status was examined, the most frequently associated genotype of HPV is HPV 11.[14]

DIFFERENTIAL DIAGNOSIS

A small and superficial biopsy of a papillary laryngeal lesion within the larynx may pose significant

△△ *Differential Diagnosis*
SQUAMOUS PAPILLOMA

- PSCC core is lined by severely dysplastic epithelium and occurs in older patients.
- Verrucous hyperplasia has extensive spires of keratinizing epithelium, is broad based, and lacks the fibrovascular cores.
- ESCC represents bulbous tumors with thick fibrovascular cores, less than 70% papillary configuration.

diagnostic challenge. The solitary papilloma is lined by an epithelium that shows normal maturation to the surface with minimal keratinization. In contrast, the RRP lesion has a nonkeratinizing surface and a suggestion of koilocytic change. A biopsy specimen demonstrating abundant orthokeratinized debris with minimal surface epithelium is suggestive of a verrucous hyperplasia. If this is accompanied by evidence of a squamous proliferation with a pronounced downward pushing advancing margin, however, then the differential diagnosis has to include verrucous carcinoma (VC) or exophytic SCC (ESCC). The architecture of papillary SCC (PSCC) resembles an SP with the exception of the surface-lining epithelium. The precise distinction between a dysplastic SP and PSCC can be nebulous because dysplastic epithelium covering a fibrovascular core may be found in both. PSCC is most common in older patients with a clinical history of smoking and alcohol abuse and infrequently associated with a prior history of papillomas (7.5%).[18] PSCC is covered by a clearly malignant epithelium, which lacks maturation, nuclear polarity, and increased mitotic activity. Approximately half of the PSCCs that have been stained with p16 immunostaining are positive. ESCC is a bulbous tumor with thick fibrovascular stalks and defined as having less than 70% papillary growth.[18]

TREATMENT AND PROGNOSIS

The clinical course of SP is unpredictable. There is no universally endorsed modality of treatment at this time. Multiple surgical procedures may be required to maintain a patent airway. As of this date, no medical modality has yet cured RRP. Reported rate of progression of SP to RRP is approximately 4% to 14%.

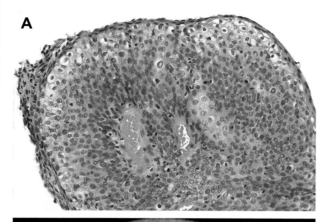

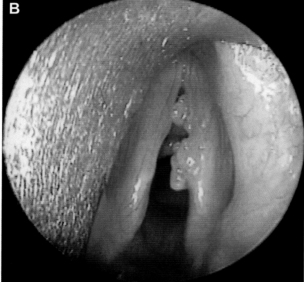

Fig. 4. Laryngeal papilloma. (A) Laryngeal cyst. This laryngeal papilloma shows hyperplasia of the parabasal layers and koilocytic changes within the superficial epithelial layers. These changes are suggestive of active disease phase for this HPV associated lesion. (B) Laryngeal papilloma as seen via the endoscopic view. (C) In situ hybridization is positive (nuclear staining) for HPV 6 and 11 in the superficial epithelial layers.

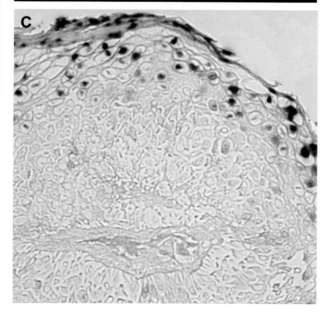

EPITHELIAL PRECURSOR LESIONS

OVERVIEW

Precursor lesions discussed in this article pertain to the larynx, because lesions of the hypopharynx commonly present as an established malignancy. Epithelial precursor lesions (EPLs), as defined by the World Health Organization (WHO), are altered epithelium with an increased likelihood for progression to SCC. EPLs are usually seen in the adult population, more commonly in men and are associated with tobacco smoking and alcohol consumption. Recent evidence suggests gastroesophageal reflux should also be regarded as a risk factor.

Histopathologic assessment of the clinically observed lesion is typically done by small biopsy. The biopsy specimen in itself poses many challenges. Among the most problematic of the challenges is attaining proper orientation for complete viewing of the epithelial-stroma interface. Confounding this challenge is the lack of a universally accepted classification schema, characterized by[19]

1. Agreement on the diagnostic criteria
2. Good intraobserver and interobserver reproducibility
3. Prognostic value.

The WHO[20] has recently adopted a system that includes tenets of three classification schemas for these lesions (**Table 1**). The 2005 WHO classification of dysplasia suggests a three-tiered system that is used for the remainder of this discussion:

mild, moderate, and severe.[20] The prognostic usefulness of the grading system naturally requires concordance between the degree of severity and the clinical risk of malignant transformation.[21–23] Several comparison and reliability studies have been published.[19,24] Lesions classified as basal-parabasal hyperplasia (mild dysplasia) show malignant transformation in approximately 1.1% and atypical hyperplasia (moderate to severe dysplasia) in 9.5%.[24,25] In a recent meta-analysis, the overall malignant transformation rate was 14%, with a mean time to transformation of 5.8 years.[26,27] Clinical management of mild to moderate dysplasia may result in close clinical follow-up whereas severe dysplasia or carcinoma in situ likely elicits therapeutic intervention.[24,27–29] Still, this area remains controversial because precursor lesions may be self-limiting and reversible whereas others may persist.

MACROSCOPIC

There is no characteristic macroscopic appearance of precursor lesions. They have a wide variety of clinical features, including leukoplakia or erythroplakia, exophytic or smooth, and diffuse or circumscribed. Bilateral disease is frequent (60% of cases) and located anywhere along the vocal cord.

MICROSCOPIC

Cellular aberrations in the form of nuclear pleomorphism and variation in nuclear size typify

---

Table 1
Classification schemes that histologically categorize precursor and related lesions (WHO 2005)

2005 WHO Classification	Squamous Intraepithelial Neoplasia	Ljubljana Classification
		Squamous intraepithelial lesions
Squamous cell hyperplasia		Squamous cell (simple)
		Hyperplasia
Mild dysplasia	SIN 1	Basal/parabasal cell
		Hyperplasia[a]
Moderate dysplasia	SIN 2	Atypical hyperplasia[b]
Severe dysplasia	SIN 3[c]	Atypical hyperplasia[b]
Carcinoma in situ	SIN 3[c]	Carcinoma in situ

Abbreviation: SIN, squamous intraepithelial neoplasia.
[a] Basal/parabasal cell hyperplasia may histologically resemble mild dysplasia, but the former is conceptually benign lesion and the latter the lower grade of precursor lesions.
[b] Risky epithelium. The analogy to moderate and severe dysplasia is approximate.
[c] The advocates of SIN combine severe dysplasia and carcinoma in situ.
Data from Gale N, Pilch BZ, Sidransky D, et al. Epithelial precursor lesions. In: Barnes EL, Eveson JW, Reichart P, et al, editors. Pathology and genetics of head and neck tumours. Kleihues P, Sobin LH, series editors. World Health Organization classification of tumours. Lyon (France): IARC Press; 2005. p. 140–3.

WHO Criteria for Diagnosing Dysplasia (2005)[20]

Architectural Disturbances

- Irregular epithelial stratification
- Loss of normal polarity of basal cells
- Increased number of mitoses beyond cells of basal one-third of the epithelium
- Atypical and superficial mitotic figures
- Premature keratosis (dyskeratosis of single cells)
- Formation of teardrop-shaped rete ridges
- Formation of keratin pearls within the rete pegs

Cytology

- Abnormal nuclear size and shape
- Cellular pleomorphism
- Increased nuclear to cytoplasmic ratio
- Atypical mitoses
- Enlarged size and increased number of nucleoli

---

encompass both architectural and cytologic deviations from the normal sequence. The lack of appropriate maturation is usually noted first in the basal and parabasal layers, with loss of nuclear polarity, increased nuclear to cytoplasmic ratio, dyskeratosis, elevated mitotic activity, and atypical mitotic figures. The cytologic and architectural alterations may be confined to the lower one-third of the epithelium (mild dysplasia) or progress to the middle (moderate dysplasia) and/or upper two-thirds (severe dysplasia). The grading of keratinizing dysplasia, as is frequently observed in the larynx, does not necessarily follow the same histologic progression of nonkeratinizing dysplasia (as seen in the uterine cervix) through all thirds of the epithelium. The extent of cytologic and architectural atypia may be confined to the lower third yet qualify as severe dysplasia and, from there, early invasion (**Figs. 6** and **7**).

DIFFERENTIAL DIAGNOSIS

Several benign processes can mimic dysplasia: regeneration, repair, reactive features, and hyperplastic epithelium (eg, presence of fungus, viral infection, ulceration, irradiation, and abscess)

what is seen in cytomorphologic atypia (**Fig. 5**). Dysplasia, however, connotes a marked loss of coordinated growth and maturation of the surface epithelium. Therefore, changes in the epithelium

---

Key Features
DYSPLASIA

- Epithelium confined above the basement membrane, which shows marked architectural disorder of basal to surface maturation and cytologic alteration
- Nuclear size inappropriate by cellular location within the epithelium
- Architectural alterations—irregular maturation, lack of nuclear polarity, dyskeratosis, and increased cellularity
- Cytologic alterations—increased nuclear to cytoplasmic ratio, nuclear hyperchromasia, nuclear pleomorphism, and increased and/or abnormal mitotic figures
- Precursor lesions may be self-limiting and reversible whereas others may persist

---

Differential Diagnosis
DYSPLASIA

- Hyperplasia—thickened epithelium due to increased number of cells >10 cells thick, may be associated with subjacent granular cell tumor
- Regeneration—proliferating epithelium with features of basal and parabasal cells lacking surface maturation
- Repair—epithelial atypia noted immediately adjacent an inflammatory reaction or ulcer
- Reactive changes—downward proliferation of epithelium but lacking branching complexity
- Irradiation changes—enlarged nucleus and cytoplasm, adjacent vessels frequently contain enlarged endothelial cells
- Necrotizing sialometaplasia—adjacent seromucous gland with infarction and retention of lobular architecture
- Intermediate epithelium of a squamociliary junctions
- Papilloma—has fibrovascular fonds covered by maturing squamous epithelium

---

Fig. 5. EPLs. (*A*) The interface between squamociliary junctions often contains a transitional zone with intermediate epithelium (*area subjacent to the arrow*). Intermediate epithelium can be misdiagnosed as dysplasia, however cytologic features of dysplasia: pleomorphic nuclei, atypical mitotic figures, and variable nuclear chromasia are absent. (*B*) Hyperplasia. Often hyperplasia is seen in response to irritants and injury. The maturation of the epithelium is only mildly altered.

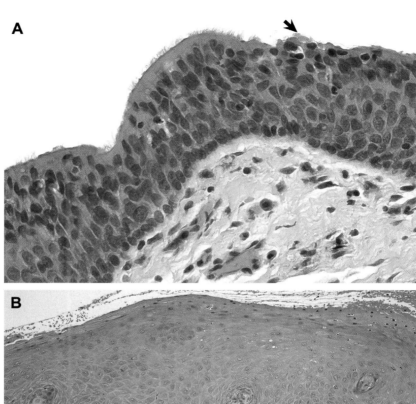

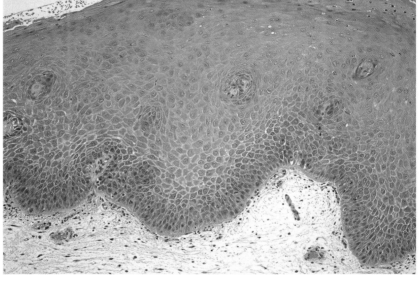

(see **Fig. 5**). Clinical history and additional finding in the adjacent tissue often assist in suggesting the changes are a tissue response to insult and not a premalignant lesion. Finding epithelial stratification with maturation and the absence of abnormal mitotic figures aid in the determining the lesion to be reactive. If, however, there is a marked difference between the clinical impression and biopsy results, then clinicians should be aware that sampling error may necessitate rebiopsy.

The vocal cord lining is consistently exposed to various forms of injury. The intermediate epithelium lines the transitional zone seen at the junction of squamous and respiratory epithelium. This metaplastic transitional zone may be misinterpreted as dysplasia on a small or limited biopsy without awareness of the location of the tissue

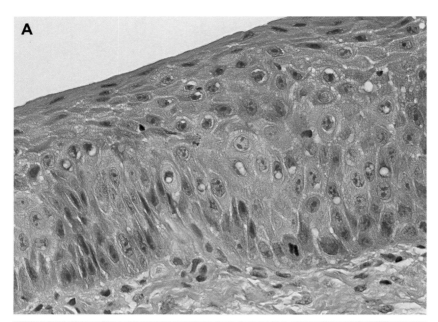

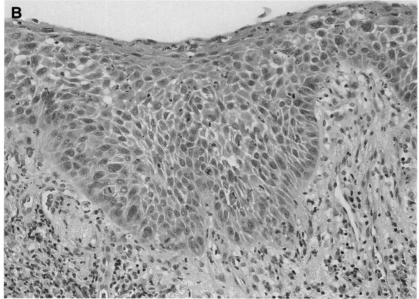

Fig. 6. Dysplasia. (*A*) Mild dysplasia. Note the mild disorder of the basal nuclei, prominent nucleioli, and lack of normal maturation. (*B*) Moderate dysplasia. The abnormalities of loss of nuclear polarity and disordered maturation are easily identified.

sampled. The epithelium shows uniform nuclear chromatin and shape but lacks normal polarity.

PROGNOSIS AND TREATMENT

The clinical management of EPL may include no follow-up, periodic observation, or treatment.[19]

The designation of the severity of the EPL is paramount to the clinical decision-making algorithm. The treatment modality varies greatly because surgical management produces scar and vocal cord morbidity. Additional scarring may compromise subsequent histopathologic evaluation of dysplasia and superficial invasion.

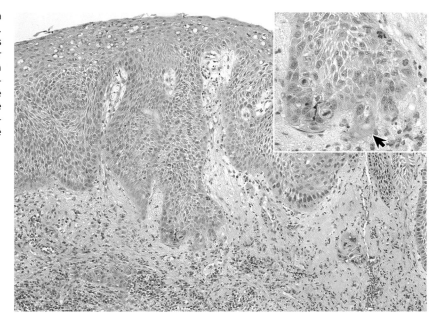

Fig. 7. EPL. Severe dysplasia with focal early invasion. The epithelium shows marked loss of cellular maturation and has begun to have downwards progression of dropping rete ridges. The arrow in the inset shows keratin production in a cell piercing the basement membrane.

SQUAMOUS CELL CARCINOMA

CONVENTIONAL TYPE

Overview

Laryngeal and hypopharyngeal carcinoma, according to the American Cancer Society, represent approximately 1% of all carcinomas. Greater than 95% of the carcinomas originating from these two sites are SCC.[2,30] The most common subsites within the larynx for SCC are the supraglottis and glottis. Within the hypopharynx, the most common subsites of involvement are the pyriform sinus followed by the posterior pharyngeal wall and postcricoid region. The vast majority of SCC at these sites is of the conventional type, although certain histologic variants of SCC have a propensity for occurrence in the larynx and hypopharynx.

The primary site for tumors in these regions carries implications for the natural history of the tumor as well as treatment options. As may be expected, glottis tumors are symptomatic and tend to present at an earlier stage when compared with the supraglottis. The tumor may remain localized because there are few lymphatics and limited mucoserous glands in this region. In contrast, SCC of the supraglottis is often clinically silent and there is an extensive network of lymphatics and mucoserous glands. Thus, glottic tumors tend to have the best survival parameters within the larynx.

Gross

The macroscopic features of SCC are variable. The glottis tumors are generally smaller than the clinically asymptomatic larger supraglottic tumors. The majority of tumors have exophytic architecture and a shaggy white surface.

Microscopic

The initial diagnosis is made on small endoscopy-derived biopsy tissue. Proper orientation for assessment of the epithelial-stromal interface is crucial. Compromised by orientation, biopsy tissue may necessitate deeper sectioning or re-biopsy before rendering a malignant diagnosis.

Early or superficially invasive SCC is defined by dysplastic squamous epithelial cells invading the stroma by disrupting the basement membrane. Foci of invasion may be identified by closely inspecting the epithelial-stroma interface in areas of abrupt or heavy inflammatory stromal response. The inflammatory foci often surround the focus of invasion before a desmoplastic stroma response is elicited by the invading cells. A downward progression of rete pegs composed of markedly atypical epithelial cells, possibly with paradoxic/premature keratinization of advancing cells at the stromal interface, is a useful indicator of imminent or early invasion (see **Fig. 7**). The designation of early invasion is not a universally defined or recognized dimension; therefore, the depth of lamina

Pitfalls

SQUAMOUS CELL CARCINOMA,
CONVENTIONAL TYPE

! Pseudoepitheliomatou hyperplasia can mimic the architectural arrangement of SCC; however, atypical cytologic features are absent.

! The following can mimic SCC and need to be excluded, the presence of deep fungal or tuberuloid infection and granular cell tumor.

propria invasion, as measured from the adjacent basement membrane, is a useful parameter to include in the diagnosis. There is also usefulness in describing the architectural features of advancing tumor margin (pushing vs tentacular strands).[31]

Differential Diagnosis

Before rendering a diagnosis of SCC in the larynx, several common histologic mimics should be excluded. The depth and size of the biopsy should allow for inspection of the stroma to aid in this process. Among those mimics is pseudoepitheliomatous hyperplasia. In pseudoepitheliomatous hyperplasia, the scanning view of the architecture suggests the pattern of the downward growth and fractured epithelial islands with squamous pearl formation, features that are typically worrisome for invasion; however, the features of marked cytologic atypia and atypical mitotic figures are absent. Conditions common to the larynx that are associated with pseudoepitheliomatous hyperplasia include chronic infection with fungus, traumatic injury, irradiation, and granular cell tumor.[30] Additional differential diagnoses are discussed in the article by Bishop and Westra elsewhere in this issue.

BASALOID SQUAMOUS CELL CARCINOMA

Overview

Basaloid SCC (BSCC) represents an infrequently encountered, aggressive, high-grade variant of SCC. BSCC is characterized by frequent nodal and distant metastases. Common sites of occurrence of BSCC are the pyriform sinus, supraglottis, and palatine tonsil. Men are more commonly affected than women, and there is a predilection for the seventh and eighth decades of life. Recent studies have searched to identify HPV in laryngeal cases of BSCC and found the majority of cases to be negative. When BSCC occurs in the oropharynx, cases are likely to be positive for HPV, show immunoreactivity for p16, and display a less-aggressive clinical course.[19,32]

Gross

There is no classical macroscopic feature of this tumor. Not surprisingly, however, the surface mucosa of BSCC may be ulcerated and friable necrotic areas are not uncommon.

Microscopic

Tumor cells can be arranged in a variety of architectural patterns (solid, lobular, cribriform, trabecular, cord-like, and cystic) and show basaloid features with abrupt transition to squamous components. The basaloid population, which should be the more prevalent pattern, is characterized by hyperchromatic, pleomorphic nuclei with high nucleus to cytoplasmic ratios and brisk mitotic activity. Peripheral palisading of nuclei is a common feature. Necrosis may be geographic or comedo-type. A peculiar stromal hyalinosis can be identified within and between islands of tumor cells in a pattern that is reminiscent of salivary gland tumors (adenoid cystic carcinoma) (**Fig. 8**). The squamous component of BSCC can be in the form of dysplasia, including carcinoma in situ, abrupt keratinization, or foci of conventional SCC. BSCC reliably expresses cytokeratins and p63, typically in diffuse and strong staining. BSCC is negative for chromogranin, synaptophysin, glial fibrillary acidic protein, and melanoma markers.

Differential Diagnosis

The growth pattern and basaloid cytology of BSCC place neuroendocrine carcinoma and adenoid cystic carcinoma in the differential diagnosis of BSCC. The immunoprofile for BSCC is negative for neuroendocrine markers. Solid adenoid cystic carcinoma may be more problematic; however, the presence of dysplasia, prominent squamous differentiation, and diffuse p63 immunostaining support the diagnosis of BSCC. Additional discussion of BSCC may be found in the article by Bishop and Westra elsewhere in the issue.

Prognosis

Laryngeal BSCC has an aggressive clinical course, often rapidly fatal even when matched stage for stage with conventional SCC.

PAPILLARY SQUAMOUS CELL CARCINOMA

Overview

PSCC, an uncommon variant of SCC, has a favorable prognosis and thus should be distinguished from conventional SCC.[2,33] This histologic variant most commonly occurs in the larynx and

Fig. 8. BSCC. (*A*) The surface epithelium is markedly dysplastic and from this surface strands of basaloid epithelium invade the stroma. One focus of abrupt keratinization can be identified. (*B*) Hyalinosis. BSCC may have areas of hyalinosis that may mimic adenoid cystic carcinoma. Overlying surface high-grade dysplasia, however, is compatible with BSCC.

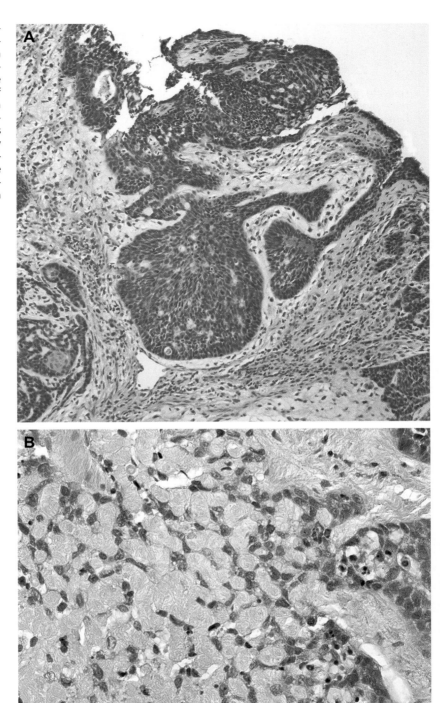

hypopharynx. The supraglottis is where PSCC is most commonly located, followed by glottis and subglottis. The lesion is usually seen in older men. Presenting symptoms include dysphagia and sore throat. The associated risk factors include smoking, alcohol abuse, and possibly HPV. The reporting of the presence of HPV (6, 11, 16, and 18) within this variant has ranged from 0 to 48% with the majority negative for HPV.[18,34] In one report, some laryngeal cases

> ### Key Features
> #### PAPILLARY SQUAMOUS CELL CARCINOMA OF THE LARYNX
>
> - Delicate fibrovascular cores covered by markedly dysplastic immature basaloid epithelium, usually seen in older adult men (sixth decade)
> - The lining epithelium of PSCC may stain positive for p16
> - Epithelium is nonkeratinizing and less commonly minimally keratinizing.
> - Definitive invasion is often difficult to identify.

(50%) of PSCC have been reported to stain with p16.[34] To this end, the precise role of HPV in this variant of SCC within the larynx is unsettled. PSCC originates de novo and only rarely has it been associated with a previous SP (carcinoma ex squamous papilloma).

Gross

The macroscopic appearance of PSCC is a characteristic delicate, often arborizing, papillary growth. The lesions may be polypoid, stalked to broad-based, or a carpet of fronds on the mucosal surface. PSCC is generally 1cm to 1.5 cm in greatest dimension.

Microscopic

The fibrovascular cores are covered by markedly dysplastic immature basaloid epithelium. The surface of the epithelium is usually nonkeratinizing or, at most, minimally keratinized. Microscopic foci of overt invasion may be difficult to identify. Invasion is frequently located in the fibrovascular stalks or near the base to the lesion (**Fig. 9**).

Differential Diagnosis

Within the larynx, two lesions are often confused with PSCC, namely, nonkeratinizing SP of RRP and ESCC. The histologic features of a recurrent respiratory papilloma resemble those of PSCC (ie, basaloid epithelium). In contrast to the SP, however, the degree of pleomorphism along the surface of PSCC is significant (severe dysplasia/carcinoma in situ).

ESCC has a papillary architecture composed of coarse fibrovascular cores covered by keratinizing SCC. The cells of ESCC lack the basaloid morphology of PSCC. Some reports have included cases with both components.[33,35]

> ### Differential Diagnosis
> #### PAPILLARY SQUAMOUS CELL CARCINOMA OF THE LARYNX
>
> - SP—epithelium of an SP shows maturing squamous epithelium with surface changes suggestive of viral cytopathic effect
> - ESCC—coarse fibrovascular cores lined by keratinizing SCC

Some investigators consider PSCC and ESCC members of the same histologic spectrum and point out that there is no clinical importance in their separation.

Prognosis

By report, the prognosis for patients with PSCC has been more favorable than conventional SCC. The favorable prognosis is postulated as related to minimally invasive growth of PSCC. Involvement of regional lymph nodes is uncommon.

SPINDLE CELL CARCINOMA

Overview

SpCC, also referred to as sarcomatoid carcinoma and spindle cell squamous cell carcinoma is defined as a biphasic malignancy composed of conventional SCC (carcinoma in situ/invasive SCC) in conjunction with a spindle cell component. The spindle cells may have a mesenchymal appearance. The larynx is one of the common sites for SpCC to occur, most frequently the true vocal cords and anterior commissure.[36] Men are more commonly affected than women and patients are usually in the sixth to seventh decade of life. Presenting symptoms include hoarseness and the sensation of airway obstruction.[35]

> ### Key Features
> #### SPINDLE CELL CARCINOMA
>
> - Biphasic malignancy composed of conventional SCC (carcinoma in situ/invasive SCC) with a spindle cell component
> - Spindle cells may be negative for cytokeratin but may stain for p63 (approximately 60%) and vimentin.
> - May show divergent differentiation with heterologous elements
> - Biopsy from the base of the polypoid mass frequently yields diagnostic tumor.

Fig. 9. PSCC. (*A*) Delicate fibrovascular cores comprise the exophytic broad-based tumor. (*B*) Markedly dysplastic immature basaloid epithelium lines the cores. Numerous mitotic figures and cellular debris are identified with the epithelium.

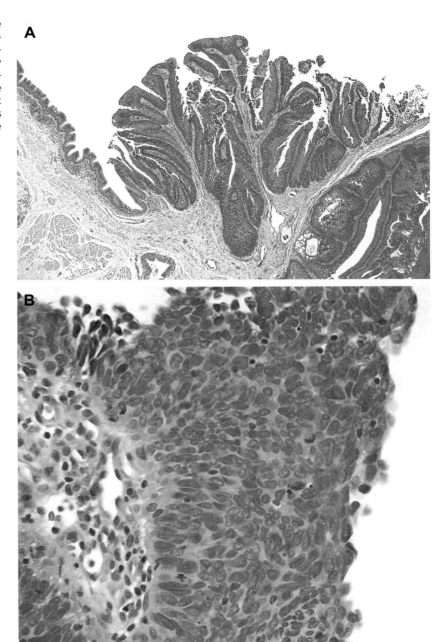

Gross

A polypoid growth of variable size is the classical appearance of SpCC (**Fig. 10**). The surface is often deeply ulcerated and covered by an exudate. The base of the lesion may be broad or pedunculated with a narrow stalk.

Microscopic

Biopsy of the surface overlying SpCC may reveal ulceration or granulation tissue. A biopsy that includes representation of the base of lesion often contains spindle cells emanating from an overlying severely dysplastic surface epithelium

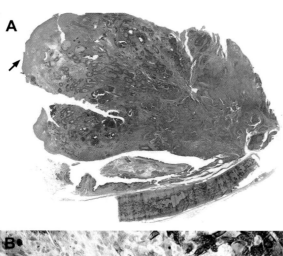

Fig. 10. SpCC. (*A*) The arrow designates the sites of biopsy attempts from a deeply ulcerated mass. Obvious SCC was seen at biopsy from the base. (*B*) Cytokeratin AE1/AE3 was positive in spindle cells, immediately dropping for the surface carcinoma. (*C*) Osteoid formation and other heterologous elements can be seen in SpCC.

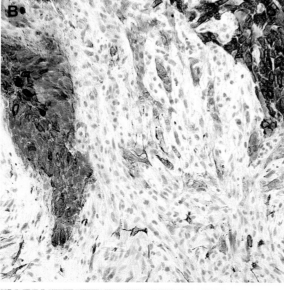

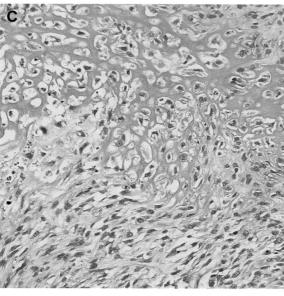

or conventional invasive SCC, enabling the diagnosis to be rendered.

The spindle cells are often cytokeratin negative or have a limited spectrum of cytokeratin staining, necessitating attempts at staining with an array of cytokeratins, vimentin, and p63.[18,36,37] Other heterologous elements, such as osteoid, cartilage, and muscle, have been reported in these tumors.[38]

Differential Diagnosis

Rendering a diagnosis of SpCC requires demonstrating both conventional SCC and malignant spindle cells. Despite negative epithelial markers, a polypoid mass in the hypopharynx or larynx with malignant spindle cells is far more likely to represent SpCC than a sarcoma. SpCC can be confused, however, with nodular fasciitis, low-grade myofibroblastic sarcoma, and myoepithelial carcinoma.

Prognosis

Several tumor features are associated with a favorable prognosis: low tumor stage, polypoid growth, and glottis origin. In one review, the 3-year survival was 90% for a polypoid glottic SpCC and 44% for a sessile glottis growth.[39] The primary mode of therapy is surgery.

VERRUCOUS CARCINOMA

Overview

VC is a recognized morphologic variant of well-differentiated SCC characterized as an exophytic, slowly growing tumor with a broad pushing margin. The larynx is the second most common site for this particular variant of SCC, with almost all reported cases in this region involving the glottis. VC represents approximately 1% to 4% of all laryngeal carcinomas.[40,41] There is a strong association with smoking. Many studies have demonstrated the presence of HPV in VC of the larynx as well as other anatomic sites (ie, oral cavity).[18]

Gross

VC is a broad-based, sharply defined exophytic mass. The surface has a shaggy appearance.

Microscopic

The microscopic hallmark of VC is the broad smooth edge of the advancing tumor front. The subjacent tissue destruction is due to a slow relentless replacement of normal tissue by thick ribbons of squamous epithelium that display minimal to no cytologic atypia (**Fig. 11**). There is marked hyperkeratosis observed in the overlying surface epithelium. The key to diagnosis of this variant is demonstration of the advancing tumor margin at a level below the adjacent uninvolved mucosa. There may be a focus of conventional SCC within a verrucous proliferation and the final diagnosis may change to conventional or hybrid (mixed) SCC after examination of the surgical resection specimen. Approximately 10–20% of tumor thought to be VC harbor foci of conventional SCC.[42]

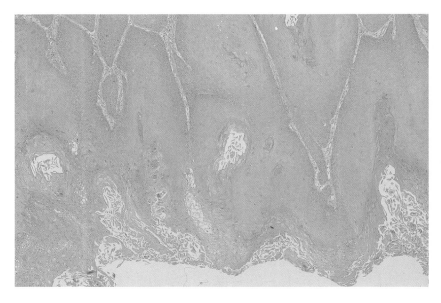

Fig. 11. Verrucous carcinoma. Exophytic and markedly keratinized tumor of well-differentiated squamous cells. The tumor shows a pushing border that is often times met with a prominent chronic inflammatory infiltrate.

Differential Diagnosis

The leading differential diagnosis for VC includes verrucous hyperplasia, verrucous vulgaris, and well-differentiated SCC. Verrucous hyperplasia, which occurs most commonly in the oral cavity and rarely in the larynx, does not show the downward push growth of VC. Verrucous vulgaris in the larynx is rare but, when it occurs, there are many parakeratotic layers, which contain large keratohyaline granules. The border of well-differentiated SCC is usually irregular and does not have a flat or smooth advancing front. More importantly, SCC has cytomorphologic atypia whereas VC does not.

Prognosis

The prognosis for VC is excellent. The slow progressive growth, however, can cause extensive tissue destruction if left untreated, but a pure VC is often considered incapable of metastasis. The reported 5-year survival for laryngeal VC is 85% to 95%.[40]

NEUROENDOCRINE NEOPLASMS OF THE LARYNX

OVERVIEW

Neuroendocrine neoplasms of the larynx represent a diverse group of tumors. They are divided into several types, paralleling pulmonary nomenclature: typical carcinoid (3%), atypical carcinoid (54%), small cell carcinoma (34%), and paraganglioma (9%).[43] The most common site for these tumors in the larynx is the supraglottis, near the aryepiglottic fold, or arytenoids. It is uncommon for these tumors to have an associated paraneoplastic syndrome.

GROSS

Most lesions present as a polypoid hemorrhagic mass and range in size from 0.5 cm to 3.0 cm in greatest dimension.

MICROSCOPIC

These tumors grow as nests, sheets, trabeculae, or a mix of architectural patterns (**Fig. 12**). Small cell carcinoma grows as ribbons and sheets of densely packed cells and almost invariably show necrosis and angiolymphatic and perineural invasion. The small cell carcinoma also rarely may be associated with a squamous or adenocarcinoma. The immunoprofile for this cohort of tumors includes positive staining for cytokeratin, synaptophysin, chromogranin A, neuron-specific enolase, calcitonin, carcinoembryonic antigen, somatostatin, serotonin, and adrenocorticotrophic hormone.

DIFFERENTIAL DIAGNOSIS

The differential diagnosis for these tumors is broad and includes SCC, melanoma, adenoid cystic carcinoma, lymphoma, and medullary carcinoma of the thyroid. A poorly differentiated SCC (BSCC

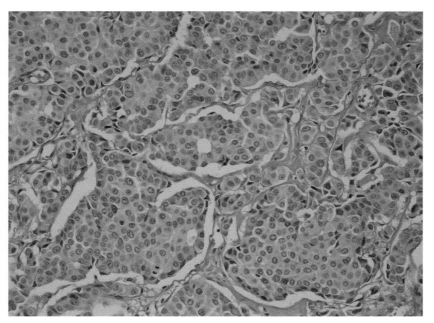

Fig. 12. Neuroendocrine carcinoma. Organoid and nested growth patterns of tumor cells within a rich fibrovascular stroma. Tumor cells have round to oval nuclei and have vesicular to hyperchromatic chromatin. Immunohistochemical stains for Cam5.2 and chromogranin confirm the diagnosis.

in particular) is negative for neuroendocrine markers and diffusely positive for cytokeratin and p63. Melanoma is S-100 and HMB-45 positive and may have a mucosa-associated lesion. Adenoid cystic carcinoma is negative for neuroendocrine markers. Lymphoma is positive lymphoid markers and negative for neuroendocrine markers. Small cell carcinoma of the lung requires additional clinical work-up because the tumor of the larynx may also be thyroid transcription factor-1 positive. Medullary carcinoma of the thyroid can have a similar immunoprofile to primary laryngeal neuroendocrine tumors, including calcitonin positivity, essentially making their distinction impossible in some circumstances.

PROGNOSIS

Laryngeal carcinoid is treated surgically and, importantly, patients have experienced distant metastasis (33%). Atypical carcinoids are aggressive tumors with a 5-year survival rate of less than 50%. Small cell carcinoma is almost invariably lethal, with a 5-year survival of 5%.[43]

REFERENCES

VOCAL CORD POLYPS

1. Werner JA, Schunke M, Rudert H, et al. Description and clinical importance of the lymphatics of the vocal fold. Otolaryngol Head Neck Surg 1990;102:13–9.
2. Barnes L. Diseases of the larynx, hypopharynx, and esophagus. In: Barnes L, editor. Surgical Pathology of the Head and Neck. 3rd edition. New York: Informa Healthcare; 2009. p. 109–200.
3. Devaney K, Rinaldo A, Ferlito A. Vocal process granuloma of the larynx-recognition, differential diagnosis and treatment. Oral Oncol 2005;41(7):666–9.

AMYLOIDOSIS

4. Penner CR, Müller S. Head and neck amyloidosis: a clinicopathologic study of 15 cases. Oral Oncol 2006;42:421–9.
5. Lewis JE, Olsen KD, Kurtin PJ, et al. Laryngeal amyloidosis: a clinicopathologic and immunohistochemical review. Otolaryngol Head Neck Surg 1992; 106(4):372–7.
6. Bartels H, Dikkers FG, van der Wal JE, et al. Laryngeal amyloidosis: localized versus systemic disease and update on diagnosis and therapy. Ann Otol Rhinol Laryngol 2004;113(9):741–8.
7. Thompson LDR, Derringer GA, Wenig BM. Amyloidosis of the larynx: a clinicopathologic study of 11 cases. Mod Pathol 2000;13(5):528–35.

CYSTS AND LARYNGOCELES

8. Celin SE, Johnson J, Curtin H, et al. The association of laryngoceles with squamous cell carcinoma of the larynx. Laryngoscope 1991;101:529–36.
9. Ramesar K, Albizzati C. Laryngeal cysts: a clinical relevance of a modified working classification. J Laryngol Otol 1980;102:923–5.
10. Newman BH, Taxy JB, Laker HI. Laryngeal cysts in adults: a clinicopathologic study of 20 cases. Am J Clin Pathol 1984;81:715–20.

PAPILLOMAS

11. Derkay CS, Wiatrak B. Recurrent respiratory papillomatosis: a review. Laryngoscope 2008;118: 1236–47.
12. Shykhom M, Kuo M, Pearman K. Recurrent respiratory papillomatosis. Clin Otolaryngol Allied Sci 2002;27:237–43.
13. Cook JR, Hill A, Humphrey PA, et al. Squamous cell carcinoma arising in recurrent respiratory papillomatosis with pulmonary involvement: Emerging common pattern of clinical features and human papillomavirus serotype association. Mod Pathol 2000;13:914–8.
14. Wiatrak BJ, Wiatrak DW, Broker TR, et al. Recurrent respiratory papillomatosis; a longitudinal study comparing severity associated with human papilloma viral types 6 and 11 and other risk factors in a large pediatric population. Laryngoscope 2004; 114(Suppl 104):1–22.
15. Kashima H, Mounts P, Leventhal B, et al. Sites of predilection in recurrent respiratory papillomatosis. Ann Otol Rhinol Laryngol 1993;102:580–3.
16. Lack EE, Jenson AB, Smith HG, et al. Immunoperoxidase localization of human papillomavirus in laryngeal papillomas. Intervirology 1980;114: 148–54.
17. Kashima HK, Shah F, Lyles A, et al. A comparison of risk factors in juvenile-onset and adult-onset recurrent papillomatosis. Laryngoscope 1992;102: 9–13.

PAPILLARY SQUAMOUS CELL CARCINOMA

18. Lewis JS. Not your usual cancer case: variants of laryngeal squamous cell carcinoma. Head Neck Pathol 2011;5:23–30.

PRECURSOR LESIONS

19. Fleskens S, Bergshoeff VE, Voogd AC, et al. Interobserver variability of laryngeal mucosal premalignant lesions: a histopathological evaluation. Mod Pathol 2011;24:892–8.

20. Gale N, Pilch BZ, Sidransky D, et al. Epithelial precursor lesions. Kleihues P, Sobin LH, series editors. World Health Organization Classification of Tumours. In: Barnes EL, Eveson JW, Reichart P, et al, editors. Pathology and Genetics of Head and Neck Tumours. Lyon (France): IARC Press; 2005. p. 140–3.

21. Crissman JD, Visscher DW, Sakr W. Premalignant lesions of the upper aerodigestive tract: pathologic classification. J Cell Biochem 1993;(Suppl 17F): 49–56.

22. Crissman JD, Zarbo RJ. Dysplasia, in situ carcinoma, and progression to invasion squamous cell carcinoma of the upper aerodigestive tract. Am J Surg Pathol 1989;13(Suppl 1):5–16.

23. Eversole LR. Dysplasia of the upper aerodigestive tract squamous epithelium. Head Neck Pathol 2009;3:63–8.

24. Gale N, Michaels L, Luzar B, et al. Current review on squamous intraepithelial lesions of the larynx. Histopathology 2009;54:639–56.

25. Hellquist H, Cardesa A, Gale N, et al. Criteria for grading in the Ljubljana classification of epithelial hyperplastic laryngeal lesions. A study by members of the Working Group on Epithelial Hyperplastic Laryngeal Lesions of the European Society of Pathology. Histopathology 1999;34:226–33.

26. Spielman PM, Palmer T, McClymont L. 15-years of laryngeal and oral dysplasias and progression to invasive carcinoma. Eur Arch Otorhinolaryngol 2010;267:423–7.

27. Weller M, Nankivell PC, McConkey C, et al. The risk and interval to malignancy of patients with laryngeal dysplasia; a systemic review of case series and meta-analysis. Clin Otolaryngol 2010;35:364–72.

28. Mehanna H, Paleri V, Robson A, et al. Consensus statement by otorhinolaryngologists and pathologists on the diagnosis and management of laryngeal dysplasia. Clin Otolaryngol 2010;35:170–6.

29. F leskens SA, van der Laak JA, Slootweg PJ, et al. Management of laryngeal premalignant lesions in the Netherlands. Laryngoscope 2010; 120:1326–35.

SQUAMOUS CELL CARCINOMA

30. Cardesa A, Gale N, Nadal A Zidar N. Squamous cell carcinoma. Kleihues P, Sobin LH, series editors. World Health Organization Classification of Tumours. In: Barnes EL, Eveson JW, Reichart P, et al, editors. Pathology and Genetics of Head and Neck Tumours. Lyon (France): IARC Press; 2005. p. 118–21.

31. Bryne M, Jenssen N, Boysen M. Histologic grading in the deep invasive front of T1and T2 glottic squamous cell carcinoma has high prognostic value. Virchows Arch 1995;427:277–81.

BASALOID SQUAMOUS CELL CARCINOMA

32. Chernock RD, Lewis JS, Zhang Q. Human papillomavirus-positive basaloid squamous cell carcinomas of the upper aerodigestive tract: a distinct clinicopathologic and molecular subtype of basaloid squamous cell carcinoma. Hum Pathol 2010;41(7):1016–23.

PAPILLARY SQUAMOUS CELL CARCINOMA

33. Cardesa A, Zidar N, Nadal A, et al. Papillary squamous cell carcinoma. Kleihues P, Sobin LH, series editors. World Health Organization Classification of Tumours. In: Barnes EL, Eveson JW, Reichart P, et al, editors. Pathology and Genetics of Head and Neck Tumours. Lyon (France): IARC Press; 2005. p. 126.

34. Jo VY, Mills SE, Stoler MH, et al. Papillary squamous cell carcinoma of the head and neck: frequent association with human papillomavirus infection and invasive carcinoma. Am J Surg Pathol 2009;33(11): 1720–4.

35. Thompson LD, Wenig BM, Heffner DK, et al. Exophytic and papillary squamous cell carcinomas of the larynx: a clinicopathologic series of 104 cases. Otolaryngol Head Neck Surg 1999;120: 718–24.

SPINDLE CELL CARCINOMA

36. Thompson LD, Wieneke JA, Miettinen M, et al. Spindle cell (sarcomatoid) carcinomas of the larynx: a clinicopathologic study of 187 cases. Am J Surg Pathol 2002;26:153–70.

37. Lewis JS, Ritter JH, El-Mofty S. Alternative epithelial markers in sarcomatoid carcinoma of the head and neck, lung and bladder-p63, MOC-31 and TTF-1. Mod Pathol 2005;18:1471–81.

38. Lewis JE, Olsen KD, Sebo TJ. Spindle cell carcinoma of the larynx: review of 26 cases including DNA content and immunohistochemistry. Hum Pathol 1997;28:664–73.

39. Lambert PR, Ward PH, Berei G. Pseudosarcoma of the larynx. A comprehensive analysis. Arch Otolaryngol 1980;106:700–8.

VERRUCOUS CARCINOMA

40. Cardesa A, Zidar N. Verrucous carcinoma. Kleihues P, Sobin LH, series editors. World Health Organization Classification of Tumours. In: Barnes EL, Eveson JW, Reichart P, et al, editors. Pathology and Genetics of Head and Neck Tumours. Lyon (France): IARC Press; 2005. p. 122–3.

41. Koch BB, Trask DK, Hoffman HT, et al. National survey of head and neck verrucous carcinoma: patterns of presentation, care, and outcome. Cancer 2001;92(1):110–20.

42. Orvidas LJ, Olsen KD, Lewis JE, et al. Verrucous carcinoma of the larynx: a review of 53 patients. Head Neck 1998;20(3):197–203.

NEUROENDOCRINE TUMORS

43. Cardesa A, Zidar N. Verrucous carcinoma. In: Barnes EL, Eveson JW, Reichart P, et al, editors. Pathology and genetics of head and neck tumours. Kleihues P, Sobin LH, series editors. World Health Organization Classification of Tumours. Lyons (France): IARC Press; 2005. p.122–3.

COMMON MALIGNANT SALIVARY GLAND EPITHELIAL TUMORS

Raja R. Seethala, MD[a],*, E. Leon Barnes, MD[b]

KEYWORDS

- Salivary gland • Malignant • Mucoepidermoid carcinoma • Adenoid cystic carcinoma
- Adenocarcinoma • Salivary duct carcinoma

ABSTRACT

Malignant salivary gland epithelial tumors are histologically diverse with at least 24 recognized distinct entities. In general, malignant tumors account for 15% to 30% of parotid tumors, 40% to 45% of submandibular tumors, 70% to 90% of sublingual tumors, and 50% of minor salivary tumors. Common malignancies include mucoepidermoid carcinoma, adenoid cystic carcinoma, acinic cell carcinoma, salivary duct carcinoma, carcinoma ex pleomorphic adenoma, polymorphous low-grade adenocarcinoma, and myoepithelial carcinoma. Each tumor type has its own unique histologic variants and prognostic pathologic features, and only mucoepidermoid carcinomas have a formalized grading system. The molecular pathogenesis of certain tumors, such as mucoepidermoid carcinoma and adenoid cystic carcinoma, has recently begun to be elucidated.

OVERVIEW

Salivary tumors are uncommon, accounting for 2.0% to 6.5% of all neoplasms of the head and neck with a worldwide incidence of about 0.4 to 6.5 cases per 100,000 population.[1] According to Ellis and Auclair,[2] approximately 60% to 80% of all primary epithelial neoplasms occur in the parotid gland, 5% to 10% in the submandibular gland, less than 1% in the sublingual gland, and 10% to 25% in the minor glands. Depending on the series, 50% to 80% of all salivary neoplasms are benign and 20% to 50% are malignant. The probability of malignancy is inversely proportional to the volume of salivary tissue. In general, malignant tumors account for 15% to 30% of parotid tumors, 40% to 45% of submandibular tumors, 70% to 90% of sublingual tumors, and 50% of minor salivary tumors.[2] A comprehensive review of all tumors is not possible but can be found in other sources.[1–4] The World Health Organization currently recognizes 13 benign and 24 malignant primary epithelial neoplasms of salivary origin.[1] The focus of this article is on the more commonly encountered malignant epithelial neoplasms (**Box 1**).

MUCOEPIDERMOID CARCINOMA

OVERVIEW

Mucoepidermoid carcinoma (MEC) is the most common salivary gland malignancy overall in adults and children, with a peak incidence in the fifth decade. As with most salivary gland tumors, there is a slight female predilection with a male: female ratio of approximately 1.5:1.0 in most series.[2,5]

It is primarily a tumor of the major salivary glands (50% to 60%), and most frequently involves the parotid gland. Of the minor salivary gland sites, the palate is by far the most common (20% to 25% of MEC overall). Of note, palate tumors tend to occur in a slightly younger age group, whereas other minor salivary sites are rarely seen

[a] Department of Pathology, University of Pittsburgh Medical Center, A614.X PUH, 200 Lothrop Street, Pittsburgh, PA 15213, USA
[b] Department of Pathology, University of Pittsburgh Medical Center, A608 PUH, 200 Lothrop Street, Pittsburgh, PA 15213, USA
* Corresponding author.
E-mail address: seethalarr@upmc.edu

doi:10.1016/j.path.2011.07.005

surgpath.theclinics.com

in patients younger than 30 years. Rare case of intraosseous or "central" mucoepidermoid carcinomas have been described and comprise only 1% to 2% of most cohorts.[2,5,6]

MEC typically presents as a well-circumscribed, painless mass that is present on average for 1.5 years in the Armed Forces Institute of Pathology (AFIP) database.[2,7,8] Longer durations of up to 20 years have been reported, suggesting that many of these tumors are quite slow growing. Pain and facial nerve paralysis can be associated with high-grade lesions, but is reported in only about 8% of all MEC.[2] Occasionally, cystic tumors may rupture, resulting in an inflammatory response that presents with pain. Superficial palate lesions may ulcerate.

MEC is also the most common salivary gland tumor seen in the postirradiation setting, both in the pediatric and adult populations comprising

almost half of postirradiation salivary gland tumors. MEC typically arises 1 to 2 decades after irradiation.[9,10] MECs are rarely multifocal or bilateral, but they have been described in association with other tumors such as pleomorphic adenoma, Warthin tumor, and oncocytoma.[11,12] The relationship between MEC and these other entities, however, is controversial.

GROSS FEATURES

The gross manifestations of MEC depend to some extent on histologic grade: low-grade MEC is often grossly cystic and well demarcated. Papillary excrescences may be noted. Intermediate-grade MEC tends to have more of a solid tan appearance, although these are still well demarcated. High-grade MEC, however, may be an infiltrative tan-white with some degree of surrounding fibrosis.[2,5] Oncocytic MEC may mimic the gross appearance of an oncocytoma or a Warthin tumor with a deeper brown cut surface.[13] Cyst contents in MECs are typically viscous and mucoid with varying degrees of hemorrhage. Subcentimeter tumors are fairly common in the minor oral salivary glands, although overall, tumors are typically 3 to 4 cm.

MICROSCOPIC FEATURES

MECs are thought to recapitulate the cell types seen in large excretory ducts, and are composed of 3 basic cell types: intermediate cells, epidermoid cells, and mucous cells (**Fig. 1**). Additionally, columnar cells comprise a minor subpopulation of tumor cells. Intermediate cells represent the most primitive phenotype: these cells have small, round dark nuclei with inconspicuous nuclei surrounded by scant pale to clear cytoplasm.[2,5] These are presumed by many to represent the "basal" cell type, which differentiates toward the other cell types.[14] Intermediate cells are often arranged in solid nests, although other elements may be interspersed. Mucous cells represent ductoacinar differentiation in MEC. They range from ovoid to columnar and characteristically line cystic spaces, although are occasionally seen singly. Epidermoid cells on the other hand represent squamous differentiation in MEC. These cells are larger and more polygonal than intermediate cells and have more densely eosinophilic cytoplasm. Well-developed squamous features, such as keratinization and prominent intercellular bridges, are highly uncommon.[6]

Columnar cells are also a form of ductal differentiation and are found only lining cysts or luminae. These are typically interspersed between mucous cells and have eosinophilic cytoplasm. In addition

Fig. 1. Cell types in MEC. MEC consist of a mixture of mucous cells (*short broad arrow, top right*), epidermoid cells (*medium arrow, bottom left*), and intermediate cells (*double long slender arrows*) (hematoxylin-eosin [H&E], original magnification ×100). Clear-cell change is fairly common.

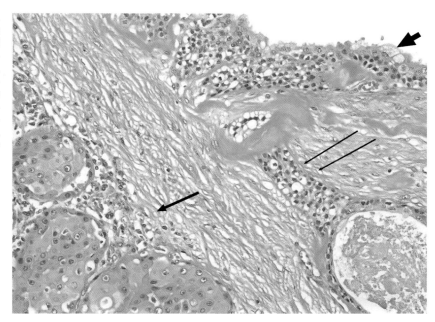

to these basic cell types, there are some fairly common modifications that can affect any cell type, namely clear-cell change and oncocytic change, leading to the designation of clear-cell MEC or oncocytic MEC variants when prominent.[13]

The stroma surrounding tumor nests is often sclerotic with varying levels of lymphoplasmacytic inflammation. Tumors with heavy sclerosis are often labeled as "sclerosing MEC."[15] Some MECs may show a prominent lymphoid stroma with germinal centers resembling that seen in Warthin tumor.

These cytoarchitectural features, along with other features of oncologic potential, such as perineural invasion, angiolymphatic invasion, tumor border, necrosis, anaplasia, and mitotic activity, are integrated into a variety of commonly used grading schemes (**Table 1**).[16] Although the specific grade of a tumor varies depending on grading system used, in general, cystic, well-demarcated tumors with a prominent mucous cell component are low grade (**Fig. 2**); solid, intermediate-cell predominant tumors are intermediate grade (**Fig. 3**); and infiltrative, anaplastic tumors with a prominent epidermoid component are high grade (**Fig. 4**).

Immunohistochemically, mucous and columnar cells show a ductal staining pattern and are positive for low molecular weight cytokeratins (CK7, CK 18, CK 19) and negative for p63, whereas the epidermoid and intermediate cells are typically positive for high molecular weight cytokeratins

(ie, CK 5/6) and p63.[2,5,13] Regarding mucin (MUC) proteins, the membrane-bound MUC1 and MUC4 are expressed in all cell types in MEC, although MUC1 increases with higher-grade tumors, whereas MUC4 decreases with higher-grade tumors. Secretory MUC proteins, such as MUC 2, 5AC, 5B, 6, and 7, are variably expressed and tend to favor mucous and intermediate cells.[17]

DIFFERENTIAL DIAGNOSIS

Classic low-grade and intermediate-grade MECs are diagnostically straightforward. However, high-grade MEC and tumors with variant morphologies may be diagnostically challenging. The main diagnostic challenges for high-grade MEC include adenosquamous carcinoma (primary or intra/peri-glandular lymph node metastases), and salivary duct carcinoma with mucin production. In the oral cavity, the overlying mucosa should be examined thoroughly to exclude the presence of a mucosal dysplasia or carcinoma in situ, which would point to a diagnosis of adenosquamous carcinoma. In the parotid, if a prior history of a cutaneous or mucosal carcinoma exists, this should be compared with the parotid lesion because it would likely represent a metastasis.[6] Adenosquamous carcinomas tend to be more pleomorphic, infiltrative, mitotically active, and heavily keratinizing (**Fig. 5**). They lack a monomorphic intermediate

Table 1
Common grading schemes in MEC

Modified Healey[22]	AFIP[21]	Brandwein[23]
Qualitative	*Point Based*	*Point Based*
Low Grade • Macrocysts, microcysts, transition with excretory ducts • Differentiated mucin-producing epidermoid cells, often in a 1:1 ratio; minimal to moderate intermediate cell population • Daughter cyst proliferation from large cysts • Minimal to absent pleomorphism, rare mitoses • Broad-front, often circumscribed invasion • Pools of extravasated mucin with stromal reaction	• Intracystic component <20% = 2 pts • Neural invasion present = 2 pts • Necrosis present = 3 pts	• Intracystic component <25% = 2 pts • Tumor invades in small nests and islands = 2 pts • Pronounced nuclear atypia = 2 pts
Intermediate Grade • No macrocysts, few microcysts, solid nests of cells • Large duct not conspicuous • Slight to moderate pleomorphism, few mitoses, prominent nuclei and nucleoli • Invasive quality, usually well defined and uncircumscribed • Chronic inflammation at periphery, fibrosis separates nests of cells and groups of nests	• Mitosis (4 or more per 10 HPF) = 3 pts • Anaplasia = 4 pts	• Lymphatic and/or vascular invasion = 3 pts • Bony invasion = 3 pts • >4 mitoses per 10 HPF = 3 pts
High Grade • No macrocysts, predominantly solid but may be nearly all glandular • Cell constituents range from poorly differentiated to recognizable epidermoid and intermediate to ductal-type adenocarcinoma • Considerable pleomorphism, easily found mitoses • Unquestionable soft tissue, perineural and intravascular invasion • Chronic inflammation less prominent, desmoplasia of stroma may outline invasive clusters		• Perineural spread = 3 pts • Necrosis = 3 pts
	Low Grade = 0–4 pts *Intermediate Grade = 5–6 pts* *High Grade = 7–14 pts*	*Low Grade = 0 pts* *Intermediate Grade = 2–3 pts* *High Grade = 4 or more pts*

Abbreviations: AFIP, Armed Forced Institute of Pathology; HPF, high-power field; pts, points.

Fig. 2. Low-grade MEC. This tumor is almost entirely cystic or even unicystic (H&E, original magnification ×40). Inset (H&E, original magnification ×100): Mucous cells predominate with underlying tufts of compressed intermediate cells.

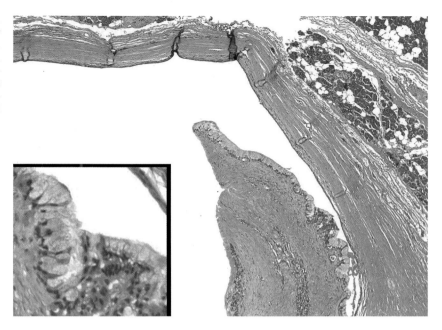

cell population. Adenosquamous carcinomas can have mucinous differentiation, but unlike high-grade MECs, adenosquamous carcinoma may have discrete gland formation, often at the base of a lesion. With modern criteria and immunohistochemistry, MEC is fairly easily distinguished from even a solid salivary duct carcinoma. Salivary duct carcinomas have a ductal and apocrine phenotype and are almost definitionally androgen receptor and gross cystic disease fluid protein 15 (GCDFP-15) positive.[18] Although CK 5/6 may be positive, p63 is not. Furthermore, these tumors tend to be far more pleomorphic and mitotically active with prominent comedonecrosis, a feature rarely seen in MEC. Oncocytic MEC may mimic oncocytoma, oncocytic cystadenoma, and Warthin

Fig. 3. Intermediate-grade MEC. This tumor is more solid with scattered microcysts only (H&E, original magnification ×40). Inset (H&E, original magnification ×200): Although the bulk of the tumor consists of intermediate cells, cysts are still lined by mucocytes.

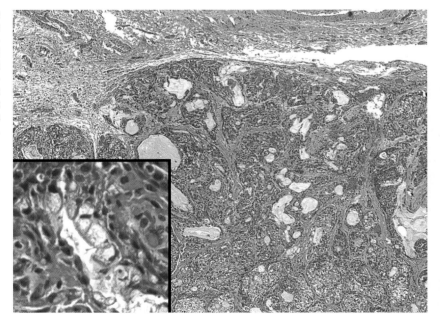

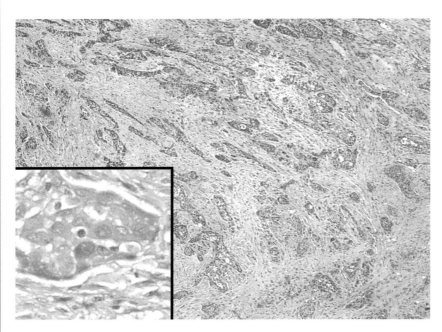

Fig. 4. High-grade MEC. This tumor is fairly infiltrative with epidermoid and intermediate cell predominance (H&E, original magnification ×40). Inset (mucicarmine, original magnification ×200): A mucicarmine stain is required to highlight the scattered mucous cells.

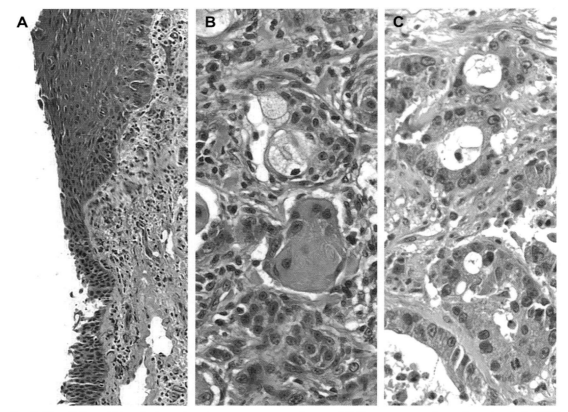

Fig. 5. Key distinguishing features in adenosquamous carcinoma. (*A*) The presence of a surface dysplasia (H&E, original magnification ×100). (*B*) Abundant keratinization, seen here in juxtaposition to mucous cell differentiation (H&E, original magnification ×200). (*C*) Discrete adenocarcinomatous foci (H&E, original magnification ×200).

△△ *Differential Diagnosis*
Mucoepidermoid Carcinoma

- Adenosquamous carcinoma
- Salivary duct carcinoma
- Oncocytoma
- Oncocystic cystadenoma
- Warthin tumor
- Hyalinizing clear-cell carcinoma
- Clear-cell myoepithelioma
- Epithelial-myoepithelial carcinoma

tumor, particularly if there is prominent lymphoid stroma. However, oncocytoma can show tubules, and tends to have less sclerosis around tumor nests. Mucous cells should not be seen in oncocytoma. By immunohistochemistry, oncocytic MEC will show more diffuse staining with p63 than oncocytoma, which is reflective of an intermediate/epidermoid phenotype.[13] Cystic oncocytic MECs are more architecturally complex than oncocytic cystadenoma or Warthin tumor and have a more prominent mucous cell component. Clear-cell MEC may mimic a variety of tumors with clear-cell change, such as epithelial myoepithelial carcinoma, hyalinizing clear-cell carcinoma, and

clear-cell myoepithelioma. Key features in distinguishing clear-cell MEC from other clear cell tumors is the recognition of a mucous cell population, and establishment of an intermediate/epidermoid phenotype (p63+ CK 5/6+, actin–, calponin–, and S100–).

Occasionally non-neoplastic conditions may be mistaken for MEC, especially on small biopsy. In the palate, necrotizing sialometaplasia, a self-limited reactive condition may resemble MEC because of the reactive squamous metaplasia of the ductoacinar units.[19] Similarly in the major salivary glands, chronic sclerosing sialadenitis may also have metaplastic changes in the ducts and may resemble a sclerosing MEC. However, these reactive conditions will retain the normal ductoacinar architecture and will not have areas of intermediate cell proliferation.

For all diagnostically challenging MECs, molecular testing for the *MECT(CRTC)1/MAML2* translocation may be useful. This is present in 40% to 80% of all MECs with a predilection for lower-grade tumors.[6] The presence of this translocation is fairly specific for MECs and can establish the diagnosis in difficult cases (**Fig. 6**); however, the absence of this translocation does not exclude MEC.

TREATMENT AND PROGNOSIS

Treatment of MEC varies depending on grade and stage. For low-grade tumors, excision with negative margins is sufficient. For high-grade tumors, patients may also undergo a neck

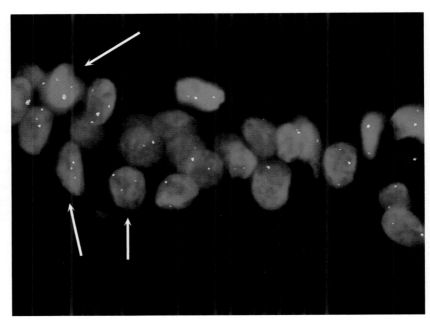

Fig. 6. Fluorescence in-situ hybridization using break-apart probes spanning the *MAML2*. Two probes (*red* and *green*) are normally juxtaposed resulting in 2 yellow signals; however in this case, there is a translocation involving one copy resulting in disruption of the probes, which flank the breakpoint, resulting in a split as indicated by a distinct red and green signal (*arrows*). This is reflective of the *MECT1-MAML2* translocation that is commonly noted in MEC.

> ⚠️ **Pitfalls**
> **MUCOEPIDERMOID CARCINOMA**
>
> ! Necrotizing sialometaplasia may mimic mucoepidermoid carcinoma on biopsy, because of the squamous metaplasia of ductoacinar units in the salivary glands of the palate.
>
> ! Distinguishing chronic sclerosing sialadenitis from sclerosing mucoepidermoid carcinoma may be difficult on biopsy.

dissection and receive postoperative radiotherapy. The treatment of intermediate-grade tumors is controversial in large part because of the variability in grading systems (see the following paragraph). Generally low-stage intermediate-grade MEC may be treated surgically, whereas higher-stage tumors may be treated with adjuvant radiotherapy and neck dissection. Only recurrent or disseminated disease (usually high-grade MEC) is treated with chemotherapy.[3,20] There is no specifically tailored regimen for MEC, and the few patients enrolled in prospective trials have shown limited objective response. The best single-agent therapy appears to be paclitaxel, with a partial response rate of 21%. Epidermal growth factor receptor (EGFR) is overexpressed by immunohistochemistry in more than two-thirds of MECs; however, activating mutations are quite rare. The rare case reports of patients treated with targeted anti-EGFR therapy show no response.[3]

Clinical parameters that correlate most strongly with disease-free and overall survival across the few studies that use multivariate analysis include age, stage, and margin status.[6,20,21] Submandibular gland tumors, floor of mouth, and base of tongue tumors may have a more aggressive behavior than parotid tumors, although this has not been as robustly validated as the other clinical prognosticators. Unlike other salivary carcinoma types, with perhaps the exception of adenoid cystic carcinoma, MEC grade is also an important prognostic factor. Low-grade tumors have a 92% to 100% 5-year survival, whereas intermediate-grade tumors have a reported 5-year survival of 62% to 100%, and high-grade tumors have a 5-year survival of 0% to 52%.[16] Whereas all grading systems correlate significantly with outcome given a sufficient sample size, the behavior of each individual grade category varies under the different grading schemes, particularly with respect to intermediate grade. Under the AFIP system, which requires more adverse parameters to move to the next grade category, intermediate-grade MEC will

behave in a similarly aggressive fashion to high-grade tumors.[21] However, under the Brandwein system, which requires fewer adverse parameters to move to the next grade, intermediate-grade tumors behave in an indolent fashion akin to low-grade MEC.[20,22] Another obstacle is the interobserver variability that may be seen when assigning a grade. Finally, one underrecognized phenomenon is the historical lack of accuracy of classification of high-grade tumors.[6] In earlier series, the terms MEC and adenosquamous carcinoma were often used interchangeably, and criteria for the delineation were not rigorously applied. More recent series likely have a more pure population of high-grade MEC, as reflected by more favorable outcomes.

Thus, in certain situations, particularly intermediate-grade MEC, more objective prognostic markers are desirable. Immunohistochemical markers of proliferation, such as Ki-67 and ploidy, correlate with histologic grade and thus outcome in a univariate fashion, but not independent of the other traditional markers. Similarly, p53 and EGFR immunoexpression are noted to correlate with grade, but do not contribute significantly as independent prognosticators.[23] The single most important molecular advance in MEC has been the description and characterization of the t(11;19)(q21;p13), which results in the fusion of CREB coactivator *MECT(CRTC)-1* and the notch signaling activator *MAML2*.[6] As mentioned previously, it is frequently found in MEC and can be used diagnostically if positive; however, perhaps an equally important role is its function as a prognosticator. Although almost 70% of low-grade and intermediate-grade MECs tested and reported in the literature are translocation positive, only 30% of high-grade MECs are reported to be positive. Okabe and colleagues[24] have demonstrated independent prognostic value of translocation status in predicting outcome. In our cohort, we were unable to establish as strong a link with prognosis, although even within the high-grade MEC subgroup, translocation-positive tumors had a more favorable outcome, although not all tumors behaved in an indolent fashion.[6] Thus, translocation status may supplement clinicopathologic parameters but will not replace them. The few translocation-positive MECs that have proven lethal in the literature have demonstrated *CDKN2A* deletions as a possible mechanism for tumor progression.[25]

ADENOID CYSTIC CARCINOMA

CLINICAL FEATURES

Adenoid cystic carcinoma (ACC) is a distinctive malignant salivary tumor described in the early

19th century as a "hetradenic tumor" by Robin and Laboulbene.[26] The relative prevalence of this tumor varies both temporally and geographically. In the United States, the incidence of ACC appears to have decreased slightly over the past decade.[2,5] This in part can be attributed to the recognition of polymorphous low-grade adenocarcinoma (see later in this article). There is a slight female predilection with a male:female ratio of approximately 1.5:1.0 in most series.

It is a tumor of minor salivary gland sites in about one-half of all cases; however, the parotid gland is still the most common single specific site. Of the specific minor salivary gland sites, the palate is the most common. ACC is typically a tumor of adults with a peak incidence in the sixth decade.[2,5]

ACC typically presents as a slow but progressively enlarging mass. Signs and symptoms, such as pain, and nerve paralysis, are more common than in other salivary gland malignancies as a result of this tumor's notorious propensity for perineural invasion. Because of the infiltrative nature of these tumors, fixation to skin, mucosa, and other soft tissue is also fairly common. Palate lesions may ulcerate.[2,5]

GROSS FEATURES

ACCs are typically firm, ill-defined, and grossly adherent to adjacent structures. Tumors may occasionally appear well demarcated when they are small or assume the contours of the structures involved (ie, bone) (**Fig. 7**). Cut surfaces are usually

Key Features
ADENOID CYSTIC CARCINOMA

- Adenoid cystic carcinoma is a slow-growing but relentless malignancy that is frequently seen at minor salivary gland sites.

- Adenoid cystic carcinoma is a biphasic tumor composed of hyperchromatic but bland angulated outer myoepithelial cells and small slightly eosinophilic inner ductules, arranged in tubular, cribriform, and solid growth patterns.

- Solid growth pattern imparts an aggressive behavior.

- Adenoid cystic carcinomas with high-grade transformation behave aggressively and unlike conventional adenoid cystic carcinomas, these tumors have a high propensity for nodal metastases.

a homogeneous gray-white.[2,27] Despite the name, ACCs are not typically cystic. Because ACC is such an infiltrative tumor, the gross impression of extent of disease is often inaccurate, which necessitates in some cases several frozen sections for margination, particularly for named nerves. Nerve segments that are submitted for intraoperative diagnosis, if involved, are often thickened and less pliable.

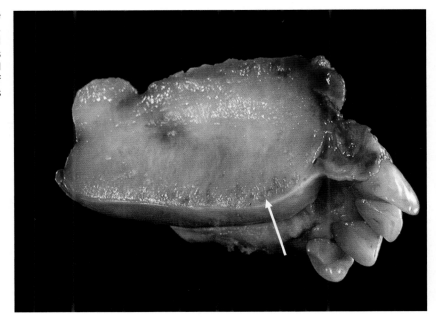

Fig. 7. Gross appearance of ACC of the palate. This tumor appears well demarcated, but this is because it has assumed the rounded contour of the hard palate, which is infiltrated (*arrow*).

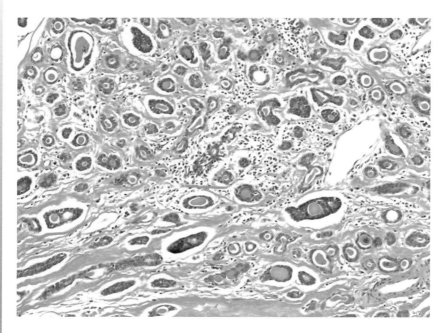

Fig. 8. ACC tubular pattern (H&E, original magnification ×100). Tubules are composed of a ductal and myoepithelial layer, both of which are composed of cells with scant cytoplasm and hyperchromatic angulated nuclei. Tubules show prominent retraction or clefting from the adjacent hyaline stroma.

MICROSCOPIC FEATURES

ACC has a very characteristic appearance. Like many salivary gland tumors, it is a biphasic tumor composed of ducts and abluminal myoepithelial cells arranged in tubular, cribriform, and solid growth patterns (**Figs. 8–10**).[2,27] The tumor nests are embedded in an acellular stroma ranging from myxoid to hyaline. The hyaline stroma is often arranged in "cylinders" within cribriform spaces (hence the archaic term "cylindroma").[28,29] A variant of ACC, the "sclerosing" variant has abundant stroma with only scattered nests of tumor embedded within (**Fig. 11**).[30] Both ductal and myoepithelial components are characterized by monomorphic hyperchromatic angulated nuclei

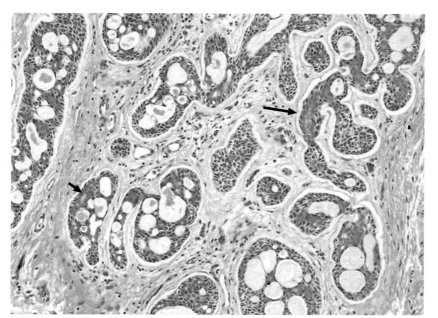

Fig. 9. ACC cribriform pattern (H&E, original magnification ×100). Tumor nests show well-demarcated spaces filled with hyaline basement membrane type material, and are also composed of cells with hyperchromatic nuclei with scant cytoplasm. Note similar retraction of the tumor nests from the stroma. True ducts are noted occasionally as well (*arrows*) within these cribriform nests.

Fig. 10. ACC solid pattern (H&E, original magnification ×100). Despite the solid growth pattern, cells contain monomorphic angulated hyperchromatic nuclei with indistinct nucleoli.

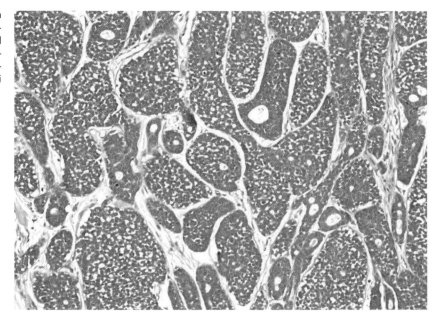

with inconspicuous nucleoli. At low-power magnification, this imparts a dark "blue" appearance to the tumor. Cytoplasm is typically scant in the myoepithelial component, although ductal elements may contain some eosinophilic cytoplasm. The proportion of these components varies with growth pattern. Solid tumors tend to have an "overgrowth" of the ductal component, whereas tubular and cribriform tumors have a high proportion of myoepithelial cells. Unlike many other salivary gland tumors, ACC is a morphologically "pure" tumor in that metaplasias (ie, squamous or oncocytic) and heterologous elements (ie, sebaceous glands) are not seen, and in fact may raise the possibility of another diagnosis when present. However, for sinonasal tumors, when they involve

Fig. 11. Sclerosing ACC (H&E, original magnification ×100). The hyaline stroma is particularly abundant with scant compressed epithelial tubules; however, the nuclei are similarly hyperchromatic as compared with usual ACC.

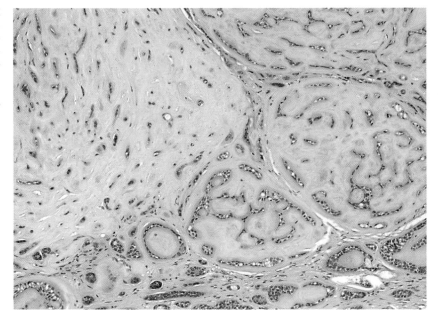

the excretory ducts as they open onto the surface mucosa,[31] slight columnar or oncocytic change may be noted, and nuclei may be slightly more vesicular and enlarged. Conventional ACC, regardless of growth pattern, does not display pleomorphism. Perineural invasion is very common in ACC, and essentially all tumors will show evidence for this with adequate sampling.

The architectural growth pattern is the main parameter used for "grading" adenoid cystic carcinomas. Generally, a predominantly tubular ACC is grade I, cribriform ACC is grade II, and solid ACC is grade III.[2,27] Other features, such as mitotic count, nuclear atypia, and necrosis, are not incorporated into this scheme, because, with the exception of solid ACC, these are rarely ever seen. Currently, this scheme is not formalized because it is not as therapeutically relevant (see later in this article), as the grading scheme for MEC for example (see previously).

Apart from the conventional ACC morphology outlined previously, a rare entity known as ACC with high-grade transformation (also known as dedifferentiated ACC) exists. This is a form of tumor progression that is characterized by a departure from the usual monomorphic biphasic appearance of conventional ACC (**Fig. 12**). The transformed areas may be localized or intermingled with any pattern of conventional ACC and are characterized by a very pleomorphic carcinoma that has lost its biphasic appearance. Nuclear size variation is often greater than 4:1, nuclei may be more vesicular, often with prominent nucleoli. The transformed component is usually a high-grade adenocarcinoma with cribriform, solid, or occasionally micropapillary areas. Squamoid areas are rare but have been described. Comedonecrosis, calcifications, and desmoplasia are also common features. High-grade transformation may occur de novo or on recurrent tumors.[32]

Immunohistochemically, the ductal component is positive for low molecular weight cytokeratins (CK7, CK 18, CK 19) and negative for p63, whereas the abluminal myoepithelial cells are positive for high molecular weight cytokeratins (ie, CK 5/6), vimentin, actin, calponin, and p63 (**Fig. 13**A, B).[2,27] S100 has low fidelity as a myoepithelial marker, and in ACC is only variably expressed in either component. Various diagnostic markers have been applied to ACC, among which the most prominent is the tyrosine receptor c-kit. C-kit shows strong immunoexpression in all ACCs, including transformed components, typically in the ductal component (see **Fig. 13**C). However, *c-kit* activating mutations are very rare.[33] Other markers such as cyclin D1, and surprisingly CD43, also expressed in ACC.[34,35] The former is not sufficiently specific, and the latter is not sufficiently sensitive as ACC markers, however.

DIFFERENTIAL DIAGNOSIS

Each pattern of ACC invokes a unique set of differential diagnostic considerations. Adding to the diagnostic challenge is that many palatal or minor salivary ACCs are encountered on biopsy rather

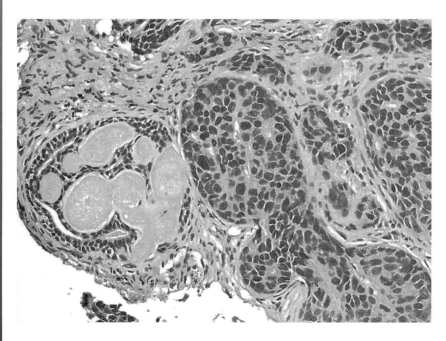

Fig. 12. ACC-HGT showing a transition from a monomorphic cribriform conventional component (*left*) to a pleomorphic high-grade adenocarcinoma (*right*) (H&E, original magnification ×200).

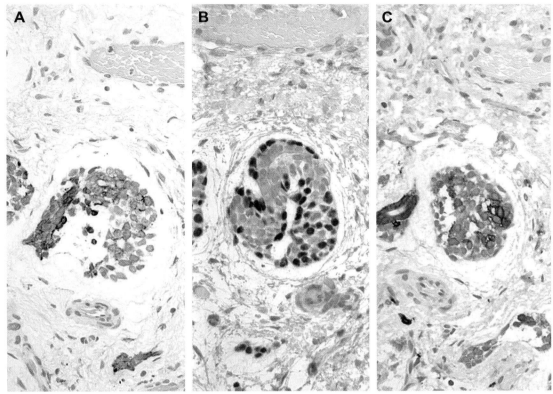

Fig. 13. Immunophenotype of ACC. (*A*) A low molecular weight pan cytokeratin cocktail highlights the ductal elements (DAB chromogen hematoxylin counterstain, original magnification ×200). (*B*) A p63 stain shows an inverse staining pattern highlighting the abluminal myoepithelial cells (DAB chromogen hematoxylin counterstain, original magnification ×200). (*C*) A c-kit immunostain shows a ductal predilection (DAB chromogen hematoxylin counterstain, original magnification ×200).

than a complete excision. For instance, pleomorphic adenomas may have ACC-like areas (**Fig. 14**). Without adequate sampling or observation of the circumscription from the surrounding normal tissue, such a pleomorphic adenoma can be mistaken as an ACC.

Perhaps the main diagnostic consideration for tubular ACC is epithelial myoepithelial carcinoma

> **△△ Differential Diagnosis**
> **ADENOID CYSTIC CARCINOMA**
>
> - Epithelial-myoepithelial carcinoma
> - Polymorphous low-grade adenocarcinoma
> - Basal cell salivary tumors (adenoma/adenocarcinoma)
> - Basaloid squamous cell carcinoma
> - Small cell neuroendocrine carcinomas

(EMCa). This may be a difficult distinction, and in some cases both tumors coexist as a hybrid tumor. Both tumors are defined by a biphasic bilayered appearance of abluminal myoepithelial cells and luminal ductal cells. However in ACC, the nuclei are more hyperchromatic and angulated than those of EMCa. Additionally, tumor nests and tubules in ACC tend to be more dyshesive and will show "stromal clefting." If there is dyshesion in EMCa, it is more commonly between tumor cells rather than between the tumor and stroma. Additionally, the tumor border for EMCa tends to be more rounded, even if permeative. Immunohistochemically, these are similar. C-kit may be useful if negative, as this argues against ACC; however, up to 75% of EMCa are c-kit positive, making this marker less useful if positive.[36]

For tubular and cribriform ACC, tumors such as polymorphous low-grade adenocarcinoma (PLGA) and basal cell salivary tumors (BCST), both adenomas and adenocarcinomas, particularly the membranous and cribriform types, are major

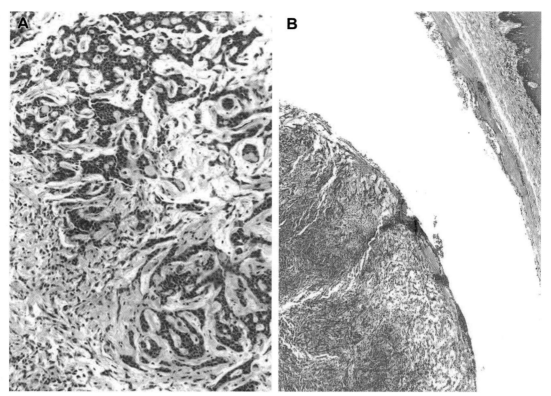

Fig. 14. ACC-like areas in a cellular pleomorphic adenoma. (*A*) Tumor nuclei are hyperchromatic and angulated with vague cribriforming reminiscent of ACC (H&E, original magnification ×100). (*B*) Taking a step back, this lesion is well demarcated and demonstrates streaming of myoepithelial cells into a myxoid stroma in other areas (H&E, original magnification ×20). This tumor was erroneously diagnosed as an ACC arising as a pleomorphic adenoma, but the patient had remained disease free at the time of last follow-up 17 years after excision.

differential diagnostic considerations. Although historically, PLGA was the leading differential diagnosis for ACC, and in fact, the decreasing prevalence of ACC may be related to the recognition of PLGA,[2] given adequate material, the challenges in distinguishing these 2 are largely exaggerated. Although PLGA can have similar myxohyaline stroma, and similar growth patterns to ACC, fundamentally this is a monophasic tumor with a ductal phenotype. Even when there is focal myoepithelial marker expression by immunostaining, it is focal and not distinctly bilayered, as in a truly biphasic tumor.[37,38] Furthermore, the nuclei of PLGA are very characteristically ovoid with vesicular, powdery almost clear chromatin, reminiscent of papillary thyroid carcinoma nuclei. By immunostaining, the distinction between the monophasic PLGA and biphasic ACC are readily apparent. Furthermore, PLGA are diffusely, strongly S100 positive, unlike ACC.[38] These are usually sufficient to resolve this differential. However, c-kit, which is strongly positive in ACC, but weak to negative in PLGA, is also

useful.[39] BCST are also biphasic and have similar myxohyaline stroma to ACC, particularly membranous variants; however, nuclei of BCST are more vesicular than those of ACC. Additionally, BCST tend to demonstrate peripheral palisading in tumor nests. BCST also may often show squamous or sebaceous metaplasia, which are rare to absent in ACC. Immunohistochemically, although the outer layers of BCST are also p63 positive like those of ACC, these tend to have only a small subpopulation of myoepithelial cells; the rest of the p63-positive cells are strictly "basal" in phenotype. Again c-kit may be expressed in some basal cell adenocarcinomas, which may lessen its utility here.[40]

Solid ACC and ACC with high-grade transformation may be confused with a variety of high-grade lesions, ranging from basaloid squamous carcinoma, or small-cell neuroendocrine carcinoma. Small-cell neuroendocrine carcinomas tend to have more of a diffuse growth pattern with a high mitotic/karyorrhectic index. These can be easily excluded with neuroendocrine markers, such as synaptophysin or chromogranin. Basaloid squamous cell carcinoma can easily mimic ACC, particularly of the solid type; however, these tumors are surface mucosa derived, and may thus show evidence of squamous dysplasia or carcinoma in situ or evidence of keratinization. Furthermore, basaloid squamous cell carcinomas are more pleomorphic, and mitotically active than solid ACC, although ACC with high-grade transformation may be equally pleomorphic and mitotically active. Perhaps the most useful ancillary stain to add in the distinction of solid ACC, and ACC with high-grade transformation from basaloid squamous cell carcinoma is p63. Basaloid squamous cell carcinomas are diffusely p63 positive. Solid ACCs are positive only in the outermost layer in tumor nests, whereas ACCs with high-grade transformation are p63 negative altogether.[32,41]

TREATMENT AND PROGNOSIS

ACC follows a slow but relentless course, with a 5-year survival of 75% to 80%, but a 15-year survival of only 35%.[42–46] ACC with high-grade transformation is a very aggressive tumor with a median survival of only 12 to 36 months, although long-term survivors have been described.[32]

Stage is perhaps the most important prognostic factor in ACC.[43] Growth pattern–based grade in most series is also important as a prognosticator, although there is some degree of controversy surrounding this parameter. Generally, any solid component suggests the possibility of an aggressive behavior, although the typical cutoff for "grade 3" tumors is a solid component of 30% or more. Using this cutoff, several studies have shown that tumors with a high solid component behave more aggressively[42,44,46]; however, Spiro and Huvos[43] suggested that pattern-based grading is not useful. The major flaw in this assertion is the use of an arbitrary grading scheme in which tumors with up to 50% of a solid component could still be considered "grade 1."

Regarding biomarkers, p53 overexpression appears to be a useful prognosticator even on multivariate analysis in one large series.[45] In fact, p53 alterations appear to be one mechanism for progression to high-grade transformation in ACC.[47] Gains on chromosome 8, particularly in the region of *c-myc,* suggest that this may also be another mechanism of tumor progression.[32] Earlier literature points to some utility in using DNA ploidy and S-phase analysis in predicting aggressiveness, but it is unclear whether these contribute beyond traditional clinicopathologic parameters. More recently, comparative genomic hybridization studies have pointed to several important regions of loss including 1p32-36, 6q23-27, and 12q12-14.[48,49] The 1p32-36 is reported to be a significant prognosticator as well.[49] Candidate tumor suppressor genes in these regions have yet to be identified. Recently, a reproducible translocation, (6;9)(q22-23;p23-24) resulting in a fusion of *MYB-NFIB* has been described in up to 25% of head and neck ACC, although its prognostic value remains to be seen.[50]

Despite the emergence of molecular prognosticators, and regardless of the debate surrounding the utility of grading of ACC, the therapeutic approach to an ACC is mainly dependent on stage. ACC, regardless of pattern and phenotype, is considered a locally aggressive tumor that requires wide resection, and radiotherapy for local control. Despite the locally aggressive nature, ACC has a fairly low propensity to metastasize to lymph nodes (5%–20%); thus, neck dissection is not routinely done at many institutions. ACC with high-grade transformation, in contrast, has a much higher propensity for lymph node metastases, which present in more than 50% of reported cases to date, suggesting a potential role for lymph node dissection for this variant of ACC.[16] On the other hand, ACC spreads hematogenously with considerable frequency. As many as one-half of patients develop metastatic disease, most commonly to lung, but other sites, such as bone, liver, and brain are also fairly common.[44] Thus, patients should have routine aggressive surveillance throughout their life. Isolated small metastases are amenable to resection in the lung and liver; however with disseminated disease, patients are typically treated with a chemotherapeutic regimen. Standard cytotoxic regimens, either single agent or in combination have been used, but typically show only partial response at best to varying degrees (0%–70%). Empiric treatment with monoclonals or inhibitors targeting EGFR and human epidermal growth factor receptor 2 (HER-2) have shown no response and may not be relevant targets. Although c-kit is overexpressed in ACC, treatment with the inhibitor imatinib mesylate has shown only partial response in a few isolated case reports.[3]

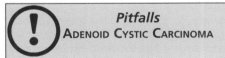

Pitfalls
ADENOID CYSTIC CARCINOMA

! Pleomorphic adenomas may have adenoid cystic carcinoma–like areas that can be mistaken on biopsies.

ACINIC CELL CARCINOMA

OVERVIEW

Acinic cell carcinoma (AciCC) is a low-grade salivary neoplasm that shows evidence, either focally or diffusely, of serous acinar differentiation.[51–55] It comprises about 10% of all malignant salivary neoplasms, occurs in all age groups, and is the second-most frequent malignant salivary tumor in children, exceeded only by mucoepidermoid carcinoma. Most large series indicate a female preference of about 60%.[52,54]

The parotid gland is, by far, the most common site of origin (85%–90% of all cases), followed by the minor salivary glands (5%–10% of all cases) and the submandibular gland (3% of all cases).[52,54] Among the minor salivary glands, the buccal mucosa and upper lip are the more common sites, whereas the sinonasal tract is rarely involved.[56]

Most tumors present as a slowly enlarging, sometimes painful mass of less than a year's duration. Facial nerve paresis or paralysis is apparent in 2% to 8% of patients.[53,55] Fixation to skin and muscle and lymph node metastasis at presentation are uncommon.

Although an infrequent occurrence, the AciCC is the third-most frequent salivary neoplasm to present with bilateral parotid involvement, exceeded in frequency by Warthin tumor and pleomorphic adenoma.[57,58] Such tumors may be either synchronous or asynchronous.

GROSS FEATURES

Most AciCCs rarely exceed 3 to 4 cm in greatest dimension. On cut surface, they are firm, tan to reddish-gray, solid to cystic, and have margins that vary from circumscribed to poorly defined (**Fig. 15**).

MICROSCOPIC FEATURES

AciCCs, histologically, are rather heterogeneous neoplasms. Five different cell types (acinar, intercalated duct, vacuolated, clear, nonspecific glandular) and 4 patterns of growth have been recognized (solid, microcystic, papillary-cystic, follicular) (**Figs. 16–20**).[51] Although the prototypic tumor is composed of acinar cells arranged in a solid pattern, tumors composed of more than one cell type and pattern of growth are almost the rule rather than the exception (see **Fig. 16**).

Acinar cells are round to polygonal with central to eccentric nuclei that vary from small, hyperchromatic to vesicular. Nucleoli are usually absent or barely discernible. The cytoplasm contains

Key Features
ACINIC CELL CARCINOMA

- Acinic cell carcinomas most frequently occur in the parotid.

- Tumors are defined by the presence of serous acinar differentiation, but can consist of up to 5 different cell types (acinar, intercalated duct, vacuolated, clear, nonspecific glandular) arranged in up to 4 different growth patterns (solid, microcystic, papillary-cystic, follicular).

- Acinic cell carcinomas are generally indolent, but some adverse prognosticators include positive margins, elevated mitotic count, necrosis, perineural and angiolymphatic invasion, and high-grade transformation.

- A subset of zymogen granule–poor and S100-positive tumors historically categorized as acinic cell carcinoma are now classified as mammary analog secretory carcinomas and are characterized by (12;15) (p13;q25) *ETV6-NTRK3* translocation.

abundant blue-purple zymogen granules (the "blue dot tumor"). Intercalated duct cells are cuboidal with eosinophilic to basophilic cytoplasm, round nuclei, and may or may not contain zymogen granules (see **Fig. 17**). Vacuolated cells, as the name implies, contain cytoplasmic vacuoles that are negative for glycogen and mucin (see **Fig. 17**). Clear cells have an optically clear cytoplasm devoid of zymogen granules, glycogen, and mucin. Nonspecific glandular cells possess eosinophilic to amphophilic cytoplasm, round nuclei, and poorly defined cell borders and are arranged in syncytial aggregates (see **Fig. 18**).

The stroma ranges from sparse to dense and sclerotic. Some tumors appear circumscribed, whereas others are infiltrative. Prominent mitotic activity, focal necrosis, and perineural invasion are variable, but, when seen, often signify a tumor with more aggressive behavior. A prominent stromal lymphoid infiltrate is a component of many tumors (**Fig. 21**).[59] A few may also contain psammoma bodies.

AciCCs can undergo high grade transformation, previously referred to as dedifferentiation and underscores the need for thorough histologic evaluation to rule out this possibility.[60] The transformation may be apparent at the time of original diagnosis or in a recurrent lesion. Such tumors are characterized by a "typical" low-grade AciCC

Fig. 15. Acinic cell carcinoma, cut surface. Tumor is reddish-tan and deceptively well circumscribed.

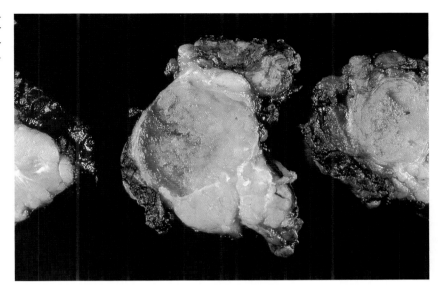

juxtaposed to a high-grade adenocarcinoma or an undifferentiated carcinoma (**Fig. 22**).

The zymogen granules, the histologic hallmark of an AciCC, are periodic acid-Schiff-positive and diastase resistant. Most tumors are either negative or weakly reactive for mucin. AciCCs are immunoreactive for cytokeratin (AE 1/3, CK5/6, CK7, CK18, CK19) and negative for P63 and other "myoepithelial markers." A few may be focally positive for S-100 protein. Antiamylase, which is reactive in normal serous acinar cells, has been found to be an unreliable indicator of acinar differentiation and is often negative in AciCC.

AciCCs with high-grade transformation show a markedly elevated Ki-67, and are positive for p53 and cyclin D1 and exhibit strong membrane staining for beta-catenin.[60]

Fig. 16. Acinic cell carcinoma composed of acinar cells arranged in a solid pattern (H&E, original magnification x100).

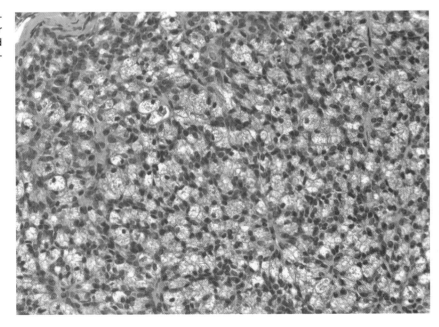

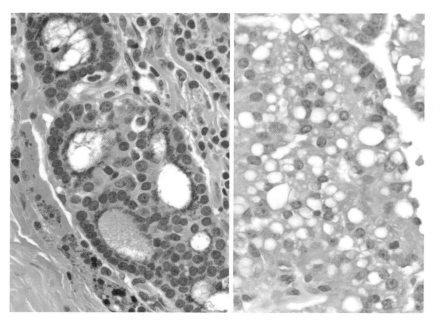

Fig. 17. Acinic cell carcinoma. Left image shows intercalated duct cells forming glands (H&E, original magnification x200). Right image shows vacuolated cells (H&E, original magnification x200).

DIFFERENTIAL DIAGNOSIS

Although the diagnosis of AciCC is usually straightforward, 6 classic potentially problematic areas exist:

1. The solid acinar variant may be difficult to recognize, especially on frozen section or limited sampling, where it is sometimes mistaken for normal parotid tissue. In normal parotid tissue, the acini are arranged in lobules and are associated with ducts, whereas in AciCC a lobular architecture and ducts are not conspicuous.

2. Because the tumor is often histologically bland and well demarcated, it is often mistaken for an "adenoma." A thorough examination for the

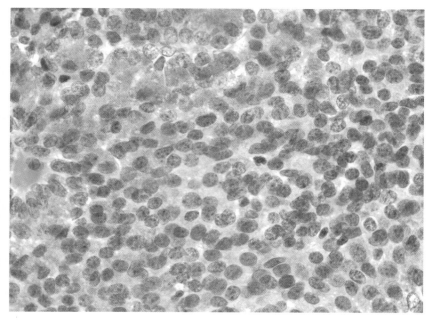

Fig. 18. Acinic cell carcinoma. Nonspecific glandular cells arranged in a syncytial pattern (H&E, original magnification x200).

Fig. 19. Acinic cell carcinoma. Left image shows microcystic pattern (H&E, original magnification x100). Right image shows follicular pattern. Note the colloidlike material with peripheral scalloping, simulating thyroid follicles (H&E, original magnification x100).

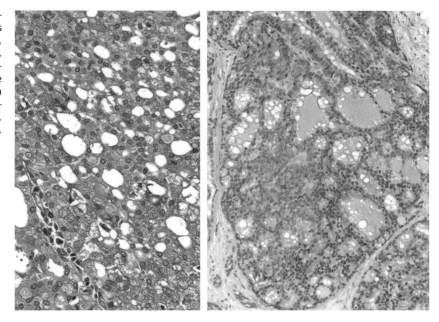

diagnostic zymogen-containing cells will confirm the diagnosis.

3. AciCC associated with a prominent lymphoid response is occasionally mistaken for lymph node metastasis. In this instance, it is important to look for a capsule around the lymphoid stroma and the presence of subcapsular and medullary sinuses, which are characteristic of a lymph node. In their absence, a tumor-associated lymphoid response is more likely.

4. Some pathologists are not familiar with the papillary-cystic variant of AciCC and mistake it for a benign salivary cyst or cystadenoma. The presence of zymogen-containing acinar cells

Fig. 20. Acinic cell carcinoma, papillary-cystic pattern (H&E, original magnification x40).

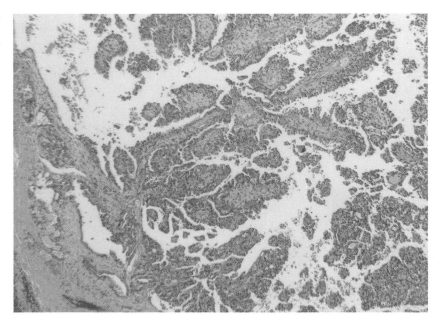

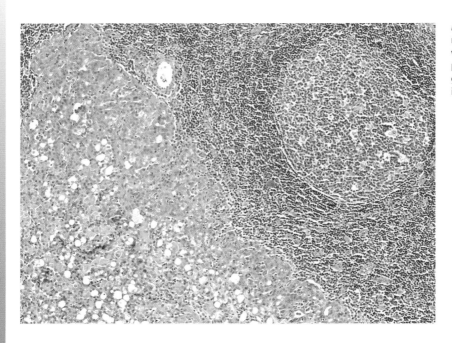

Fig. 21. Acinic cell carcinoma, microcystic pattern with tumor-associated lymphoid response. Note germinal center (H&E, original magnification x40).

lining the cyst, either focally or diffusely, should suggest the proper diagnosis. Additionally, papillary cystic AciCC often show hobnailed epithelium in the cyst lining.

5. Although AciCC may contain clear cells, such cells are very focal and never dominate the tumor. As such, a clear cell variant of AciCC for all practical purposes does not exist and should not be confused with other clear cell–dominant tumors.

6. The high-grade transformed component of an AciCC can be very focal, representing in some cases only 5% of the total tumor volume.[60] Thorough sampling of all AciCCs, therefore, is essential to avoid missing these more aggressive variants.

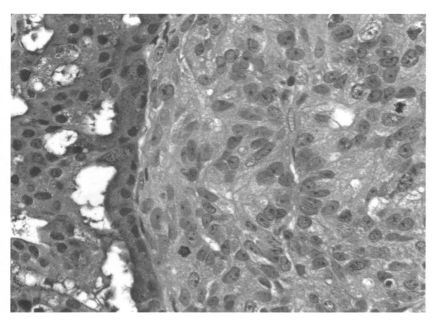

Fig. 22. Acinic cell carcinoma with high-grade transformation. Left image shows typical low-grade acinic cell component. Right image shows undifferentiated component. Note nuclear pleomorphism and mitoses (H&E, original magnification x400).

> ## Differential Diagnosis
> ### ACINIC CELL CARCINOMA
>
> - Metastatic adenocarcinoma
> - Cystadenoma
> - Clear-cell salivary gland tumors
> - Mammary analog secretory carcinoma

Molecular advances have resulted in yet another differential diagnostic consideration. A subset of AciCC, composed of intercalated and nonspecific ductal cells often arranged in a microcystic pattern showing strong S100 positivity, are now known to be characterized by a (12;15) (p13;q25) ETV6-NTRK3 translocation identical to that seen in juvenile secretory carcinoma of breast.[61] It is not clear whether clinical behavior of this newly recognized entity, dubbed mammary analog secretory carcinoma, is different from AciCC, but it appears biologically distinct. Thus, any zymogen-poor, strongly S100-positive acinar microcystic-patterned tumor should raise this entity as a potential diagnostic consideration.

TREATMENT AND PROGNOSIS

The standard treatment of AciCC is local resection with tumor free margins without a neck dissection. In the parotid gland, a superficial lobectomy is sufficient, rarely a total parotidectomy. Postoperative radiation and/or a neck dissection should be considered only for those patients with positive margins or other adverse indicators, such as greater than 2 mitoses per 10 high-power fields,

> ## Pitfalls
> ### ACINIC CELL CARCINOMA
>
> ! Distinguishing normal acini from acinic cell carcinoma by the presence of lobular architecture and presence of central ducts
>
> ! Acinic cell carcinomas may be well demarcated and mimic a benign neoplasm or "adenoma"; however, examination for serous acinar differentiation (ie, zymogen granules) will exclude benign lesions.
>
> ! Acinic cell carcinoma with high-grade transformation may not be recognizable as acinic cell carcinoma unless carefully examined for a "differentiated" component.

Ki-67 greater than 10%, necrosis, perineural and angiolymphatic invasion, recurrent tumors, and high-grade transformation.[55,60,62]

The 5-year, 10-year, and 20-year determinant survival rates for the "usual" AciCC are 90%, 83%, and 67%, respectively.[53] Approximately 35% to 45% of patients will develop local recurrences, with the median time from diagnosis to first recurrence being 3 years[53,63]; 15% to 20% will also develop cervical lymph node or more distant metastases (lungs, bones). High-grade transformed tumors are much more aggressive. In a report of 9 transformed tumors, Skalova and colleagues[60] observed that 56% developed lymph node metastases and 66% developed distant dissemination to various sites, especially lungs and brain. Six of the 9 patients died of their tumor, all within an overall median survival of 4.3 years.[60] The propensity for lymph node metastases for this variant of tumor indicates the need for a neck dissection at the time of diagnosis.

Although grading systems for AciCC have been proposed, all are controversial and rarely used.[64] All agree that cell type and pattern of growth have no prognostic significance.[53,55] It has been suggested that those AciCCs that are well circumscribed, arranged in a microcystic pattern with a low Ki-67 proliferative index, and completely surrounded by a heavy lymphoid infiltrate with germinal centers tend to be less aggressive than other tumors.[65]

Whether DNA ploidy analysis of AciCCs has any clinical relevance is debatable.[66] Some of the aneuploid tumors, alleged to be more aggressive than diploid tumors, have had areas that are probably best classified as foci of high-grade transformation.

In general, AciCCs arising in minor salivary glands are less aggressive than those occurring in the major glands. Tumors of the submandibular gland, although rare, also tend to be more aggressive than those of the parotid gland.[63]

SALIVARY DUCT CARCINOMA

OVERVIEW

Salivary duct carcinoma (SDC) is a relatively uncommon, clinically aggressive adenocarcinoma of salivary origin that is histologically similar to carcinoma of the breast.[67–72] It was first recognized by Kleinsasser and colleagues in 1968.[73] In a review of 104 cases, Barnes and colleagues[68] noted that the tumor was 3 times more common in men and occurred primarily in patients older than 50 years (range 22–91 years). The tumor occurs mainly in the parotid gland, infrequently in the submandibular gland, and rarely in the minor salivary glands.

Most patients present with a progressively, sometimes rapidly, enlarging mass, with or without evidence of positive cervical lymph nodes. Pain and facial nerve paralysis are additional features.

GROSS FEATURES

The tumor may arise de novo or in a pleomorphic adenoma (salivary duct carcinoma ex pleomorphic adenoma). Most vary from a few millimeters up to 7 cm and on cross section are gray-white to yellow-tan with borders that range from well to poorly defined. Some have a uniform, firm solid appearance, and others have both solid and cystic components. The cysts range up to 1.5 cm and are filled with either serous fluid or necrotic tumor.

MICROSCOPIC FEATURES

SDCs are characterized by both intraductal and infiltrating ductal carcinoma (**Fig. 23**). The tumor grows in papillary, cribriform, and/or solid patterns, with central (comedo) necrosis. In other instances, the infiltrating tumor forms small ducts or cords of cells with a desmoplastic stromal resection, such as seen in scirrhous carcinoma of the breast. The tumor cells have amphophilic to pink cytoplasm and large, pleomorphic, vesicular nuclei with prominent nucleoli. Some have an apocrine appearance, replete with apical snouts. Occasionally the tumor cells are more uniform and composed of small, hyperchromatic nuclei. Mitoses, lymph node metastases (59%), and vascular (31%) and peri-intraneural invasion (60%) are common.[74] Dystrophic calcification may also be seen, sometimes even on imaging, which masquerades as calculi. Rare sarcomatoid, mucin-rich, micropapillary, and intraductal variants have also been described.[74–77]

The presence of a uniform layer of cells around tumor islands that are positive for cytokeratin 14 and/or p63 is useful in identifying an in-situ (intraductal) component of the tumor (**Fig. 24**). Immunohistochemical evaluation of SDC shows that it shares many features in common with breast carcinoma, especially with regard to carcinoembryonic antigen and gross cystic disease fluid protein; however, with regard to hormonal receptors, there

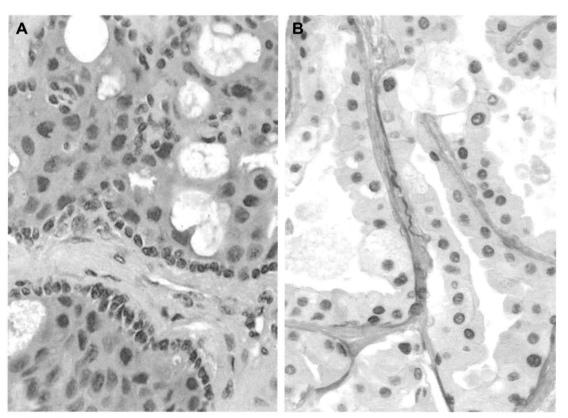

Fig. 23. Salivary duct carcinoma. (*A*) Intraductal component. Note prominent layer of peripheral myoepithelial cells (H&E, original magnification x400). (*B*) Tumor is positive for androgen receptor (DAB chromogen hematoxylin counterstain, original magnification x400).

Key Features
SALIVARY DUCT CARCINOMA

- Salivary duct carcinomas are highly aggressive malignancies that resemble ductal carcinoma of the breast.

- Salivary duct carcinoma shows frequent calcifications and comedonecrosis.

- Variants include micropapillary, sarcomatoid, and mucin-rich tumors.

- Essentially all tumors have an apocrine morphology and are positive for androgen receptor and GCDFP-15.

- Unlike ductal carcinoma of the breast, HER-2/neu amplification is not prognostically or therapeutically relevant, although not uncommonly seen.

are distinct differences. In contrast to breast carcinomas, which are frequently positive for estrogen (ER) and progesterone (PR) receptors, only 2% and 14% of SDCs are respectively positive for these markers.[18,67,78–81] Interestingly, 80% to 90% are positive for androgen receptors.[18]

HER-2/neu overexpression has been found in 25% to 88% of SDCs. Whether it has prognostic significance, however, is controversial. In one of the best studies of HER-2/neu and SDC, Skalova and colleagues[82] observed that 8 of 11 cases showed strong distinct membrane staining for this marker (score 3+) with immunohistochemistry, whereas the remaining 3 cases were inconclusive with scores of 1+ to 2+. Using fluorescence in situ hybridization, they observed that 4 of the 10 cases that were analyzed showed HER-2/neu gene amplification. They, however, observed no differences in prognosis between amplified and nonamplified tumors.

P53 positivity was found in 58% of SDCs studied by Felix and colleagues,[83] but did not correlate with the clinical course. Reviews indicate that 21% to 42% of SDCs are diploid and 58% to 79% are aneuploid. All conclude that tumor ploidy has no predictive value.

DIFFERENTIAL DIAGNOSIS

Although one should consider metastatic breast carcinoma in a woman and, possibly, even metastatic prostatic carcinoma in a man, these possibilities are distinctly uncommon. According to Gnepp,[84] only 2% to 3% of all metastatic tumors to the parotid gland are from the breast and only 0.5% from the prostate. These events would be even more unlikely if the parotid mass is also associated with enlarged cervical lymph nodes. The absence of a breast mass on physical or mammographic examination, coupled with a tumor that is negative for estrogen receptor, would also favor an SDC rather than a metastasis from the breast. The finding of unequivocal in situ ductal carcinoma would also indicate a primary parotid tumor.

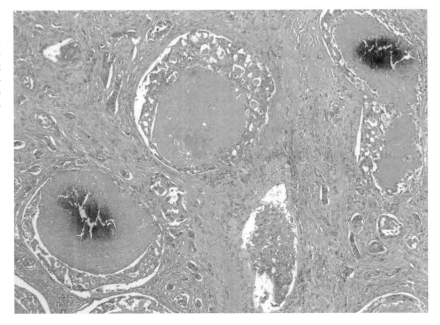

Fig. 24. Salivary duct carcinoma showing both intraductal and infiltrating carcinoma. Note the comedonecrosis with dystrophic calcification and the desmoplastic stromal response (H&E, original magnification x40).

△△ **Differential Diagnosis**
SALIVARY DUCT CARCINOMA

- Metastatic ductal carcinoma of breast
- Metastatic prostatic adenocarcinoma
- Oncocytic carcinoma
- Mucoepidermoid carcinoma
- Adenocarcinoma, not otherwise specified
- Low-grade salivary duct carcinoma (low-grade cribriform cystadenocarcinoma)

 Pitfalls
SALIVARY DUCT CARCINOMA

! Salivary duct carcinoma may express PSA, which may raise confusion with metastatic prostatic adenocarcinoma.

Caution must be exercised in distinguishing an SDC from metastatic prostatic carcinoma based on the results of an immunoperoxidase stain for prostatic-specific antigen (PSA).[85] James and colleagues[86] reported an SDC that was not only immunopositive for PSA but was also associated with an elevated serum PSA level. The absence of a palpable lesion of the prostate on physical examination and the simultaneous presence of a parotid mass and enlarged cervical lymph nodes would, of course, favor the diagnosis of an SDC.

Other entities that have been mentioned in the differential diagnosis include oncocytic carcinoma (OCa), mucoepidermoid carcinoma (MEC), and adenocarcinoma not otherwise specified type (ANOS). Because of the eosinophilic or apocrinelike appearance of tumor cells, SDC may be mistaken for an OCa. OCa, however, does not exhibit prominent comedonecrosis or papillary intraductal projections of tumor cells. OCa, furthermore, are packed with mitochondria, whereas in SDC they are less conspicuous. Stains for mitochondria, such as the phosphotungstic acid hematoxylin or an immunoperoxidase stain for cytochrome-c-oxidase, may be helpful in distinguishing the 2.

The absence of epidermoid cells and the overall resemblance to a breast carcinoma respectively exclude an MEC and an ANOS from consideration.

Delgado and colleagues[81] reported 10 cases of "low-grade salivary duct carcinoma," which, according to them, represented the low-grade end of a spectrum of salivary duct carcinoma. The World Health Organization has recently renamed this tumor as "low-grade cribriform cystadenocarcinoma."

TREATMENT AND PROGNOSIS

Complete surgical excision with removal of regional lymph nodes and postoperative irradiation is the preferred treatment. Systemic metastases, unfortunately, are common and are directed primarily to the lungs and bones. Chemotherapy is largely ineffective.

Because SDCs are rarely positive for estrogen receptor and progesterone receptor, one would expect antiestrogen therapy, as used in breast cancer, would have little if any, therapeutic value in the management of the vast majority of patients. The observation that 80% to 90% of SDCs are positive for androgen receptor raises the question of whether antiandrogen therapy, such as flutamide, might have merit. Because 25% to 88% of SDCs are positive for HER-2/neu, one might also speculate on whether or not trastuzumab (Herceptin) might be beneficial.

SDC is very aggressive. Most patients die of their disease within 4 years of diagnosis. The incidence of local recurrence, cervical lymph node metastases, and distant metastases are, respectively 33%, 59%, and 46%.[68]

CARCINOMA EX PLEOMORPHIC ADENOMA

OVERVIEW

The risk of malignant transformation in a pleomorphic adenoma increases with the longevity of the tumor. According to Eneroth and colleagues,[87] the incidence of malignancy in a pleomorphic adenoma of 5 years or less duration is 1.6% but increases to 9.6% for those present for more than 15 years.

Auclair and Ellis[88] indicate that pleomorphic adenomas that show prominent zones of hyalinization and moderate mitotic activity (mean 1.5 mitoses/10 high-power fields [HPFs]) have a 13.8% chance of malignant transformation. Clinical findings at diagnosis that point toward a greater tendency of malignant change include an origin in the submandibular gland, older age (mean 62 years), and large tumor size (mean 4 cm).

Malignant neoplasms arising in pleomorphic adenomas are collectively referred to as malignant mixed tumors and can be divided into 3 categories:

1. carcinoma ex pleomorphic adenoma (CXPA)
2. carcinosarcoma (true malignant mixed tumor)
3. metastasizing pleomorphic adenoma.

CXPA accounts for more than 90% of these tumors and is defined as a carcinoma arising in a primary or recurrent pleomorphic adenoma. As such, only the epithelial component can metastasize, as opposed to the carcinosarcoma in which both epithelial and mesenchymal components can disseminate, either simultaneously or independently.

The term "CXPA" includes a heterogeneous group of carcinomas that vary from in situ to widely invasive and from low to high grade. Accordingly, "CXPA" cannot be used as a histologic diagnosis without further qualification. The World Health Organization has recently proposed that CXPAs be divided into 3 categories[89] (**Fig. 25**):

1. noninvasive
2. minimally invasive
3. invasive.

NONINVASIVE CXPA

Noninvasive CXPA, also known as in situ or intracapsular CXPA, is a pleomorphic adenoma that shows either focal or diffuse cellular pleomorphism, increased mitotic activity, prominent stromal hyalinization, and/or necrosis, but no capsular, vascular, or lymphatic invasion.[88–90] The earliest changes are usually observed in the luminal duct cells, which may or may not be surrounded by myoepithelial cells. Needless to say, the tumor must be thoroughly sampled, preferably totally submitted for microscopic evaluation, to make this diagnosis.

Assessment of androgen receptor, HER-2/neu, and P53 in evaluating the malignant potential of pleomorphic adenomas must be interpreted with caution, as these markers can be seen focally in 5% to 10% of otherwise benign pleomorphic adenomas.[91]

If the margins of resection are free of tumor, no further treatment is warranted and the prognosis is similar to an ordinary pleomorphic adenoma; however, rare recurrences and metastases have been reported.[92,93] Perhaps the only thoroughly documented case, however, is that of Felix and colleagues[92] in which "missed capsule infiltration

Fig. 25. Diagram showing progression of pleomorphic adenoma (PA) from intracapsular (*white area*) to minimally invasive (MIC) to invasive carcinoma (IC) based on presence or absence of capsular invasion (*yellow border*) and extent of invasion beyond the capsule.

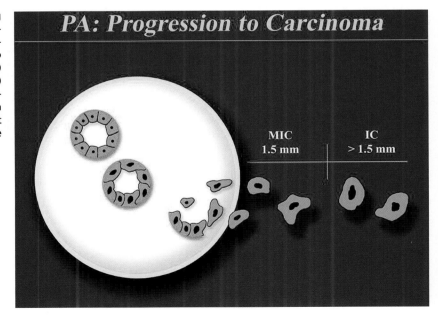

and lymphatic permeation were excluded since the neoplasm was totally submitted and serial recuts done."

MINIMALLY INVASIVE CXPA

There are many histologic indices of CXPA that affect survival. Among these include the proportion of carcinoma, histologic type, surgical margins, perineural and angiolymphatic invasion, and the extent of invasion.[4,7–9,90,94–96] Tortoledo and colleagues[95] observed that when CXPAs did not exceed 8 mm of invasion from the capsule of a pleomorphic adenoma, no patients died of their tumor. When the microscopic invasion exceeded 6 mm, the local recurrence was 70.5%, whereas when it was less than 6 mm, the recurrence rate was only 16.5%.

Lewis and colleagues[96] described 4 patients with CXPA in which the extent of invasion was only 5 mm from the capsule of the pleomorphic adenoma. Of these 4 patients, 2 had no progression of disease and 2 died of disease. The investigators stated that they would cautiously predict a favorable prognosis in cases of less than 5 mm invasion.

Brandwein and colleagues[90] studied 12 CXPAs that were either noninvasive or exhibited capsular invasion of no more than 1.5 mm. DNA ploidy was performed on 7 of these and 5 were found to be aneuploid and 2 diploid. Ploidy had no predictive value. The tumors in their series ranged from 0.8 to 3.5 cm (mean 1.8 cm). Some cases showed

"occasional perineural or perivascular tumor outside nearby the capsule." No recurrences or metastases were seen in 11 patients available for follow-up (mean 4.2 years; range 15 months to 13 years).

Based on the aforementioned, the World Health Organization has recently endorsed 1.5 mm as the cutoff between "minimally invasive" and "invasive" CXPA (see **Fig. 25**; **Fig. 26**).[89] Using the 1.5-mm definition, Katabi and colleagues[93] described 12 cases of noninvasive and minimally invasive CXPA. With a median follow-up of 30 months, 3 of the 12 (2 noninvasive and 1 minimally invasive) recurred. Distant metastasis occurred in 3 of 12 tumors (not indicated if these were noninvasive or minimally invasive). One minimally invasive tumor resulted in death.

How then should minimally invasive (1.5 mm or less) CXPA be treated? If the margins are free and no perineural and/or angiolymphatic invasion is seen, we believe that no additional therapy is warranted other than periodic follow-up. If, on the other hand, the margins are positive and/or perineural neural or angiolymphatic invasion is apparent, then additional surgery and/or radiation must be considered. There are several problematic issues in the diagnosis of minimally invasive CXPA:

First, pathologists must be aware that the capsule around a pleomorphic adenoma is often focally absent, even in tumors of the major salivary glands. Just because a pleomorphic

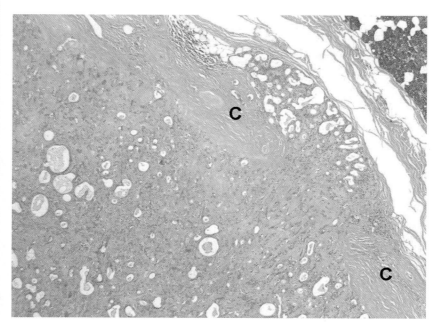

Fig. 26. Minimally invasive carcinoma arising in a pleomorphic adenoma. The tumor has completely breached the capsule (C) of the adenoma and extents laterally on the surface (H&E, original magnification x40).

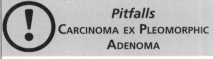

Differential Diagnosis
CARCINOMA EX PLEOMORPHIC ADENOMA

- Pleomorphic adenoma with pseudopodia
- De novo salivary carcinomas of all types

adenoma abuts normal salivary parenchyma without a capsular interface does not always indicate invasion.

Second, capsular invasion like in the thyroid can be very subjective. Not infrequently, small foci of tumor cells can be seen in the capsule of an otherwise benign pleomorphic adenoma and should not be mistaken for invasion. To qualify for invasion, tumor should completely penetrate the capsule and, ideally, extend laterally over the capsular surface in a "mushroom" fashion.

Third, distinguishing pseudopods of a pleomorphic adenoma from microinvasion can be difficult. Recuts may be helpful. In addition, look for a desmoplastic reaction and/or a condensation of myofibroblasts (supplemented with an alpha smooth muscle actin stain), which is more compatible with invasion than a pseudopod.[97]

Fourth, the carcinomas, by definition, are small and often difficult to subclassify. In these instances, a diagnosis of carcinoma, not otherwise specified type, either low or high grade, may have to suffice.

INVASIVE CXPA

Invasive CXPA is defined as a carcinoma that extends more than 1.5 mm from the capsule of a pleomorphic adenoma.[89] They represent 5% to 10% of all pleomorphic adenomas and, on the average, occur in individuals who are 10 to 15 years older than those with benign pleomorphic adenomas. Most studies indicate a female predilection. Approximately two-thirds of all invasive CXPAs occur in the parotid gland, with the rest about

Pitfalls
CARCINOMA EX PLEOMORPHIC ADENOMA

! An acellular sclerotic calcific nodule within a carcinoma may be the only residual evidence of a preexisting pleomorphic adenoma.

equally divided between the submandibular and minor salivary glands.[98] The typical history is that of a patient with a long-standing salivary neoplasm that starts to rapidly increase in size and is associated with pain and occasionally facial palsy.

Although any of the salivary carcinomas may arise in a pleomorphic adenoma, in our experience most are high grade and are usually an adenocarcinoma not otherwise specified, salivary duct carcinoma, or a myoepithelial carcinoma. In most cases, the carcinoma comprises more than half of the tumor volume. In some instances, the only histologic evidence of an underlying pleomorphic adenoma may be a residual sclerotic, hyalinized nodule.

Treatment and prognosis depend on stage and histologic type, but treatment usually necessitates wide excision with removal of regional lymph nodes often supplemented by postoperative radiation. In a review of 66 cases with a mean follow-up of 3.2 years, Lewis and colleagues[96] observed that 23% developed local recurrences, 56% developed regional metastasis, 44% developed distant metastasis, and 53% died of disease with an overall 5-year survival rate of 30%. Based on the types of carcinoma arising in a pleomorphic adenoma, Tortoledo and colleagues[95] observed the 5-year survival rate to be 30% for undifferentiated carcinomas, 50% for myoepithelial carcinomas, 62% for ductal carcinomas, and 96% for terminal duct carcinoma.

POLYMORPHOUS LOW-GRADE ADENOCARCINOMA

OVERVIEW

Polymorphous low-grade adenocarcinoma (PLGA) was the term given by Evans and Batsakis in 1984[99] to describe this distinct salivary gland tumor, although it was described earlier as "terminal duct carcinoma" and "lobular carcinoma," and may have even composed a subset of earlier papillary adenocarcinomas.[100–102] The increasing recognition of this tumor has led to its increasing prevalence in series, and comprises approximately 20% of all malignant tumors. There is a female predilection with a female:male ratio of approximately 2:1 in most series.[38,103–105]

PLGA is a tumor that occurs almost exclusively in the minor salivary glands, and of these, 60% to 80% arise in the palate. Other common sites include the lip and buccal mucosa. PLGA is a tumor of adults, with a wide age range, although the peak incidence in the sixth decade.[2]

PLGA typically presents as a nontender swelling at the hard-soft palate junction. Erythema and even ulceration of the mucosa may occur. Palate tumors are typically smaller than extrapalatal tumors. Pain and nerve paralysis are not common findings with PLGA. Bone erosion/involvement may be seen in approximately one-quarter of palate tumors, and virtually all nasopharyngeal PLGAs will show bone involvement.[37]

GROSS FEATURES

PLGA are usually firm, ovoid, white masses. Although they are not encapsulated, they often appear well delineated. Gross cystic change is not common.

MICROSCOPIC FEATURES

PLGA, as its name would suggest, has a great variety of growth patterns: solid, tubular, cribriform, and papillary. Although grossly not extremely infiltrative, microscopically, a highly permeative border is typical of PLGA. PLGA often replaces and permeates adjacent seromucinous acini. Tubules may stream, giving the appearance of a single-file growth pattern similar to lobular carcinoma of the breast (hence the earlier name for PLGA). Often within a tumor, targetoid whorls of infiltrating cells can be seen. Despite the variety of growth patterns this tumor displays (**Fig. 27**), the cytomorphologic features of the tumor cells are, in contrast, monomorphic. Tumor cells have varying degrees of eosinophilic cytoplasm. Nuclei are ovoid, with delicate powdery, often cleared chromatin reminiscent of papillary thyroid carcinoma nuclei. Although it is an adenocarcinoma, PLGA can deposit myxohyaline matrix in a similar fashion to tumors with myoepithelial cells such as adenoid cystic carcinoma (ACC). Tyrosinelike

---

Key Features
POLYMORPHOUS LOW GRADE ADENOCARCINOMA

- Polymorphous low-grade adenocarcinoma arises mainly in the minor salivary glands and is historically confused with adenoid cystic carcinoma because of similarities in growth pattern and propensity for perineural invasion.

- Polymorphous low-grade adenocarcinomas show a variety of growth patterns (solid, tubular, cribriform, and papillary), but consist of one basic cell type with ovoid nuclei and vesicular chromatin.

- Papillary predominant tumors are generally more aggressive, as are extrapalatal tumors.

---

crystals can be seen in 3% to 5% of PLGAs. Papillary patterned tumors may show psammoma bodies as well. Angiolymphatic invasion is not common, and it tends to occur more frequently in papillary predominant PLGA. Mitotic rates are low, and tend to be less than 3 per 10 high power fields.[2,37,38,105]

Immunohistochemically, this is a "monophasic" tumor, composed of a ductal phenotype. As such, PLGA will be positive for low molecular weight cytokeratins (CK7, CK 18, CK 19). Very focally, there may be some phenotypic divergence with a few cells, particularly those embedded in myxohyaline stroma, showing focal myoepithelial marker expression, namely for p63, actin, or calponin. One useful marker for PLGA is S100, which shows a diffuse, strong reactivity in tumor cells (**Fig. 28**A).[38,105] C-kit is usually negative and, when present, only focally positive (see **Fig. 28**B).[39]

DIFFERENTIAL DIAGNOSIS

Historically, PLGA has been vastly underrecognized as a diagnostic category, although recognition of this diagnostic category has improved[2,5,105]; however, in one recent series, overdiagnosis has now emerged as the more frequent problem.[37] It is also important to note that this danger of overdiagnosis of PLGA is more prominent in uncommon sites (ie, parotid). The main diagnostic considerations include ACC, pleomorphic adenoma (PA), and epithelial-myoepithelial carcinoma (EMCa). The specific distinction from each of these tumors is outlined in the following paragraphs, but briefly, PLGA is separated based on: (1) the recognition of the PLGA characteristic nuclear features, and (2) recognition of the monophasic ductal phenotype in PLGA (in contrast to the biphasic nature of these other diagnostic considerations).

When PLGA was described, the classic "misdiagnosis" for this tumor was ACC. This distinction can indeed be a troublesome one on biopsy, but with adequate material, this differential diagnosis is fairly simple. PLGA is a composed of cells with ovoid vesicular nuclei, whereas ACC is composed of angulated hyperchromatic nuclei (**Fig. 29**). As

---

△△ Differential Diagnosis
POLYMORPHOUS LOW-GRADE ADENOCARCINOMA

- Adenoid cystic carcinoma
- Pleomorphic adenoma
- Epithelial-myoepithelial carcinoma

Fig. 27. Different patterns in PLGA. (*A*) Tubular pattern percolating through normal salivary acini (*arrow*) (H&E, original magnification ×200). (*B*) Cribriform pattern (H&E, original magnification ×200).

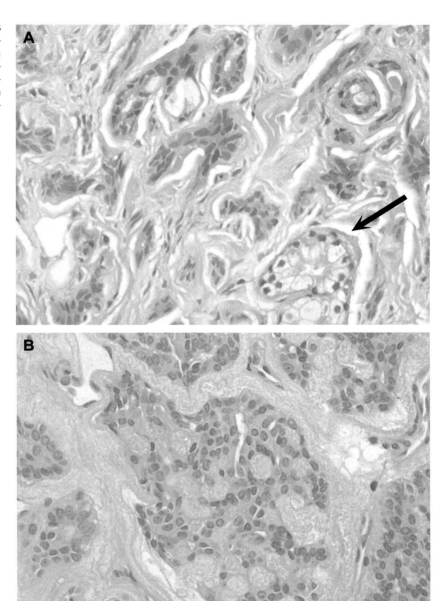

mentioned, PLGA is a monophasic tumor composed of cells with a ductal phenotype, whereas ACC is a clearly biphasic tumor with a dual population of ducts and myoepithelial cells. When this is not readily apparent on light microscopy, immunostains can highlight the presence of abluminal myoepithelial cells (p63 and actin) in ACC. Furthermore, PLGAs are strongly S100 positive, whereas ACCs are variably positive to negative.[37,38] Conversely, ACC is diffusely strongly positive for c-kit, whereas PLGA is variably positive to

negative.[39] Thus, with adequate sampling, this distinction can be readily resolved.

The distinction of PLGA from PA can also be troublesome, as both can produce myxohyaline stroma and can even demonstrate tyrosinelike crystals. Furthermore, PAs in the palate, although well demarcated, are not always encapsulated. However, PLGA is a carcinoma; thus, any evidence of perineural or angiolymphatic invasion is useful in the distinction from PA. More specifically, however, despite the morphologic diversity in PA,

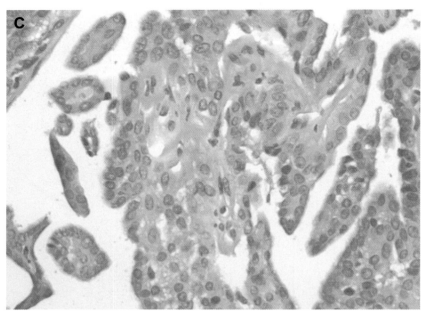

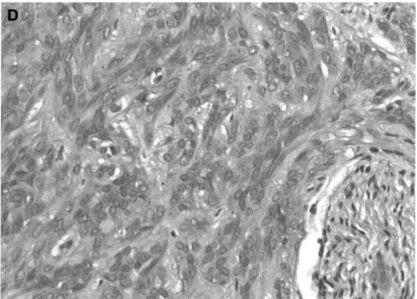

Fig. 27. (*C*) Papillary pattern (H&E, original magnification ×200). (*D*) Solid pattern (H&E, original magnification ×200) with perineural invasion (*right*). Regardless of pattern, all tumor cells are monomorphic, bland, and composed of ovoid nuclei with vesicular to cleared chromatin reminiscent of papillary thyroid carcinoma nuclei.

it is still a biphasic tumor with ducts and myoepithelial cells, unlike PLGA.[105]

In one recent series, EMCa was the most common named tumor type misdiagnosed as PLGA.[37] Both share several similarities in that they are low-grade carcinomas that can be arrayed in a variety of patterns and contain myxohyaline stroma. Although the prototypical EMCa has large polygonal clear myoepithelial cells, many EMCa may show less of a clear-cell component, which

can lead to confusion with PLGA. The key to distinction is the recognition of a biphasic appearance on light microscopy or immunohistochemistry in EMCa.

TREATMENT AND PROGNOSIS

PLGAs tend to behave quite favorably, with deaths from disease rare. However, PLGA can recur locoregionally in about one-third of cases.[37,104]

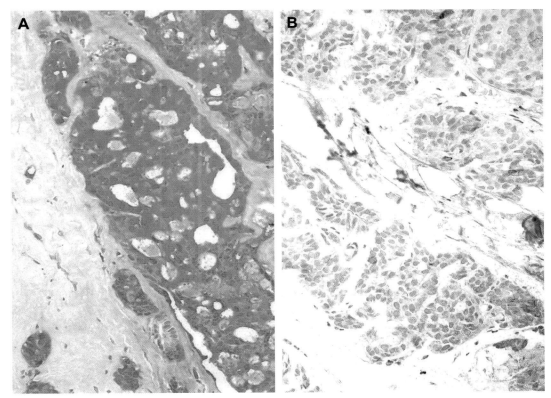

Fig. 28. (*A*) S100 showing strong positivity in PLGA (FAST RED chromogen hematoxylin counterstain, original magnification ×200). (*B*) C-kit when present is only focal (DAB chromogen hematoxylin counterstain, original magnification ×200).

Lymph node metastases are uncommon, ranging from 0% to 17%, and distant metastases are rare. Recurrences may be late, with a median disease survival ranging from 7 to 12 years. Factors reported to predict an aggressive behavior include margin status, vascular invasion, extrapalatal site, and papillary growth.[37,104] Although perineural invasion is a frequent finding in PLGA, it may not be a significant predictor of recurrence, although large-nerve perineural invasion may be important.

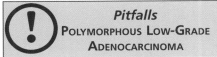

Pitfalls
POLYMORPHOUS LOW-GRADE ADENOCARCINOMA

! Small biopsies may not show adequate distinguishing features between adenoid cystic carcinoma and polymorphous low-grade adenocarcinoma.

! Major salivary gland polymorphous low-grade adenocarcinomas are rare, and other diagnoses should be considered before entertaining this possibility in the parotid or submandibular gland.

The presence of a papillary component in some PLGAs raises an important controversy. Some believe that tumors are different entities than PLGA with tubular or solid growth; however, given the large degree of morphologic overlap and absence of additional biologic understanding, papillary predominant tumors are kept as variants of PLGA.[105] Similarly, cribriform adenocarcinoma of the tongue has been proposed as an entity distinct from PLGA, because of its prominent cribriform growth, and high propensity for lymph node metastases. Again, there is too much morphologic overlap between this entity and standard PLGA to currently warrant classification as a distinct tumor.[106] Additionally, it must be noted that 3 additional noncribriform PLGAs of the tongue have been reported, all with lymph node metastases, suggesting that it is the location rather than tumor type that is responsible for this "unique" behavior.[37]

Very rarely, PLGA may progress or transform to a high-grade carcinoma, which can be potentially lethal.[107] It is also noted that almost one-half of PLGA recurrences show an "intermediate-grade" morphology, with increased mitotic activity and nuclear pleomorphism (**Fig. 30**).

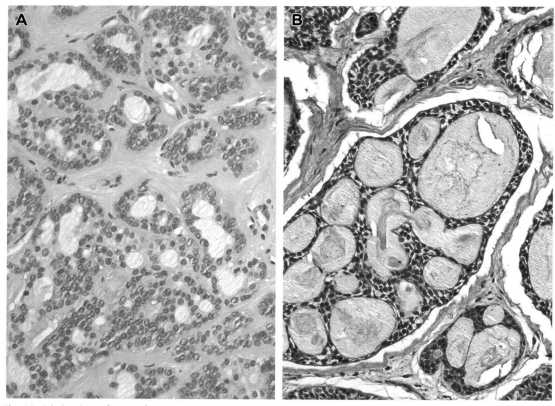

Fig. 29. Distinction of PLGA from ACC. (*A*) This PLGA shows ovoid vesicular nuclei, including some with clearing (H&E, original magnification ×200). (*B*) ACC, on the other hand, is composed of dark, angulated, hyperchromatic nuclei (H&E, original magnification ×200).

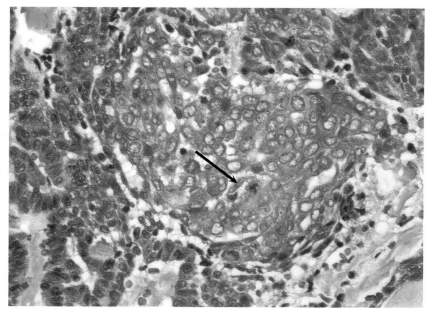

Fig. 30. Recurrent PLGA may show "intermediate-grade" features, such as nuclear atypia and increased mitotic activity (*arrow*, H&E, original magnification ×400).

Treatment of PLGA is mainly surgical with negative margins. Although this is readily feasible in palatal and oral tumors, it may be more difficult in the oropharynx and nasopharynx. Given the presence of bone invasion in one-quarter of tumors, the resection of sizeable palate tumors may include a portion of bone. Although radiotherapy is given for nasopharyngeal PLGA, these tumors recur despite this treatment suggesting that this is not particularly useful. Most tumors do not require a neck dissection[37,108]; however, some advocate that base of tongue tumors receive a neck dissection because of the high propensity for nodal metastases. Recurrent tumors can also be managed successfully by surgical excision. Adjuvant therapy may be warranted in rare cases with transformation to high-grade carcinoma.

MYOEPITHELIAL CARCINOMA

OVERVIEW

Myoepithelial carcinoma (MyoCA) is the term preferred by the World Health Organization to describe the malignant counterpart of myoepithelioma.[109] Malignant myoepithelioma is another popular synonym.

Although uncommon, MyoCAs are being recognized more frequently, and currently comprise about 10% to 30% of all myoepithelial neoplasms. They may arise de novo or in a pleomorphic adenoma (MyoCA ex pleomorphic adenoma). The mean age at diagnosis is about 50 to 60 years (range 16–85 years) with a male:female ratio of 1.0:1.0 to 1.3:1.0.[2–6,110–114] Approximately 55% arise in the parotid gland, 15% in the submandibular gland, and 30% in minor salivary glands (especially the palate).

Although most patients present with a relatively asymptomatic mass, pain and rapid enlargement may be seen.

GROSS FEATURES

Although tumors as large as 20 cm have been described, most are in the 3 to 5 cm range. On cut surface, the tumors are tan, yellow, white, or gray, often with areas of necrosis and margins that vary from well to poorly defined. More than 50% of MyoCAs are stated to arise from pleomorphic adenomas or preexisting myoepitheliomas and, accordingly, areas of blue-white opalescent cartilage may also be apparent.

MICROSCOPIC FEATURES

MyoCAs exhibit varying degrees of cellular pleomorphism, increased mitotic activity, perineural-

> **Key Features**
> **MYOEPITHELIAL CARCINOMA**
>
> - Myoepithelial carcinomas may arise de novo or from pleomorphic adenoma.
> - Cell types (spindled, epithelioid, clear cell, plasmacytoid) are identical to their benign counterparts in myoepitheliomas.
> - Myoepithelial carcinoma is immunophenotypically confirmed by the expression of keratins, and one or more smooth muscle–type markers, such as actin or calponin.
> - S100, p63, and vimentin can also be used to confirm a myoepithelial carcinoma diagnosis in the appropriate morphologic context.
> - Fifty percent to 60% of myoepithelial carcinomas will develop local recurrences, 30% to 50% will metastasize, and 30% to 45% of patients will die of their disease.

angiolymphatic invasion, necrosis and/or local invasion (**Figs. 31** and **32**). Occasionally, a tumor will be invasive yet show little evidence of pleomorphism or mitotic activity. Tumors with more than 7 mitoses/10 HPFs and a Ki-67 index greater than 10% are generally malignant, according to Nagao and colleagues.[111]

The range of cell types and growth patterns reflect those seen in their benign counterparts (see next section on "myoepithelioma"). Clear-cell myoepithelial neoplasms should always be viewed with skepticism. In our experience, this variant often appears deceptively benign but clinically over a period of time often recurs and may be locally aggressive. A "dedifferentiated" MyoCA has also been described.[115]

As with all myoepithelial neoplasms, there is no one immunohistochemical marker that is specific for myoepithelial lineage. As such, multiple stains may be necessary to establish a specific diagnosis. In a review of 18 MyoCAs, Savera and colleagues[112] observed that 89% expressed CAM 5.2, 100% AE 1/3, 92% 34BE12, 21% CK7, 53% CK14, 100% vimentin, 100% S-100 protein, 50% smooth muscle actin, 75% calponin, 31% muscle-specific actin, 31% glial fibrillary acidic protein, 0% carcinoembryonic antigen, and 21% epithelial membrane antigen.

DIFFERENTIAL DIAGNOSIS

The first order of business is distinguishing a myoepithelioma from a MyoCA. Features that are useful

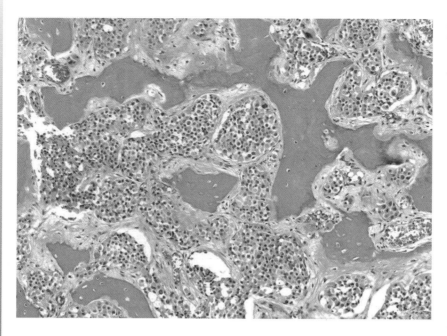

Fig. 31. Myoepithelial carcinoma, plasmacytoid variant, of palate invading bone (H&E, original magnification x100).

are listed previously. It must be emphasized again that some MyoCAs are low grade and may not exhibit all of the findings described. In this case, look for unequivocal evidence of invasion (angiolymphatic, perineural and/or parenchyma, soft tissue, bone), which is the sine qua non for distinguishing benign from malignant tumors.

The differential diagnosis varies according to the cellular composition of the MyoCA. For spindle-cell MyoCAs, amelanotic melanoma, monophasic synovial carcinoma, malignant peripheral nerve sheath tumor, and leiomyosarcoma must be considered. For the clear-cell MyoCA, clear-cell carcinoma of salivary origin, epithelial-myoepithelial carcinoma, and possibly even metastatic renal cell carcinoma should be excluded. The plasmacytoid MyoCA, especially on small biopsies, may be confused with an extramedullary plasmacytoma, whereas the epithelioid MyoCA can be mistaken for a variety of metastatic carcinomas.

Once the differential diagnosis is considered, a battery of appropriate immunostains, coupled with the clinical history, can usually point toward the correct diagnosis.

TREATMENT AND PROGNOSIS

MyoCAs should be widely excised with ample margins.[110–112] Because data indicate that cervical lymph node metastasis is uncommon, a neck dissection may not be warranted. Chemotherapy and radiation are largely untested.

Current experience indicates that about 50% to 60% of MyoCAs will develop local recurrences, 30% to 50% will metastasize, and 30% to 45% of patients will die of their disease.[110–112] Most metastases are directed to the lungs, liver, bones, kidneys, and occasionally regional lymph nodes. Most deaths occur within 5 years. There is no

 Differential Diagnosis
MYOEPITHELIAL CARCINOMA

- Myoepithelioma
- True sarcomas (synovial sarcoma, malignant peripheral nerve sheath tumor)
- Spindle-cell melanoma
- Epithelial-myoepithelial carcinoma
- Extramedullary plasmacytoma
- Metastatic carcinomas

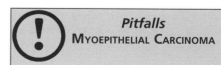 *Pitfalls*
MYOEPITHELIAL CARCINOMA

! The biologic behavior of clear-cell myoepithelial tumors may not be predictable on histologic features alone.

Fig. 32. Myoepithelial carcinoma, plasmacytoid variant. Higher magnification of **Fig. 31** showing cellular pleomorphism and 3 mitoses (H&E, original magnification x400).

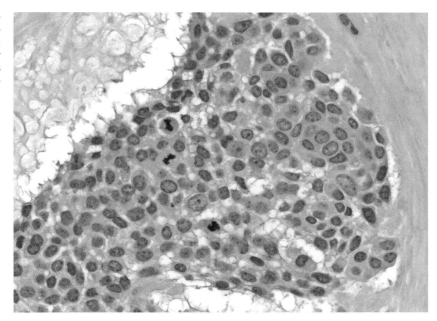

correlation with cell type and biologic behavior and no difference in clinical outcome of "de novo" MyoCAs versus those that arise in pleomorphic adenomas and/or myoepitheliomas.[109]

REFERENCES

1. Eveson JW, Auclair PL, Gnepp DR, et al. Tumors of the salivary glands: introduction. In: Barnes EL, Eveson JW, Reichart P, et al, editors. World Health Organization classification of tumours: pathology & genetics. Head and neck tumours. Lyon (France): IARCPress; 2005. p. 221–2.

2. Ellis G, Auclair PL. Tumors of the salivary glands. 4th series ed. Washington, DC: Armed Forces Institute of Pathology; 2008.

3. Myers EN, Ferris RL, editors. Salivary gland disorders. Berlin: Springer; 2007.

4. Eveson JW, Nagao T. Diseases of the salivary glands. In: Barnes L, editor. Surgical pathology of the head and neck, vol. 1. New York: Informa; 2009. p. 475–648.

5. Ellis G, Auclair P, editors. Tumors of the salivary glands. 3rd series edition. Washington, DC: Armed Forces Institute of Pathology; 1996. Atlas of tumor pathology; No. 17.

6. Seethala RR, Dacic S, Cieply K, et al. A reappraisal of the MECT1/MAML2 translocation in salivary mucoepidermoid carcinomas. Am J Surg Pathol 2010; 34(8):1106–21.

7. Auclair PL, Goode RK, Ellis GL. Mucoepidermoid carcinoma of intraoral salivary glands. Evaluation and application of grading criteria in 143 cases. Cancer 1992;69(8):2021–30.

8. Goode RK, Auclair PL, Ellis GL. Mucoepidermoid carcinoma of the major salivary glands: clinical and histopathologic analysis of 234 cases with evaluation of grading criteria. Cancer 1998;82(7): 1217–24.

9. Rutigliano DN, Meyers P, Ghossein RA, et al. Mucoepidermoid carcinoma as a secondary malignancy in pediatric sarcoma. J Pediatr Surg 2007; 42(7):E9–13.

10. Rahbar R, Grimmer JF, Vargas SO, et al. Mucoepidermoid carcinoma of the parotid gland in children: a 10-year experience. Arch Otolaryngol Head Neck Surg 2006;132(4):375–80.

11. Batsakis JG. Carcinoma ex papillary cystadenoma lymphomatosum. Malignant Warthin's tumor. Ann Otol Rhinol Laryngol 1987;96(2 Pt 1):234–5.

12. Pires FR, Alves Fde A, de Almeida OP, et al. Synchronous mucoepidermoid carcinoma of tongue and pleomorphic adenoma of submandibular gland. Oral Surg Oral Med Oral Pathol Oral Radiol Endod 2003;95(3):328–31.

13. Weinreb I, Seethala RR, Perez-Ordonez B, et al. Oncocytic mucoepidermoid carcinoma: clinicopathologic description in a series of 12 cases. Am J Surg Pathol 2009;33(3):409–16.

14. Luna MA. Salivary mucoepidermoid carcinoma: revisited. Adv Anat Pathol 2006;13(6):293–307.

15. Veras EF, Sturgis E, Luna MA. Sclerosing mucoepidermoid carcinoma of the salivary glands. Ann Diagn Pathol 2007;11(6):407–12.

16. Seethala RR. An update on grading of salivary gland carcinomas. Head Neck Pathol 2009;3(1): 69–77.

17. Alos L, Lujan B, Castillo M, et al. Expression of membrane-bound mucins (MUC1 and MUC4) and secreted mucins (MUC2, MUC5AC, MUC5B, MUC6 and MUC7) in mucoepidermoid carcinomas of salivary glands. Am J Surg Pathol 2005;29(6):806–13.

18. Kapadia SB, Barnes L. Expression of androgen receptor, gross cystic disease fluid protein, and CD44 in salivary duct carcinoma. Mod Pathol 1998;11(11):1033–8.

19. Carlson DL. Necrotizing sialometaplasia: a practical approach to the diagnosis. Arch Pathol Lab Med 2009;133(5):692–8.

20. Nance MA, Seethala RR, Wang Y, et al. Treatment and survival outcomes based on histologic grading in patients with head and neck mucoepidermoid carcinoma. Cancer 2008;113(8):2082–9.

21. Aro K, Leivo I, Makitie AA. Management and outcome of patients with mucoepidermoid carcinoma of major salivary gland origin: a single institution's 30-year experience. Laryngoscope 2008; 118(2):258–62.

22. Brandwein MS, Ivanov K, Wallace DI, et al. Mucoepidermoid carcinoma: a clinicopathologic study of 80 patients with special reference to histological grading. Am J Surg Pathol 2001;25(7):835–45.

23. Seethala RR. Histologic grading and prognostic biomarkers in salivary gland carcinomas. Adv Anat Pathol 2011;18(1):29–45.

24. Okabe M, Miyabe S, Nagatsuka H, et al. MECT1-MAML2 fusion transcript defines a favorable subset of mucoepidermoid carcinoma. Clin Cancer Res 2006;12(13):3902–7.

25. Anzick SL, Chen WD, Park Y, et al. Unfavorable prognosis of CRTC1-MAML2 positive mucoepidermoid tumors with CDKN2A deletions. Genes Chromosomes Cancer 2010;49(1):59–69.

26. Robin C, Laboulbene A. Memoire sur trois productions morbides non decrites. Compte Rend Soc Biol 1853;5(1):185–96.

27. el-Naggar AK, Huvos AG. Adenoid cystic carcinoma. In: Barnes EL, Eveson JW, Reichart P, et al, editors. World Health Organization classification of tumours: pathology & genetics. Head and neck tumours. Lyon (France): IARCPress; 2005. p. 221–2.

28. Foote FW Jr, Frazell EL. Tumors of the major salivary glands. Cancer 1953;6(6):1065–133.

29. Tauxe WN, Mc DJ, Devine KD. A century of cylindromas. Short review and report of 27 adenoid cystic carcinomas arising in the upper respiratory passages. Arch Otolaryngol 1962;75:364–76.

30. Albores-Saavedra J, Wu J, Uribe-Uribe N. The sclerosing variant of adenoid cystic carcinoma: a previously unrecognized neoplasm of major salivary glands. Ann Diagn Pathol 2006;10(1):1–7.

31. Gnepp DR, Heffner DK. Mucosal origin of sinonasal tract adenomatous neoplasms. Mod Pathol 1989; 2(4):365–71.

32. Seethala RR, Hunt JL, Baloch ZW, et al. Adenoid cystic carcinoma with high-grade transformation: a report of 11 cases and a review of the literature. Am J Surg Pathol 2007;31(11):1683–94.

33. Moskaluk CA, Frierson HF Jr, El-Naggar AK, et al. C-kit gene mutations in adenoid cystic carcinoma are rare. Mod Pathol 2010;23(6):905–6 [author reply: 906–7].

34. Greer RO Jr, Said S, Shroyer KR, et al. Overexpression of cyclin D1 and cortactin is primarily independent of gene amplification in salivary gland adenoid cystic carcinoma. Oral Oncol 2007;43(8): 735–41.

35. Seethala RR, Pasha TL, Raghunath PN, et al. The selective expression of CD43 in adenoid cystic carcinoma. Appl Immunohistochem Mol Morphol 2008;16(2):165–72.

36. Seethala RR, Barnes EL, Hunt JL. Epithelial-myoepithelial carcinoma: a review of the clinicopathologic spectrum and immunophenotypic characteristics in 61 tumors of the salivary glands and upper aerodigestive tract. Am J Surg Pathol 2007;31(1):44–57.

37. Seethala RR, Johnson JT, Barnes EL, et al. Polymorphous low-grade adenocarcinoma: the University of Pittsburgh experience. Arch Otolaryngol Head Neck Surg 2010;136(4):385–92.

38. Castle JT, Thompson LD, Frommelt RA, et al. Polymorphous low grade adenocarcinoma: a clinicopathologic study of 164 cases. Cancer 1999; 86(2):207–19.

39. Beltran D, Faquin WC, Gallagher G, et al. Selective immunohistochemical comparison of polymorphous low-grade adenocarcinoma and adenoid cystic carcinoma. J Oral Maxillofac Surg 2006; 64(3):415–23.

40. Andreadis D, Epivatianos A, Poulopoulos A, et al. Detection of C-KIT (CD117) molecule in benign and malignant salivary gland tumours. Oral Oncol 2006;42(1):57–65.

41. Emanuel P, Wang B, Wu M, et al. p63 Immunohistochemistry in the distinction of adenoid cystic carcinoma from basaloid squamous cell carcinoma. Mod Pathol 2005;18(5):645–50.

42. Perzin KH, Gullane P, Clairmont AC. Adenoid cystic carcinomas arising in salivary glands: a correlation of histologic features and clinical course. Cancer 1978;42(1):265–82.

43. Spiro RH, Huvos AG. Stage means more than grade in adenoid cystic carcinoma. Am J Surg 1992;164(6):623–8.

44. Fordice J, Kershaw C, El-Naggar A, et al. Adenoid cystic carcinoma of the head and neck: predictors of morbidity and mortality. Arch Otolaryngol Head Neck Surg 1999;125(2):149–52.

45. da Cruz Perez DE, de Abreu Alves F, Nobuko Nishimoto I, et al. Prognostic factors in head and neck adenoid cystic carcinoma. Oral Oncol 2006; 42(2):139–46.

46. Szanto PA, Luna MA, Tortoledo ME, et al. Histologic grading of adenoid cystic carcinoma of the salivary glands. Cancer 1984;54(6):1062–9.

47. Nagao T, Gaffey TA, Serizawa H, et al. Dedifferentiated adenoid cystic carcinoma: a clinicopathologic study of 6 cases. Mod Pathol 2003;16(12): 1265–72.

48. Vekony H, Ylstra B, Wilting SM, et al. DNA copy number gains at loci of growth factors and their receptors in salivary gland adenoid cystic carcinoma. Clin Cancer Res 2007;13(11):3133–9.

49. Rao PH, Roberts D, Zhao YJ, et al. Deletion of 1p32-p36 is the most frequent genetic change and poor prognostic marker in adenoid cystic carcinoma of the salivary glands. Clin Cancer Res 2008;14(16):5181–7.

50. Mitani Y, Li J, Rao PH, et al. Comprehensive analysis of the MYB-NFIB gene fusion in salivary adenoid cystic carcinoma: incidence, variability and clinicopathological significance. Clin Cancer Res 2010;16(19):4722–31.

51. Abrams AM, Cornyn J, Scofield HH, et al. Acinic cell adenocarcinoma of the major salivary glands. A clinicopathologic study of 77 cases. Cancer 1965;18:1145–62.

52. Ellis GL, Corio RL. Acinic cell adenocarcinoma. A clinicopathologic analysis of 294 cases. Cancer 1983;52(3):542–9.

53. Lewis JE, Olsen KD, Weiland LH. Acinic cell carcinoma. Clinicopathologic review. Cancer 1991;67(1): 172–9.

54. Hoffman HT, Karnell LH, Robinson RA, et al. National Cancer Data Base report on cancer of the head and neck: acinic cell carcinoma. Head Neck 1999;21(4):297–309.

55. Gomez DR, Katabi N, Zhung J, et al. Clinical and pathologic prognostic features in acinic cell carcinoma of the parotid gland. Cancer 2009;115(10): 2128–37.

56. Neto AG, Pineda-Daboin K, Spencer ML, et al. Sinonasal acinic cell carcinoma: a clinicopathologic study of four cases. Head Neck 2005;27(7):603–7.

57. Gnepp DR, Schroeder W, Heffner D. Synchronous tumors arising in a single major salivary gland. Cancer 1989;63(6):1219–24.

58. Di Palma S, Corletto V, Lavarino C, et al. Unilateral aneuploid dedifferentiated acinic cell carcinoma associated with bilateral-low grade diploid acinic cell carcinoma of the parotid gland. Virchows Arch 1999;434(4):361–5.

59. Auclair PL. Tumor-associated lymphoid proliferation in the parotid gland. A potential diagnostic pitfall. Oral Surg Oral Med Oral Pathol 1994;77(1):19–26.

60. Skalova A, Sima R, Vanecek T, et al. Acinic cell carcinoma with high-grade transformation: a report of 9 cases with immunohistochemical study and analysis of TP53 and HER-2/neu genes. Am J Surg Pathol 2009;33(8):1137–45.

61. Skalova A, Vanecek T, Sima R, et al. Mammary analogue secretory carcinoma of salivary glands, containing the ETV6-NTRK3 fusion gene: a hitherto undescribed salivary gland tumor entity. Am J Surg Pathol 2010;34(5):599–608.

62. Skalova A, Leivo I, Von Boguslawsky K, et al. Cell proliferation correlates with prognosis in acinic cell carcinomas of salivary gland origin. Immuno-histochemical study of 30 cases using the MIB 1 antibody in formalin-fixed paraffin sections. J Pathol 1994;173(1):13–21.

63. Ellis G, Simpson RH. Acinic cell carcinoma. In: Barnes EL, Eveson JW, Reichard P, et al, editors. World Health Organization classification of tumors. Pathology and genetics. Head and neck tumors. Lyon (France): IARC Press; 2005. p. 216–8.

64. Batsakis JG, Luna MA, el-Naggar AK. Histopathologic grading of salivary gland neoplasms: II. Acinic cell carcinomas. Ann Otol Rhinol Laryngol 1990;99(11):929–33.

65. Michal M, Skalova A, Simpson RH, et al. Well-differentiated acinic cell carcinoma of salivary glands associated with lymphoid stroma. Hum Pathol 1997;28(5):595–600.

66. el-Naggar AK, Batsakis JG, Luna MA, et al. DNA flow cytometry of acinic cell carcinomas of major salivary glands. J Laryngol Otol 1990;104(5): 410–6.

67. Barnes L, Rao U, Contis L, et al. Salivary duct carcinoma. Part II. Immunohistochemical evaluation of 13 cases for estrogen and progesterone receptors, cathepsin D, and c-erbB-2 protein. Oral Surg Oral Med Oral Pathol 1994;78(1):74–80.

68. Barnes L, Rao U, Krause J, et al. Salivary duct carcinoma. Part I. A clinicopathologic evaluation and DNA image analysis of 13 cases with review of the literature. Oral Surg Oral Med Oral Pathol 1994;78(1):64–73.

69. Afzelius LE, Cameron WR, Svensson C. Salivary duct carcinoma—a clinicopathologic study of 12 cases. Head Neck Surg 1987;9(3):151–6.

70. Brandwein MS, Jagirdar J, Patil J, et al. Salivary duct carcinoma (cribriform salivary carcinoma of excretory ducts). A clinicopathologic and immuno-histochemical study of 12 cases. Cancer 1990; 65(10):2307–14.

71. Lewis JE, McKinney BC, Weiland LH, et al. Salivary duct carcinoma. Clinicopathologic and immunohistochemical review of 26 cases. Cancer 1996;77(2): 223–30.

72. Williams MD, Roberts D, Blumenschein GR Jr, et al. Differential expression of hormonal and growth

factor receptors in salivary duct carcinomas: biologic significance and potential role in therapeutic stratification of patients. Am J Surg Pathol 2007; 31(11):1645–52.

73. Kleinsasser O, Klein HJ, Hubner G. Salivary duct carcinoma. A group of salivary gland tumors analogous to mammary duct carcinoma. Arch Klin Exp Ohren Nasen Kehlkopfheilkd 1968;192(1): 100–5 [in German].

74. de Araujo VC, Kowalski LP, Soares F, et al. Salivary duct carcinoma: cytokeratin 14 as a marker of in-situ intraductal growth. Histopathology 2002; 41(3):244–9.

75. Nagao T, Gaffey TA, Serizawa H, et al. Sarcomatoid variant of salivary duct carcinoma: clinicopathologic and immunohistochemical study of eight cases with review of the literature. Am J Clin Pathol 2004;122(2):222–31.

76. Simpson RH, Prasad AR, Lewis JE, et al. Mucin-rich variant of salivary duct carcinoma: a clinicopathologic and immunohistochemical study of four cases. Am J Surg Pathol 2003;27(8):1070–9.

77. Nagao T, Gaffey TA, Visscher DW, et al. Invasive micropapillary salivary duct carcinoma: a distinct histologic variant with biologic significance. Am J Surg Pathol 2004;28(3):319–26.

78. Dimery IW, Jones LA, Verjan RP, et al. Estrogen receptors in normal salivary gland and salivary gland carcinoma. Arch Otolaryngol Head Neck Surg 1987;113(10):1082–5.

79. Nasser SM, Faquin WC, Dayal Y. Expression of androgen, estrogen, and progesterone receptors in salivary gland tumors. Frequent expression of androgen receptor in a subset of malignant salivary gland tumors. Am J Clin Pathol 2003;119(6):801–6.

80. Hoang MP, Callender DL, Sola Gallego JJ, et al. Molecular and biomarker analyses of salivary duct carcinomas: comparison with mammary duct carcinoma. Int J Oncol 2001;19(4):865–71.

81. Delgado R, Klimstra D, Albores-Saavedra J. Low grade salivary duct carcinoma. A distinctive variant with a low grade histology and a predominant intraductal growth pattern. Cancer 1996;78(5):958–67.

82. Skalova A, Starek I, Vanecek T, et al. Expression of HER-2/neu gene and protein in salivary duct carcinomas of parotid gland as revealed by fluorescence in-situ hybridization and immunohistochemistry. Histopathology 2003;42(4):348–56.

83. Felix A, El-Naggar AK, Press MF, et al. Prognostic significance of biomarkers (c-erbB-2, p53, proliferating cell nuclear antigen, and DNA content) in salivary duct carcinoma. Hum Pathol 1996;27(6): 561–6.

84. Gnepp DR. Metastatic disease to the major salivary glands. In: Ellis G, Auclair PL, Gnepp DR, editors. Surgical pathology of the salivary glands. Philadelphia: WB Saunders; 1991. p. 560–9.

85. Fan CY, Wang J, Barnes EL. Expression of androgen receptor and prostatic specific markers in salivary duct carcinoma: an immunohistochemical analysis of 13 cases and review of the literature. Am J Surg Pathol 2000;24(4):579–86.

86. James GK, Pudek M, Berean KW, et al. Salivary duct carcinoma secreting prostate-specific antigen. Am J Clin Pathol 1996;106(2):242–7.

87. Eneroth CM, Blanck C, Jakobsson PA. Carcinoma in pleomorphic adenoma of the parotid gland. Acta Otolaryngol 1968;66(6):477–92.

88. Auclair PL, Ellis GL. Atypical features in salivary gland mixed tumors: their relationship to malignant transformation. Mod Pathol 1996;9(6):652–7.

89. Gnepp DR, Brandwein-Gensler MS, el-Naggar AK, et al. Carcinoma ex pleomorphic adenoma. In: Barnes EL, Eveson JW, Reichart P, et al, editors. World Health Organization classification of tumours: pathology & genetics. Head and neck tumours. Lyon (France): IARCPress; 2005. p. 242–3.

90. Brandwein M, Huvos AG, Dardick I, et al. Noninvasive and minimally invasive carcinoma ex mixed tumor: a clinicopathologic and ploidy study of 12 patients with major salivary tumors of low (or no?) malignant potential. Oral Surg Oral Med Oral Pathol Oral Radiol Endod 1996;81(6):655–64.

91. DeRoche TC, Hoschar AP, Hunt JL. Immunohistochemical evaluation of androgen receptor, HER-2/neu, and p53 in benign pleomorphic adenomas. Arch Pathol Lab Med 2008;132(12):1907–11.

92. Felix A, Rosa-Santos J, Mendonca ME, et al. Intracapsular carcinoma ex pleomorphic adenoma. Report of a case with unusual metastatic behaviour. Oral Oncol 2002;38(1):107–10.

93. Katabi N, Gomez D, Klimstra DS, et al. Prognostic factors of recurrence in salivary carcinoma ex pleomorphic adenoma, with emphasis on the carcinoma histologic subtype: a clinicopathologic study of 43 cases. Hum Pathol 2010;41(7):927–34.

94. LiVolsi VA, Perzin KH. Malignant mixed tumors arising in salivary glands. I. Carcinomas arising in benign mixed tumors: a clinicopathologic study. Cancer 1977;39(5):2209–30.

95. Tortoledo ME, Luna MA, Batsakis JG. Carcinomas ex pleomorphic adenoma and malignant mixed tumors. Histomorphologic indexes. Arch Otolaryngol 1984;110(3):172–6.

96. Lewis JE, Olsen KD, Sebo TJ. Carcinoma ex pleomorphic adenoma: pathologic analysis of 73 cases. Hum Pathol 2001;32(6):596–604.

97. de Araujo VC, Furuse C, Cury PR, et al. Desmoplasia in different degrees of invasion of carcinoma ex-pleomorphic adenoma. Head Neck Pathol 2007; 1(2):112–7.

98. Gnepp DR. Malignant mixed tumors of the salivary glands: a review. Pathol Annu 1993;(28 Pt 1): 279–328.

99. Evans HL, Batsakis JG. Polymorphous low-grade adenocarcinoma of minor salivary glands. A study of 14 cases of a distinctive neoplasm. Cancer 1984;53(4):935–42.

100. Allen MS Jr, Fitz-Hugh GS, Marsh WL Jr. Low-grade papillary adenocarcinoma of the palate. Cancer 1974;33(1):153–8.

101. Batsakis JG, Pinkston GR, Luna MA, et al. Adeno-carcinomas of the oral cavity: a clinicopathologic study of terminal duct carcinomas. J Laryngol Otol 1983;97(9):825–35.

102. Freedman PD, Lumerman H. Lobular carcinoma of intraoral minor salivary gland origin. Report of twelve cases. Oral Surg Oral Med Oral Pathol 1983;56(2):157–66.

103. Perez-Ordonez B, Linkov I, Huvos AG. Polymor-phous low-grade adenocarcinoma of minor sali-vary glands: a study of 17 cases with emphasis on cell differentiation. Histopathology 1998;32(6): 521–9.

104. Evans HL, Luna MA. Polymorphous low-grade adenocarcinoma: a study of 40 cases with long-term follow up and an evaluation of the importance of papillary areas. Am J Surg Pathol 2000;24(10): 1319–28.

105. Luna MA, Wenig BM. Polymorphous low-grade adenocarcinoma. In: Barnes EL, Eveson JW, Sidransky D, editors. Pathology and genetics of head and neck tumors. Lyons (France): World Health Organization; 2005. p. 223–4.

106. Michal M, Skalova A, Simpson RH, et al. Cribriform adenocarcinoma of the tongue: a hitherto unrecog-nized type of adenocarcinoma characteristically occurring in the tongue. Histopathology 1999; 35(6):495–501.

107. Simpson RH, Pereira EM, Ribeiro AC, et al. Poly-morphous low-grade adenocarcinoma of the sali-vary glands with transformation to high-grade carcinoma. Histopathology 2002;41(3):250–9.

108. Pogodzinski MS, Sabri AN, Lewis JE, et al. Retro-spective study and review of polymorphous low-grade adenocarcinoma. Laryngoscope 2006; 116(12):2145–9.

109. Skalova A, Jakel KT. Myoepithelial carcinoma. In: Barnes EL, Eveson JW, Reichart P, et al, editors. World Health Organization classification of tumours: pathology & genetics. Head and neck tumours. Lyon (France): IARCPress; 2005. p. 240–1.

110. Alos L, Cardesa A, Bombi JA, et al. Myoepithelial tumors of salivary glands: a clinicopathologic, immu-nohistochemical, ultrastructural, and flow-cytometric study. Semin Diagn Pathol 1996;13(2):138–47.

111. Nagao T, Sugano I, Ishida Y, et al. Salivary gland malignant myoepithelioma: a clinicopathologic and immunohistochemical study of ten cases. Cancer 1998;83(7):1292–9.

112. Savera AT, Sloman A, Huvos AG, et al. Myoepithe-lial carcinoma of the salivary glands: a clinicopath-ologic study of 25 patients. Am J Surg Pathol 2000; 24(6):761–74.

113. Yu G, Ma D, Sun K, et al. Myoepithelial carcinoma of the salivary glands: behavior and management. Chin Med J (Engl) 2003;116(2):163–5.

114. Bellizzi AM, Mills SE. Collagenous crystalloids in myoepithelial carcinoma: report of a case and review of the literature. Am J Clin Pathol 2008; 130(3):355–62.

115. Ogawa I, Nishida T, Miyauchi M, et al. Dedifferenti-ated malignant myoepithelioma of the parotid gland. Pathol Int 2003;53(10):704–9.

RARE MALIGNANT AND BENIGN SALIVARY GLAND EPITHELIAL TUMORS

Raja R. Seethala, MD[a],*, E. Leon Barnes, MD[b]

KEYWORDS

- Salivary gland • Malignant • Benign • Epithelial-myoepithelial carcinoma • Pleomorphic adenoma
- Adenoma • Basal • Oncocytoma • Warthin

ABSTRACT

Although at least 24 distinct histologic salivary gland carcinomas exist, many of them are rare, comprising only 1% to 2% of all salivary gland tumors. These include epithelial-myoepithelial carcinoma, (hyalinizing) clear cell carcinoma, basal cell adenocarcinoma, cystadenocarcinoma, low-grade salivary duct carcinoma (low-grade cribriform cystadenocarcinoma), oncocytic carcinoma, and adenocarcinoma not otherwise specified. Few tumors (clear cell carcinoma and basal cell adenocarcinoma) have unique molecular correlates. Benign tumors, although histologically less diverse, are far more common, with pleomorphic adenoma and Warthin tumor the most common salivary gland tumors. Many benign tumors have malignant counterparts for which histologic distinction can pose diagnostic challenge.

OVERVIEW

The World Health Organization currently recognizes 13 benign and 24 malignant primary epithelial neoplasms of salivary origin.[1] Many carcinomas are rare, comprising less than 3% of all tumors in most series.[1–4] Their recognition is important, however, because they often enter into the differential diagnosis of the more common salivary gland carcinomas and, in some cases, benign tumors. Benign tumors, alternatively, although less histologically diverse, are far more common that their malignant counterparts, with pleomorphic adenoma (PA) and Warthin tumor the most common. The focus of this review is on rare malignant epithelial neoplasms and benign tumors (**Box 1**).

RARE MALIGNANT TUMORS

EPITHELIAL-MYOEPITHELIAL CARCINOMA

Overview

Epithelial-myoepithelial carcinoma (EMCa) is a tumor that was described in 1972 by Donath and colleagues,[5] but like other salivary tumors, it has existed in the literature under a variety of different names, including adenomyoepithelioma, clear cell adenoma, and glycogen-rich adenoma.[6,7] This tumor is rare and comprises only 1% to 2% of all salivary tumors in most series. Gender distribution is nearly equal, although in some series there is a slight female predilection.[8,9]

EMCa is primarily a tumor of the parotid gland although can occur in minor salivary sites and the submandibular gland. EMCa has a wide age range and can occasionally be seen in the pediatric population. Similar to many other tumors, the peak incidence is the sixth decade.[9]

EMCa usually has an indolent presentation as a painless slowly growing swelling of the parotid gland. Pain and nerve paralysis are not common findings with EMCa.

[a] Department of Pathology, University of Pittsburgh Medical Center, A614.X PUH, 200 Lothrop Street, Pittsburgh, PA 15213, USA
[b] Department of Pathology, University of Pittsburgh Medical Center, A608 PUH, 200 Lothrop Street, Pittsburgh, PA 15213, USA
* Corresponding author.
E-mail address: seethalarr@upmc.edu

Surgical Pathology 4 (2011) 1217–1272
doi:10.1016/j.path.2011.07.006

surgpath.theclinics.com

Gross Features

EMCa is deceptively well circumscribed and may display a capsule. This tumor often is multinodular and, despite the nonaggressive border to these nodules, EMCa can be permeative in some cases (**Fig. 1**). Cystic change, although not common, can be seen. Approximately 2% of EMCa cases arise

from PAs; thus, evidence of lobular gray chondromyxoid stroma or areas of ossification may be seen.[8] On average, an EMCa is less than 3 cm.

Microscopic Features

EMCa tends to infiltrate in a multinodular fashion—tumor nests have a pushing rather than an angulated border. Partial encapsulation of one or more of these nodules is common. As the name suggests, EMCa is a prototypical biphasic tumor. Classically this tumor is composed of tubules and nests of cells with an outer layer consisting of large polygonal clear cells and an inner layer of small cuboidal eosinophilic ductal cells.[8,9] The ratio of myoepithelial cells to ductal cells is approximately 2:1 to 3:1 although overgrowth of either component may be seen. Tumor nests are often embedded in a myxohyaline stroma (**Fig. 2**). Occasionally, the myoepithelial component is so prominent that the ductal elements are compressed and not readily apparent by light microscopy (**Fig. 3**).

More recently, several variant morphologies have been described. Two of the named variants include oncocytic-sebaceous EMCa and apocrine EMCa.[10] These variants challenge the notion that clear cell change is a requisite for the diagnosis of EMCa. In oncocytic-sebaceous EMCa, both components may show oncocytic change. Bilayered papillae are common, and tubules are of larger caliber than in classic EMCa (**Fig. 4**). Unlike the flat cuboidal cells in the ducts of classic EMCa, oncocytic-sebaceous EMCa often has columnar eosinophilic ductal cells. Sebaceous metaplasia is common in this variant. Apocrine EMCa has an oncocytoid or pink appearance. This variant often has an overgrowth of the ductal element in either a solid or cribriform pattern. But these areas are surrounded by an outer polygonal myoepithelial cell layer. The ductal cells show apocrine features, namely decapitation secretions and vacuolated cytoplasm.

Aside from these variants, other changes may be seen. The myoepithelial cells may have a spindled appearance (**Fig. 5**) and display verocay-like palisading. Degenerative atypia or ancient change may be observed. Other changes, such as squamous metaplasia, are also common. Rarely, not only is the myoepithelial component clear in appearance but also the ductal component (ie, double-clear EMCa).[8]

EMCa is typically bland with low mitotic activity. Approximately one-third of cases show perineural invasion; angiolymphatic invasion and necrosis are rare. EMCa occasionally progresses to a high histologic grade. This progression can involve either cell type (**Fig. 6**). Occasionally, the

Fig. 1. EMCa gross appearance. This tumor is a homogenous tan white and has a well-demarcated border. Despite this innocuous pushing border, this tumor has infiltrated the adjacent skeletal muscle (*left*).

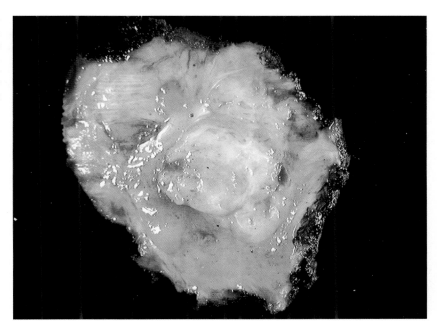

myoepithelial component shows severe atypia or anaplasia with overgrowth.[8] Conversely, EMCa with high-grade transformation, similar to other low-grade carcinomas with high-grade transformation, involves tumor progression of the ductal component, although Roy and colleagues[11] use this term to include transformation of either component.

Immunohistochemically, this is the prototypical biphasic tumor. The ductal component is positive for low molecular weight cytokeratins (CK7, CK18, and CK19) whereas the myoepithelial cells are positive for p63, actin, calponin, and vimentin (**Fig. 7**). For the myoepithelial markers, p63 and vimentin have the best performance. When applying a pankeratin cocktail, both the ductal and

Fig. 2. Classic EMCa. Even at this magnification the bilayered appearance is readily visible. This tumor is composed of a back-to-back tubular proliferation with a polygonal clear cell outer layer and a cuboidal inner ductal layer with pale eosinophilic cytoplasm ($\times$100). These are embedded in a sclerotic stroma (*upper left*).

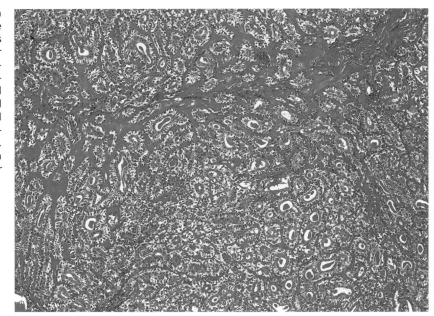

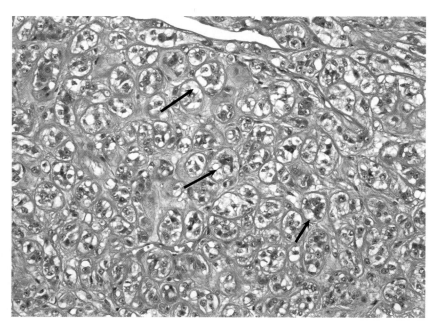

Fig. 3. EMCa with myoepithelial overgrowth. In this tumor the ductal elements are compressed and difficult to visualize (*arrows*) on routine hematoxylin-eosin–stained sections (×200).

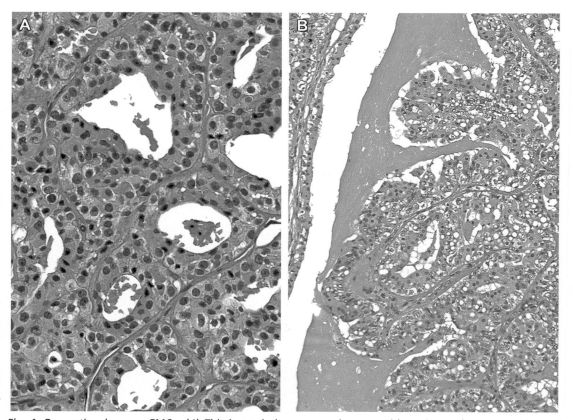

Fig. 4. Oncocytic-sebaceous EMCa. (*A*) This is a tubular patterned tumor with an intensely oncocytic luminal ductal layer. The outer myoepithelial layer is also eosinophilic although slightly paler (×200). (*B*) Bilayered papillary growth is common in oncocytic-sebaceous EMCa (×100).

Fig. 5. EMCa with spindled myoepithelial component. Within this spindled proliferation, scattered compressed tubules are noted (*arrows*) (×200).

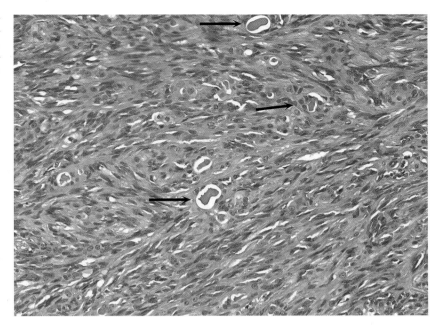

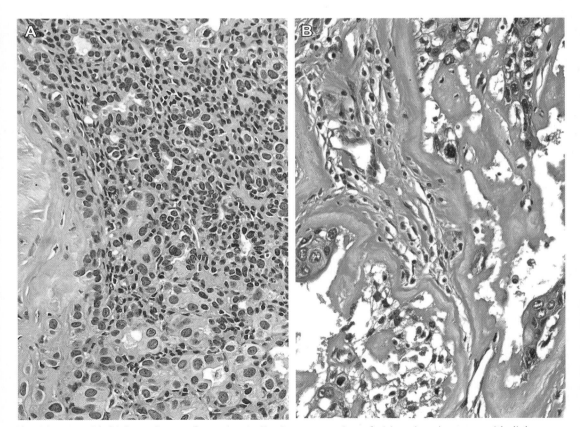

Fig. 6. EMCa with high-grade transformation indicating progression of either ductal or myoepithelial components. (*A*) Progression of the ductal component to a high-grade adenocarcinoma (*bottom*) (×200). (*B*) Anaplasia in the myoepithelial component with focal squamous metaplasia (×200).

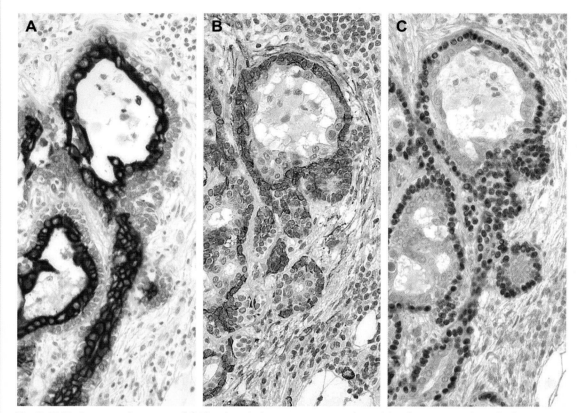

Fig. 7. EMCa immunophenotype. (*A*) The ductal elements are strongly positive for CAM 5.2 (×200). The myoepithelial elements are positive for (*B*) actin and (*C*) p63 (×200).

myoepithelial cells are positive, but ductal structures are more strongly positive than the myoepithelial components. S-100 may stain either the ductal or myoepithelial component and is thus not particularly useful for highlighting the biphasic nature of this tumor.[8] Oncocytic-sebaceous EMCa stains strongly for histochemical stains, such as Mallory phosphotungstic acid–hematoxylin stain (PTAH), or immunostains, such as antimitochondrial antibody. The ductal components of apocrine EMCa are positive for apocrine markers, such as gross cystic disease fluid protein 15 (GCDFP-15) and androgen receptor (AR).[10] Sebaceous elements may be positive for adipophilin or perilipin.[12]

Differential Diagnosis

Classic EMCa has a differential diagnosis that is different from the variants. Because classic EMCa is a clear cell predominant tumor, other clear cell tumors enter the differential diagnosis. EMCa is distinguished from clear cell myoepithelioma/myoepithelial carcinoma by the presence of ductular structures. In some situations, immunostaining is necessary to highlight the compressed ductules

in EMCa. From a purist perspective, myoepitheliomas should not have any ductular structures, although some accept a small ductal component.[9] Clear cell carcinoma (CCC) (also known as hyalinizing CCC) is a rare salivary carcinoma that may also be mistaken for EMCa. This tumor is monophasic; unlike EMCa, it can show extension along the outside of normal ducts, thus giving the semblance of a biphasic tumor. Current understanding of CCC is that this is a well-differentiated glycogenated squamous carcinoma of salivary type supported by ultrastructural and immunohistochemical evidence.[13] As such, CCCs are p63 and CK5/6 positive; unlike the clear cells in EMCa, these tumors are negative for actin, S-100, and calponin.[14] Other tumors, such as clear cell mucoepidermoid carcinoma (CCMEC) and metastatic renal cell carcinoma (RCC), may enter into the differential for EMCa, but these can be readily distinguished using immunostains to highlight the biphasic pattern in EMCa.

Oncocytic-sebaceous EMCa, alternatively, is a variant that can be confused with other oncocytic tumors. Again the key to distinction from other oncocytic or oncocytoid tumors is the recognition of a biphasic growth pattern. Oncocytoma and oncocytic carcinoma may show an attenuated layer of p63-positive tumor cells surrounding tumor nests, but these tumors are not arranged in a prominent bilayer as seen in oncocytic-sebaceous EMCa. Apocrine EMCa may be mistaken for salivary duct carcinoma, because salivary duct carcinoma is essentially an apocrine ductal carcinoma. There are rare EMCA salivary duct carcinoma hybrids described, suggesting that this variant is related to these hybrids. The apocrine components of a salivary duct carcinoma, however, are overtly malignant with mitoses and necrosis. Furthermore, these components are not surrounded by a myoepithelial component.[10]

Occasionally, EMCa may be difficult to differentiate from a cellular PA. PAs often have areas that mimic EMCa. With adequate material, EMCa is distinguished by the presence of invasion. The tumor normal interface may not be present on a biopsy, which renders this distinction virtually impossible. Some additional subtle features include the size of the myoepithelial cells. In EMCA, the myoepithelial component is composed of cells larger than the ductal cells. The nuclei often have an activated appearance with round contours and more vesicular chromatin. Additionally, the myoepithelial component does not blend into the surrounding stroma. In contrast, in cellular PA, the myoepithelial cells are often smaller than the ductal cells and may blend into a more chondromyxoid stroma than seen in EMCa.

Finally, in the sinonasal tract, EMCa can be confused with tubular adenoid cystic carcinoma (ACC) (as discussed in article elsewhere in this issue). Briefly, EMCa does not show as much clefting of tumor from the surrounding stroma and displays less nuclear angulation and hyperchromasia compared with tubular ACC. Altemani and

Pitfalls
EPITHELIAL-MYOEPITHELIAL CARCINOMA

! Because up to three-quarters of EMCa show c-kit immunopositivity, this marker alone cannot be used to distinguish this tumor from ACC.

---

colleagues[15] have suggested that CD10 positivity in EMCa can be used to distinguish this tumor from ACC. Up to three-quarters of EMCa may express c-kit; thus, this is not necessarily a useful marker for the distinction. ACC and EMCa may coexist as hybrids, and, beyond that, occasional ACC may show EMCa-like areas and vice versa. The convention in these cases is to classify the tumor according to predominant morphology.

Treatment and Prognosis

EMCa has an excellent prognosis with a 5-year survival rate of 94% and a 10-year survival rate of 86%.[8] Recurrences are frequent, present in almost 40%, but these usually occur late, on average 11 years after diagnosis.[8] In some cohorts, the EMCa is more aggressive, possibly due to selection bias for cases with adverse histologic parameters.[16–18] Myoepithelial anaplasia/overgrowth, margin status, necrosis, and vascular invasion are the strongest predictors of recurrence. Both lymph node metastases and distant metastases are rare.

Most cases of EMCa are treated surgically with complete excision. Adjuvant therapy is usually not given unless a tumor is not completely resectable. A neck dissection is typically not warranted because the frequency of lymph node metastases is low.

EMCas with high-grade transformation, alternatively, represent an aggressive group of tumors that may be rapidly lethal. As such, aggressive management of this variant may be warranted.[11]

(HYALINIZING) CLEAR CELL CARCINOMA

Overview

CCC—also known as CCC not otherwise specified, clear cell adenocarcinoma, and hyalinizing CCC—is an uncommon tumor with a predilection for older adults (median 53 years; range 1–86 years) and female gender (1.6:1).[19–22] In a review of 103 cases, Wang and colleagues[22] observed that 67% arose from the minor salivary glands of the oral cavity, 21% from the parotid gland, 8% from the submandibular gland, and 4% in

---

Differential Diagnosis
EPITHELIAL-MYOEPITHELIAL CARCINOMA

- Clear cell myoepithelioma/myoepithelial carcinoma
- Hyalinizing CCC
- Metastatic RCC
- Oncocytoma/oncocytic carcinoma
- Salivary duct carcinoma
- Cellular pleomorphic adenoma
- ACC (tubular)

miscellaneous sites. In the oral cavity, almost half of all cases involve the palate.

Most patients present with a localized submucosal painless mass of several months to years duration covered by an intact, rarely ulcerated surface. Metastases at the time of diagnosis are uncommon.

Gross Features

CCCs are firm and gray-white and rarely exceed 3 cm. Although some may appear circumscribed, closer inspection reveal infiltrating margins.

Microscopic Features

CCCs are composed of solid sheets, nests, and cords of round to polygonal cells with optically clear cytoplasm (**Fig. 8**). The nuclei are predominately round with smooth to slightly irregular nuclear membranes and are moderately chromatic and may contain small nucleoli (**Fig. 9**). The clear appearance of the cytoplasm is due mainly to a large content of glycogen. Small groups of cells with pale eosinophilic cytoplasm are occasionally seen scattered among the more typical clear cells as well as small foci of squamous metaplasia (**Fig. 10**). Ducts are not observed and mitoses are sparse to absent. Involvement of nerves and invasion of adjacent soft tissue and/or bone are common. Some tumors contain thick bands of collagen, which often appear hyalinized (so-called hyalinizing CCC) (see **Fig. 10**).

Key Features
CLEAR CELL CARCINOMA

- CCC is a rare low-grade salivary gland malignancy that is most common in the oral cavity, often in the palate.

- CCC is composed of infiltrative cords and nests of clear to eosinophilic cells embedded in a fibrosclerotic stroma.

- Current understanding of this tumor suggests a well-differentiated squamous phenotype as supported by frequent squamous metaplasia and p63 and CK5/6 positivity.

- Recently a novel fusion of *EWSR1-ATF1* has been found in almost all CCCs.

CCCs are devoid of intracytoplasmic mucin and, on immunostaining, are positive for cytokeratin (AE 1/3 and CAM 5.2); variably reactive for epithelial membrane antigen, carcinoembryonic antigen, and S-100 protein; and negative for myoepithelial markers.[20,23] One common misconception regarding CCC is that it is an adenocarcinoma. Immunophenotypic and morphologic evidence (discussed previously) support the notion that this is a well-differentiated squamous tumor because these tumors are uniformly p63 and CK5/6 positive.[13,14] Most are also negative for vimentin.

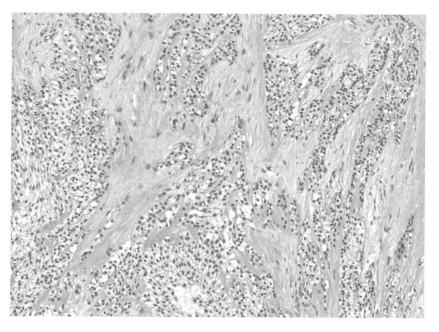

Fig. 8. CCC with dense bands of collagen (hyalinizing CCCs).

Fig. 9. CCC, high magnification. The cytoplasm is clear and well defined. The nuclei are basically round with smooth to irregular nuclear membranes. Some cells contain nucleoli.

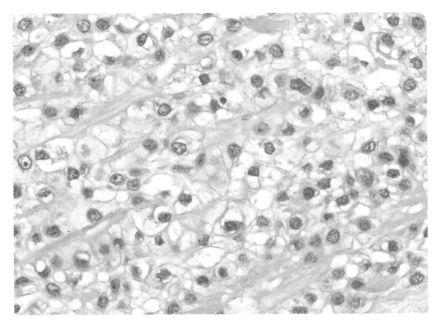

Ultrastructural studies also support a squamous phenotype, including tight junctions, desmosomal attachments, tonofilaments, microvilli, and basal lamina.[13] No evidence of myoepithelial derivation has been observed. Glycogen is usually conspicuous but zymogen granules, fat, mucin, and neurosecretory granules are not.

Recently, a novel fusion of *EWSR1-ATF1* has been found in almost all CCC.[24]

Differential Diagnosis

Salivary tumors, both primary and secondary, composed either focally or predominantly of clear

Fig. 10. CCC. Some tumors contain an admixture of cells with eosinophilic cytoplasm. Note the perineural invasion.

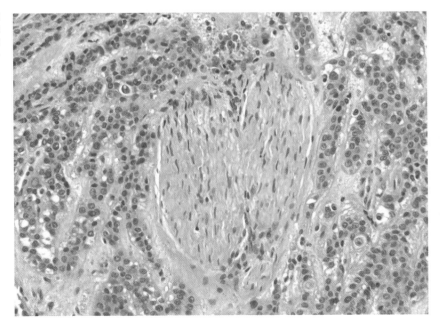

cells, are not uncommon.[21,22] In most cases, the diagnosis can be "clearly" established by clinical correlation, more thoroughly sampling of the tumor, and the use of histochemical and immuno-histochemical stains. Some tumors may be more problematic. Among these include clear cell myoepithelial carcinoma, EMCa, clear cell odontogenic carcinoma (CCOC), and metastatic RCC.

Distinguishing CCC from clear cell myoepithelial carcinoma is straightforward. The only problem is failing to consider it in the differential diagnosis. Clear cell myoepithelial carcinoma is composed of a monomorphic population of myoepithelial cells that happen to be clear (usually due to glycogen content) and, accordingly, are positive not only for cytokeratin but also for a variety of my-oepithelial muscle markers.[21,22,25] CCC is devoid of myoepithelial cells.

EMCa is a biphasic neoplasm composed of my-oepithelial and epithelial cells arranged in a charac-teristic pattern—ducts lined by cuboidal epithelial cells surrounded by multiple layers of optically clear myoepithelial cells that are absent in CCC. Distinguishing CCC from CCOC can be difficult or impossible at times. CCOC is a rare intraoss-eous tumor of the jaws that predilects the mandible over the maxilla by a ratio of 2–5:1.[14,26] It has been described in patients from age 17 to 89 years (mean 65 years) and is 2 to 3 times more common in women. Clinically, it is locally aggressive with a propensity for multiple local recurrences (55%) and may metastasize to regional lymph nodes (21%) or more distant sites (17%). Immunophenotypically and morphologi-cally, there is significant overlap between CCC and CCOC, although CCOC tends to have more prominent peripheral palisading reminiscent of ameloblastoma.[14] Ultimately a predominant intra-osseous location is the most important criteria for distinction of CCOC from CCC. It is unknown at this point whether *EWSR1-ATF1* is useful for separation of these tumors.

Differential Diagnosis
Clear Cell Carcinoma

- EMCa
- Clear cell myoepithelioma/myoepithelial carcinoma
- Metastatic RCC
- CCMEC
- CCO

Pitfalls
Clear Cell Carcinoma

! CCC and CCOC cannot reliably be distin-guished by morphology alone, location is required.

Metastatic RCC of the clear cell type is usually associated with necrosis, prominent vascular lakes, and occasionally papillary structures. As opposed to CCC, RCC is positive for CD10, RCC antigen, and vimentin. CCC is also positive for high molecular weight cytokeratin 903 whereas RCC is negative.[27]

Treatment and Prognosis

CCC is a low-grade neoplasm with an excellent prognosis usually managed by wide local excisim. Low recurrence (10%–15%) and regional lymph node metastasis (15%–20%) may be observed but dissemination below the clavicles is exceptional.[14,20–22]

BASAL CELL ADENOCARCINOMA
Overview

Basal cell adenocarcinoma (BCAC) is an un-common, low-grade salivary neoplasm considered the malignant counterpart of basal cell adenoma (BCA). It occurs almost exclusively in adults aver-aging age 60 years (range 27–92 years) and affects both genders equally.[3] Approximately 80% arise in the parotid gland, 10% in the submandibular gland and 10% in minor salivary glands (palate, tongue, cheek, and sinonasal tract).[3,28,29]

Most present as an asymptomatic, slowly enlarging mass. Tenderness and pain are uncommon. Like BCAs, approximately 15% of BCACs are associated with multiple cutaneous adnexal tumors, especially cylindromas and trichoepitheliomas.[3]

Gross Features

BCACs average 2 cm to 3 cm (range 0.7–7 cm) and on cut surface are uniformly tan or gray-white (**Fig. 11**). Necrosis and cyst formation are uncommon. Although some are well demarcated, most BCACs have gross tumor margins that are either partially or totally poorly defined and blend into the adjacent nontumorous parenchyma.

Microscopic Features

BCACs are essentially caricatures of BCAs and, as such, are composed of aggregates of basaloid

Fig. 11. Gross Appearance of a BCAC. The tumor shows a fibrous tan cut surface with only a slightly irregular interface with the surrounding parotid tissue.

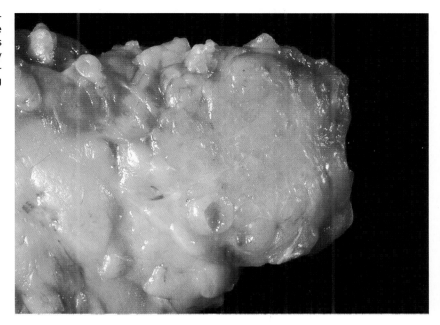

cells arranged in solid, trabecular, tubular, and membranous patterns. Although some appear partially encapsulated, suggesting an origin from a pre-existing BCA, all BCACs by definition are invasive (**Fig. 12**).

The basaloid cells are of 2 types: a small cell with a hyperchromatic round nucleus and sparse cytoplasm and a larger, more polygonal cell with a pale, basophilic round nucleus often with a nucleolus and more ample basophilic to slightly eosinophilic cytoplasm. The larger cells tend to occupy the center of the tumor clusters whereas the smaller cells are more apparent at the periphery where they frequently palisade (**Fig. 13**). The ratio of these 2 cells in any given tumor is highly variable,

and in some tumors, one cell type dominates to the exclusion of the others. Sporadic squamous eddies, occasional ducts, mitoses (typically 3 or more per 10 high-power fields), angiolymphatic and perineural invasion, focal necrosis, and mild cellular pleomorphic are often apparent (see **Fig. 13; Fig. 14**).

Immunohistochemical reactivity is variable among tumors. Similar to BCAs, BCACs also show a distinctive pattern of staining. The outermost small or dark basal cells are vimentin, p63, high molecular weight keratin, and actin positive, indicating myoepithelial differentiation. The adjacent large or pale basal cells are only p63, high molecular weight keratin, and vimentin positive, indicating a purely basal phenotype. Finally the ductules that are present to varying degrees are positive only for lower molecular weight keratins.[29] BCAC may also be focally positive for S-100 protein, epithelial membrane antigen, and carcinoembryonic antigen.

Differential Diagnosis

The differential diagnosis includes BCA, ACC, basaloid squamous cell carcinoma, and cutaneous basal cell carcinoma.

BCA is an encapsulated, noninvasive tumor with no plemorphism, sparse to absent mitotic activity, low Ki-67 proliferative index (mean 2%), and absent p53 immunoreactivity.[30] BCAC, alternatively, is invasive and occasionally exhibits mild pleomorphism and mitoses (usually 3 or more

Key Features
BASAL CELL ADENOCARCINOMA

- BCACs most frequently occur in the parotid gland and occasionally are associated with multiple skin adnexal tumor syndromes: cylindromas and trichoepitheliomas.

- BCACs show growth patterns that are similar to their benign counterparts, including tubulotrabecular, membranous, and solid.

- BCACs are usually low grade with an indolent behavior with only rare cases with distant metastases and lethal outcomes.

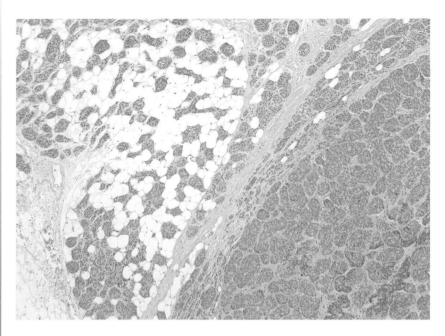

Fig. 12. Growth pattern of BCAC (×40). Although bland, BCAC are defined by their infiltrativeness, as seen here.

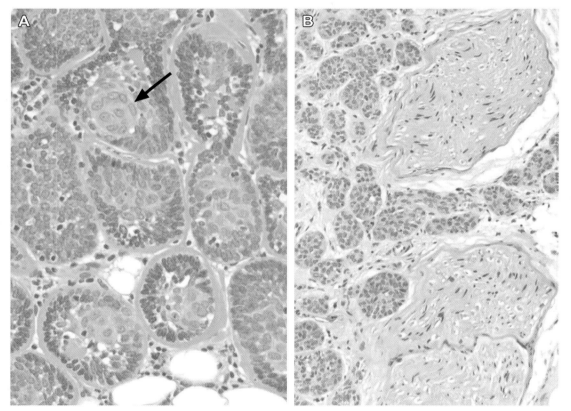

Fig. 13. (*A*) Squamous pearls (*arrow*) in BCAC (×100); note the peripheral palisading of the outermost dark layer. (*B*) Perineural invasion by a tubular patterned BCAC (×100).

Fig. 14. BCAC (200) may have an increased mitotic count (*arrows*).

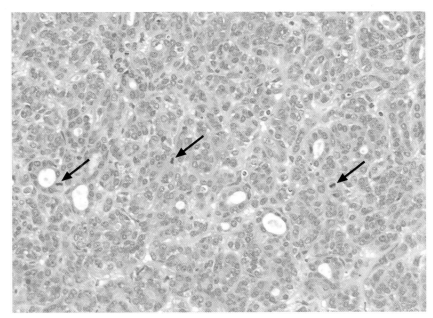

per 10 high-power fields) with a Ki-67 proliferation of 5% or more. It is also positive for p53 in approximately half the cases. In contrast to the findings of Nagao and colleagues,[30] the authors have not found immunostaining for bcl-2 and epidermal growth factor receptor helpful in separating these 2 lesions.

ACC can usually be distinguished by the cytologic appearance of the tumor cells. In ACC, the cells have nuclei that are small, hyperchromatic, and angulated whereas the nuclei in BCAC are round and less chromatic. ACC also has a greater Ki-67 proliferative index than BCAC (usually 20% or higher). Biopsies of ACC, even of the solid variant, frequently exhibit a classic cribriform pattern not seen in BCAC. Squamous eddies and peripheral palisading of nuclei, likewise, are more characteristic of BCAC. Although both tumors may be positive for c-kit, the staining is more diffuse and intense in ACC and only focal in BCAC.

Basaloid squamous cell carcinoma is a variant of squamous cell carcinoma and not a salivary neoplasm. It is characterized by prominent comedonecrosis, frequent mitoses, and an in situ mucosal origin.

Distinguishing a cutaneous basal cell carcinoma with secondary involvement of the parotid gland from a BCAC can be problematic, especially if the cutaneous lesion has been previously excised without knowledge of the pathologist. The presence of extensive scarring (from previous surgery) should alert the pathologist to this possibility and the need to inquire and review previous biopsies. In lieu of this, look for a dual population of basaloid cells, scattered ducts among the basaloid cells, and basaloid cells with myoepithelial differentiation.

Treatment and Prognosis

Local excision with tumor-free margins is the treatment of choice. A neck dissection is not indicated. In a review of 72 BCACs with a mean follow-up of 54 months, the incidence of local recurrence, positive cervical lymph nodes, and distant metastasis

---

△△ **Differential Diagnosis**
BASAL CELL ADENOCARCINOMA

- BCA
- ACC
- Basaloid squamous cell carcinoma
- (Cutaneous) basal cell carcinoma

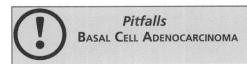

(!) **Pitfalls**
BASAL CELL ADENOCARCINOMA

! BCACs can have squamous and sebaceous elements.

was 37%, 8%, and 4%, respectively.[3] Only one patient (2%) actually died of disease. Whether BCACs that arise in minor salivary glands are more aggressive than those of the major salivary glands, as suggested by some investigators, is debatable.

CYSTADENOCARCINOMAS

Overview

Similar to their benign counterparts, cystadeno-carcinomas represent a group of cystic malignant salivary tumors that do not fit into other named categories. These are tumors with no particular gender predilection. Approximately 60% of cysta-denocarcinomas occur in the parotid gland, with the palate the second most common site. Cysta-denocarcinoma is one of the more frequent sali-vary gland tumors found in the sublingual gland. Cystadenocarcinomas are predominantly a tumor found in the fifth to eighth decades.[3,31]

Cystadenocarcinomas typically present as slow-growing painless masses, although a subset may have pain and facial nerve paralysis. Palatal tumors may erode bone.

Gross Features

These tumors are typically well demarcated, although not encapsulated, and are typically multi-cystic. The solid components are typically a homogenous tan white.

Key Features
CYSTADENOCARCINOMA

- Although many salivary gland carcinomas can have cystic predominance, cystadenocar-cinomas are cystic salivary gland malignan-cies that do not otherwise fit into named tumor category.

- Cystadenocarcinomas often grow in an arborizing pattern and often contain a complex papillary architecture regardless of histologic grade.

- Cystadenocarcinomas may have an intraduc-tal component as highlighted by p63 immu-nostaining.

Microscopic Features

Cystadenocarcinomas demonstrate diverse mor-phologies and cell types. One common feature, however, is the complex arborizing papillary growth pattern, often with micropapillae (**Fig. 15**). Tumor nests may be embedded in a sclerotic stroma. Tubular and cribriform growth may be noted focally but should not be prominent. Luminal calcifications are common. The cells lining these cysts range from small and cuboidal (**Fig. 16**) to tall and columnar. Cystadenocarcinomas may be composed mainly of oncocytes but more frequently contain cells with slightly eosinophilic

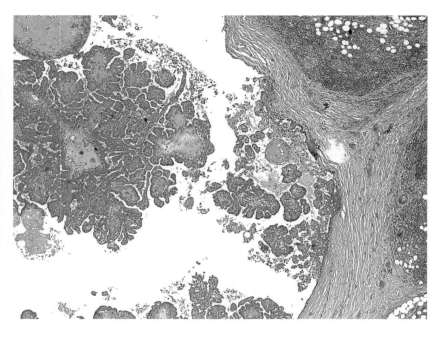

Fig. 15. Complex papil-lary and micropapillary growth in cystadenocar-cinoma (×40).

Fig. 16. Cytomorphologic features in cystadenocarcinoma (×100). This tumor is composed of monomorphic, multilayered cuboidal cells with slightly eosinophilic cytoplasm.

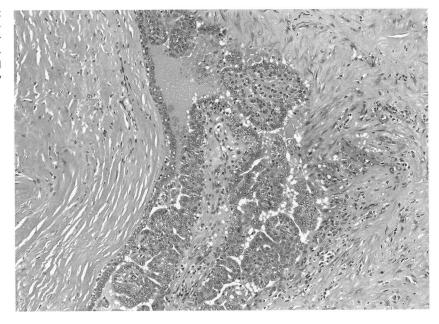

cytoplasm. When columnar cell predominate, there is often stratification of this columnar layer (**Fig. 17**). Mucocytes and epidermoid areas may be scattered throughout in some tumors designated as cystadenocarcinomas. Although not universal, a subset of cystadenocarcinomas has an indistinct delimiting basal layer similar to low-grade salivary duct carcinoma (LGSDC) (or low-grade cribriform cystadenocarcinoma).[32] Tumors are typically low grade, although approximately 5% may be high grade.

Immunohistochemical stains are similar to those seen in LGSDC. Many cystadenocarcinomas are in part surrounded by a delimiting p63, CK5/6-positive basal layer, although higher-grade lesions are often negative. The luminal cuboidal to

Fig. 17. Columnar cell predominant cystadenocarcinoma (×200). This tumor has an almost enteric appearance with higher-grade cytology and stratification of columnar cells.

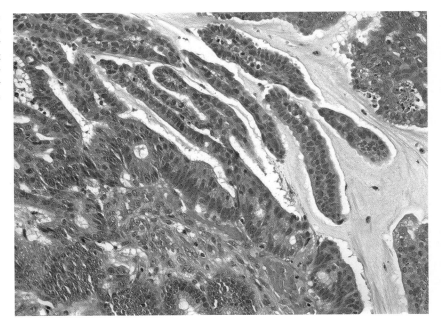

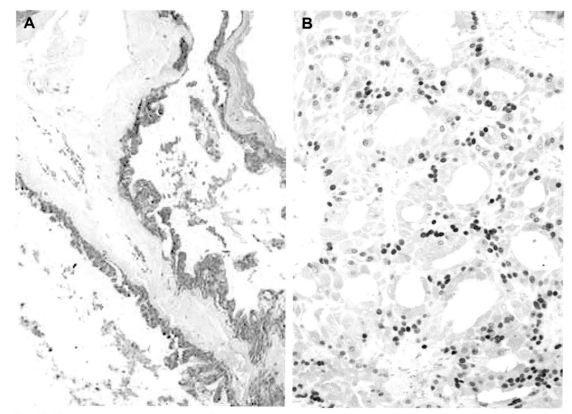

Fig. 18. Common immunophenotype of cystadenocarcinoma. (*A*) This tumor is S-100 positive (×100). (*B*) p63 shows a delimiting cell layer similar to LGSDC.

columnar cells are positive for low molecular weight keratins, such as CK7, CK8, and CK18, and, like LGSDC, are often strongly positive for S-100, although S-100 negative cases occur (**Fig. 18**).[32] Areas of oncocytic change may be highlighted by antimitochondrial antibody stains.

Differential Diagnosis

Cystadenocarcinomas are distinguished from LGSDC by morphologic heterogeneity of cell types and occurrence outside the parotid gland. Additionally, cribriform growth in cystadenocarcinomas is only focal; instead, papillary growth predominates, unlike LGSDC. Also, higher-grade cystadenocarcinomas may have no evidence of a delimiting basal layer nor are necessarily S-100 positive.[32] Cystadenocarcinomas are distinguished from cystadenoma by architectural complexity and evidence for infiltration.[31]

Cystadenocarcinomas should also be distinguished from the papillary cystic growth pattern of other named tumor types, such as acinic cell carcinoma. Acinic cell carcinomas with this growth

pattern show a characteristic hobnailed appearance to the vacuolated cells lining papillae and cysts and, additionally, acinar cell may be demonstrated on careful examination or using periodic acid–Schiff stains after diastase treatment.[31] On the high-grade end of the spectrum, cystadenocarcinomas must be distinguished from cystic salivary duct carcinomas. The latter tend to have

△△ **Differential Diagnosis**
CYSTADENOCARCINOMA

- Cystadenoma
- LGSDC (low-grade cribriform cystadenocarcinoma)
- Acinic cell carcinoma (papillary cystic variants)
- Salivary duct carcinoma
- Mucoepidermoid carcinoma

Pitfalls
CYSTADENOCARCINOMA

! Oncocytic cystadenocarcinomas can show scattered mucous cells mimicking MEC.

Key Features
LOW-GRADE SALIVARY DUCT CARCINOMA

- LGSDCs (low-grade cribriform cystadenocarcinomas) resemble low-grade ductal carcinoma in situ or atypical ductal hyperplasia of the breast.

- These tumors are characteristically predominantly intraductal with an attenuated delimiting p63-positive peripheral cell layer.

- Tumors are typically S-100 positive but may rarely show apocrine areas and transition to conventional salivary duct carcinoma.

a more vacuolated oncocytoid cytoplasm and may show decapitation secretions. Furthermore, nuclei are more vesicular with prominent nucleoli in salivary duct carcinoma. Finally, immunostains for apocrine markers, such as GCDFP-15 and AR, are positive in salivary duct carcinomas but negative in cystadenocarcinomas.[33] Oncocytic cystadenocarcinomas with mucous cells may be difficult do discriminate from oncocytic MECs. Oncocytic cystadenocarcinomas, however, do not show areas of epidermoid or intermediate cell subpopulations. In difficult cases, assessment for the *MECT1-MAML2* translocation may resolve these two because this translocation is diagnostic of MEC.[34,35]

Treatment and Prognosis

As a group, cystadenocarcinomas tend to be indolent and behave favorably with complete surgical excision. Recurrences and regional metastases occur in approximately 10%. Distant metastases and a lethal course for cystadenocarcinomas are rare.[3,31]

LOW-GRADE SALIVARY DUCT CARCINOMA (LOW-GRADE CRIBRIFORM CYSTADENOCARCINOMA)

Overview

LGSDC, also known as low-grade cribriform cystadenocarcinoma, was first described by Delgado and colleagues[36] in 1996. This is a tumor with approximately equal gender predilection.[36,37] LGSDCs arise almost exclusively in the parotid gland, although one case has been described in the submandibular gland.[37] Typically, these are tumors of the sixth to seventh decades. LGSDC are typically painless slow growing masses. Pain and facial nerve paralysis are generally not seen.

Gross Features

These tumors are typically well demarcated, although not encapsulated, with a uniform tan to white cut surface. These tumors range from solid to cystic.

Microscopic Features

This tumor is typically composed of an unencapsulated solid to cribriform to cystic proliferation of bland tumor cells (**Fig. 19**) resembling low-grade ductal carcinoma in situ or atypical ductal hyperplasia of breast. Micropapillary and tubular growth patterns may be seen. Tumor cells are round with scant cytoplasm and monomorphic nuclei with indistinct nucleoli. Careful examination of the outer layer of tumor nests reveal a flattened attenuated basal layer around the majority of nests. As the alternate designation of low-grade cribriform cystadenocarcinoma indicates, cystic change is common, and subsequent hemosiderosis of the epithelium may be observed. Many of these tumors may show areas of moderate cytologic atypia and oncocytic change with nuclear enlargement, vesicular chromatin, and nucleolation, although increased mitotic activity and necrosis are not seen (**Fig. 20**). Rarely, apocrine rather than oncocytic change, may be observed, suggesting the capability of transition to conventional salivary duct carcinoma.[38] Perineural and angiolymphatic invasion are rare. Many investigators regard this tumor as an in situ or intraductal carcinoma because of this general lack of infiltrative parameters.

Immunohistochemical stains support that LGSDC are in situ, meaning that the majority of tumor nests are surrounded by a delimiting p63, CK5/6, actin positive basal/myoepithelial layer. Aside from this layer, the tumor is a ductal neoplasm showing positivity for low molecular weight keratins, such as CK7, CK8, and CK18. Additionally, LGSDC are strongly positive for S-100 (**Fig. 21**). Histochemical stains show intraepithelial iron deposition in many cases. Areas of oncocytic change may be highlighted by antimitochondrial antibody stains.

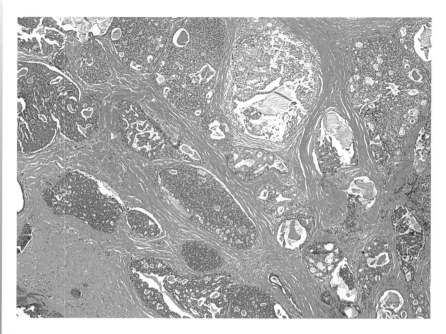

Fig. 19. LGSDC showing a cribriform and cystic proliferation in a sclerotic stroma (×40).

Rarely, apocrine areas are observed, and these may be positive for AR and GCDFP-15.[38]

Differential Diagnosis

It is important to distinguish LGSDC from its far more aggressive conventional counterpart. In most cases this is straightforward since conventional salivary duct carcinomas are high grade, infiltrative, and have high mitotic activity and necrosis. Purely in situ forms of conventional salivary duct carcinoma exist, however, which may be confusing because they also have a delimiting outer basal layer, although these have more pronounced atypia than LGSDC.[39] Both invasive and in situ conventional salivary duct carcinoma are tumors with an

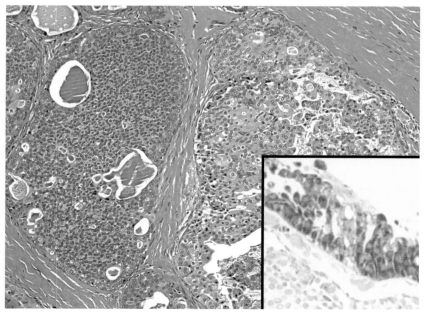

Fig. 20. Tumor cells are typically a monomorphic bland tumor composed of small cuboidal cells with scant eosinophilic cytoplasm (*left*), although oncocytic change and modest nuclear atypia may be seen (*right*) (×200). Inset (×200): iron stain highlighting intraepithelial hemosiderin deposits in a cystic area.

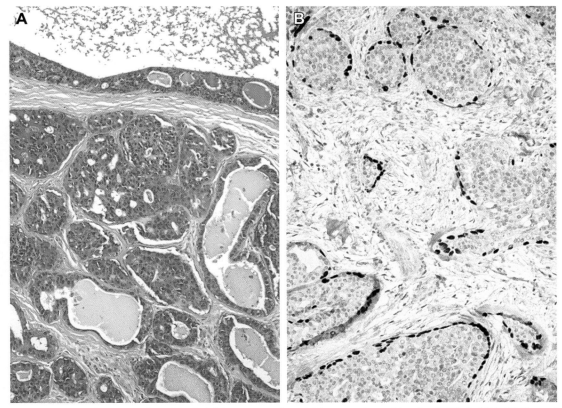

Fig. 21. Immunophenotype for LGSDC. (*A*) Tumors are invariably strongly positive for S-100 (×100). (*B*) There is a delimiting basal/myoepithelial layer around most tumor nests as highlighted by this p63 immunostain (×100), which has led many to designate this tumor as a low-grade intraductal carcinoma (×200).

apocrine predominant phenotype, unlike LGSDC, which usually has only focal apocrine change. The apocrine phenotype is characterized immunohisto-chemically by GCDFP-15 and AR.[33] Conventional salivary duct carcinoma is also often positive for Her-2/neu and almost always negative for S-100. Tumors with both an LGSDC and apocrine phenotype have been described.[38]

LGSDCs may resemble polymorphous low-grade adenocarcinoma (PLGA) in that both are bland and low-grade malignancies. Additionally both are S-100 positive. PLGA, however, does not have a delimiting basal/myoepithelial cell layer and is more infiltrative than LGSDC. LGSDC has an alternate designation of low-grade cribriform cystadenocarcinoma and as such may be confused with other cystadenocarcinomas. Cystadenocarcinomas can more frequently occur outside the parotid gland and may be composed of more heterogeneous cell types ranging from columnar to oncocytic to mucinous. Additionally, cystadenocarcinomas may be intermediate or high grade.[31] Occasionally, acinic cell carcinomas with a predominance of intercalated duct type

Differential Diagnosis
LOW-GRADE SALIVARY
DUCT CARCINOMA

- Conventional salivary duct carcinoma in situ
- Polymorphous low-grade adenocarcinoma
- Cystadenocarcinoma
- Acinic cell carcinom

Pitfalls
LOW-GRADE SALIVARY DUCT
CARCINOMA

! Oncocytic change in LGSDC may result in moderate nuclear enlargement and pleomorphism, which may raise concern for a higher-grade tumor; however, these areas do not have mitoses or necrosis.

cells may resemble LGDSC and may be S-100 positive. These show evidence of acinar differentiation on careful examination. Additionally, acinic cell carcinomas do not have a delimiting p63-positive outer layer.

Treatment and Prognosis

LGSDCs have a favorable prognosis with no recurrences reported to date. Treatment is purely surgical with compete excision curative.

ONCOCYTIC CARCINOMA

Overview

Oncocytic carcinomas are the malignant counterparts of oncocytoma and are among the rarest of salivary gland carcinomas, comprising less than 1% of all salivary gland carcinomas. Similar to oncocytomas, these are typically tumors of the elderly usually occurring in the sixth decade and beyond.[3] Aside from these points, understanding of oncocytic carcinomas based on prior studies is likely incorrect in that many of these tumors are more accurately classified as solid salivary duct carcinomas.

The vast majority of oncocytic carcinomas occur in the parotid gland, although other sites have been described. Unlike oncocytomas, an antecedent radiation history is not as commonly observed. Oncocytic carcinomas have presentation that ranges from indolent akin to oncocytoma to highly aggressive.[3] One-third of patients are

Key Features
ONCOCYTIC CARCINOMA

- Oncocytic carcinoma is among the rarest of salivary gland malignancies and mainly a parotid tumor seen in the elderly.

- Oncocytic carcinomas often resemble oncocytomas but show infiltration.

- The biologic behavior of oncocytic carcinoma is obscured by the likely inclusion of solid salivary duct carcinomas within this category.

reported to have facial nerve paralysis or pain. Many patients have bulky lymphadenopathy. Unlike oncocytomas, bilateral masses are not common.

Gross Features

Oncocytic carcinomas are typically more fibrotic and paler than oncocytomas. Although some are well demarcated, oncocytic carcinomas tend to be more infiltrative. Multinodularity may be observed.

Microscopic Features

Oncocytic carcinomas are also composed of polygonal oncocytes that may be arranged in solid, trabecular, and occasionally a compressed

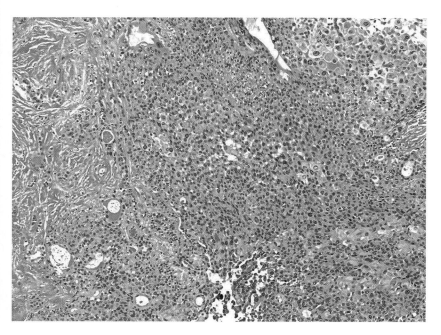

Fig. 22. Oncocytic carcinoma showing an irregular border and sclerosis (×100).

Fig. 23. Oncocytic carcinoma showing areas of cytologic atypia (×400).

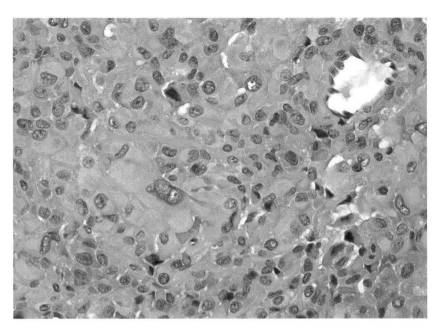

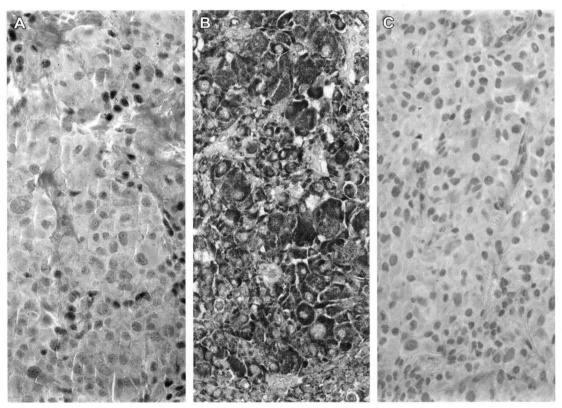

Fig. 24. Immunophenotype of oncocytic carcinoma. Similar to oncocytoma, solid growth in oncocytic carcinoma often represents compressed solid trabeculae. (*A*) As such, the periphery of such trabeculae often retain p63 positivity (×200) similar to their benign counterparts. (*B*) Oncocytic carcinomas are also strongly positive for antimitochondrial antibody (×200) and (*C*) negative for AR (×200).

tubular growth pattern. Unlike oncocytomas, on-cocytic carcinomas may have more interstitial sclerosis and infiltration of their capsule (**Fig. 22**). Nuclei are larger with more prominent nucleoli and membrane irregularities than seen in oncocytoma (**Fig. 23**).[40] Mitoses may be present. The darker cells in the periphery of oncocytomas are often seen in oncocytic carcinoma. Similar to oncocytoma, clear cell change may be prominent. Many prior reports of oncocytic carcinoma indicate a highly infiltrative growth pattern with high mitotic rates and necrosis.[3,41,42] This has not been the authors' experience, however, and all such cases of aggressive oncocytic carcinoma in the authors' files have shown foci of apocrine differentiation and been positive for AR and GCDFP-15, indicating that these are better regarded as solid salivary duct carcinomas. The authors suspect that many oncocytic carcinomas previously reported are actually solid salivary duct carcinomas.

Similar to oncocytomas, oncocytic carcinomas also show a striated duct phenotype. In areas, a p63-positive outer layer is retained suggesting that oncocytic carcinomas are related to their benign counterparts (**Fig. 24**A). Alternatively, the majority of tumor cells are more of a ductal luminal phenotype (CK7, CK18, and CK19 positive). Oncocytic carcinomas also demonstrate abundant cytoplasmic often ultrastructurally abnormal mitochondria and are strongly positive for PTAH and antimitochondrial antibody (see **Fig. 24**B). AR should be negative (see **Fig. 24**C).

Differential Diagnosis

Oncocytic carcinomas are distinguished from their benign counterparts by the presence of infiltration or perineural or angiolymphatic invasion. Oncocytic carcinomas also have more nuclear atypia and mitotic activity. As alluded to previously, however, the major problematic area is the

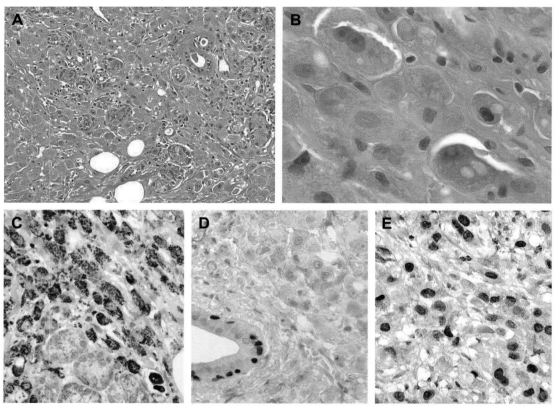

Fig. 25. Solid salivary duct carcinoma misdiagnosed as oncocytic carcinoma. (*A*) The tumor shows diffuse permeative growth infiltrating normal acini and resembles oncocytic carcinoma (×100). (*B*) Many of the cells have a microvacuolated appearance (×100). (*C*) Salivary duct carcinomas may be very oncocytoid and have abundant mitochondria as seen on this antimitochondrial antibody stain (×200); (*D*) p63, however, shows no peripheral staining (left normal striated duct internal control). (*E*) AR is diffusely strongly positive.

distinction of oncocytic carcinoma from solid salivary duct carcinomas. Solid salivary duct carcinomas often have an oncocytoid appearance, which is likely the reason for misclassification in the authors' files (**Fig. 25**). Apocrine cells may actually have abundant mitochondria and may be positive for PTAH or antimitochondrial antibody. The apocrine cells of salivary duct carcinoma tend to have more of a microvacuolated appearance than true oncocytes.[10] The ultrastructural correlate is the presence of numerous secretory vacuoles. Solid salivary duct carcinomas are strongly GCDFP-15 and AR positive in contrast to true oncocytic carcinoma. Furthermore, in solid salivary duct carcinoma, there is no p63-positive peripheral component. Unlike the compressed tubulotrabecular solid growth of oncocytic carcinoma, solid salivary duct carcinomas are often more diffuse and sheetlike in growth. One likely limitation of prior series of oncocytic carcinoma is that this distinction is not made rigorously.[43]

Similar to oncocytoma, oncocytic carcinoma should be distinguished from metastatic RCC. The nuclei of oncocytic carcinoma may equate to Fuhrman grade III but, unlike RCC, these do not typically have blood lakes or the same vascular pattern. p63 is also useful as a discriminatory marker between RCC and oncocytic carcinoma. Although CD10 is more supportive of RCC, oncocytic carcinomas of the salivary gland are also occasionally positive.

Treatment and Prognosis

The reported prognosis for oncocytic carcinoma is poor, with a metastatic rate greater than 50% and a mortality rate greater than 33%. Deaths from disease typically occur within 2 years. Distant metastases have been reported and include lung, mediastinum, and bone. Lymph node metastases are frequent in reported series.[3,41–43] Given the confusion with solid salivary duct carcinoma, it is unclear whether this is an accurate assessment of biologic behavior. In the authors' experience, after these solid salivary duct carcinomas are excluded, oncocytic carcinoma has a far more indolent behavior.[40] Given the assumed biologic behavior resported in literature, oncocytic carcinomas are treated aggressively with surgery, neck dissection, and radiotherapy. Lower-grade oncocytic carcinomas, which are actually more likely the norm, may be treated by surgical excision alone.

ADENOCARCINOMA NOT OTHERWISE SPECIFIED

Overview

Adenocarcinoma not otherwise specified (ANOS) is a malignant salivary neoplasm that exhibits glandular or ductal differentiation but lacks histomorphologic features that characterize more traditional (named) carcinomas.[44] The phrase, *not otherwise specified*, is added to distinguish it from other well-defined salivary adenocarcinomas.

Although reported as representing 8% to 17% of all salivary epithelial malignancies, little information is currently available regarding its biologic behavior.[3,45,46] Older studies, no doubt, have included under the rubric ANOS many neoplasms that by current standards are best classified as PLGA, EMCa, and low-grade cribriform cystadenocarcinoma.[47]

Critical evaluation in recent literature indicates that ANOS occurs more often in older adults, averaging approximately ages 60 to 70 years, and is rare in children.[3,44,46] The gender distribution varies according to study. Some investigators have found that 54% occur in women whereas others have observed a male predominance of 4:1.[3,46] Approximately 60% of cases arise in the major salivary glands and 40% in the minor glands, especially the palate, buccal mucosa, tongue, and lips.[3]

The tumors range from small, nonulcerated, and relatively asymptomatic to large and aggressive with pain, facial paresis, fixation to surrounding tissues, and/or lymph node metastasis.

Gross Features

Although most ANOSs have poorly defined margins, a few are relatively circumscribed. On cut surface, they appear tan, yellow, or white, often with foci of hemorrhage and necrosis. Scar-like areas are sometimes apparent, raising the probability of an underlying PA.

Microscopic Features

Other than the presence of glands/ducts and an infiltrative growth, there are no characteristic histologic features of ANOS (**Fig. 26**). The glands/ducts vary in frequency from tumor to tumor and from different areas in the same tumor and may be arranged in a cribriform, papillary, cystic, solid, lobular, and/or cord-like configuration. Most cells are cuboidal, columnar, or polygonal and contain nuclei that vary from bland to pleomorphic. Oncocytic, mucous, sebaceous, and plasmacytoid cells are not uncommon although usually sparse and randomly distributed. May arise de novo or from a PA. Finding remnants

of the underlying adenoma, therefore, is not uncommon.

Most ANOSs are high grade, but low-grade to intermediate-grade tumors also exist. These are distinguished on the presence or absence of the usual histologic features, such as cellular pleomorphism, increased mitotic activity, atypical mitoses, necrosis, and perineural/angiolymphatic invasion.

Differential Diagnosis

ANOS, by definition, does not have classic features of any of the usual salivary adenocarcinomas. One named entity that often comes into the differential is PLGA—which may be a problem separating it from ANOS low-grade.[48] Despite the multitude of patterns, PLGA is characterized by cytologically uniform, bland, round nuclei with open chromatin sometimes resembling the orphan Annie nuclei of papillary thyroid carcinoma. Mitoses are sparse (usually fewer than 3 per 10 high-power fields) to absent. In addition, PLGA usually has a mucohyaline matrix and exhibits prominent targetoid perineural invasion. If PLGA and ANOS low-grade are confused, that generally has little consequence for patients because treatments are the same (wide excision).

Perhaps the biggest issue for high-grade ANOS is distinction from a metastatic adenocarcinoma and salivary duct carcinoma. Salivary duct carcinoma has an apocrine phenotype and is AR and GCDFP-15 positive, unlike ANOS. With regards to metastases, a review of the medical history

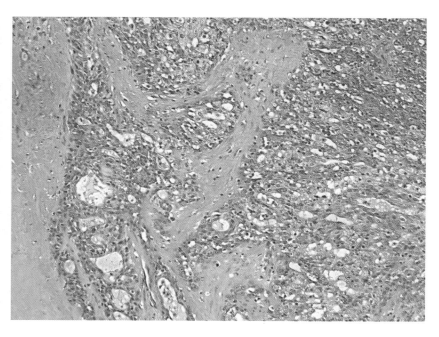

Fig. 26. ANOS. Note the solid component with the focal gland formation. The stroma is fibrotic. The carcinoma is nonspecific and does not resemble any of the named or more traditional salivary carcinomas.

Differential Diagnosis
ADENOCARCINOMA NOT
OTHERWISE SPECIFIED

- PLGA
- Salivary duct carcinoma
- Metastatic carcinoma

and thorough clinical examination are essential. Immunohistochemical markers for specific tumor sites, such as prostate specific antigen, may be helpful. The transformed components of acinic cell carcinoma, ACC, and EMCa with high-grade transformation have the appearance of a high-grade ANOS.[11,49,50] Identification of a differentiated component is necessary to distinguish these from pure ANOS. Finally, ANOS often represents the carcinomatous component of a carcinoma ex PA (CAxPA).[51]

Treatment and Prognosis

Prognosis depends on clinical stage, site of origin, and histologic grade. Although the study of Spiro and colleagues[47] is dated, it provides some insight into the biologic behavior of ANOS. According to these investigators, the 15-year survival rates for low-grade, intermediate-grade, and high-grade tumors are 54%, 31%, and 3%, respectively. Wahlberg and colleagues[45] observed a relative 5-year rate of 63% for those tumors arising in the parotid gland and 43% for those involving the submandibular gland. In general, tumors of the minor salivary glands have a better prognosis than those of the major glands.[44]

Low-grade ANOS has been stated to have a prognosis similar to acinic cell carcinoma and

is usually managed by wide excision.[3] Patients with high-grade ANOS, in contrast, often need a neck dissection and possibly postoperative radiation.

BENIGN TUMORS

PLEOMORPHIC ADENOMA

Overview

PA is, by far, the most frequent salivary gland tumor, accounting for 45% to 60% of all benign and malignant salivary neoplasms.[52–54] Approximately 80% occur in the parotid gland, 15% in the submandibular gland, and 10% in the minor salivary glands.[52,53] In the parotid gland, the most common site of origin is the superficial lobe, especially the lower pole, whereas in the oral cavity, the preferred site is the palate followed by the upper lip and buccal mucosa.[55]

PAs are more frequent in women and occur in all age groups, although uncommon in individuals below 10 years of age.[56] The mean age is approximately 45 years. The majority grow slowly and are relatively asymptomatic but can reach enormous size if neglected. Most parotid tumors are well defined and mobile as opposed to those of the palate, which are frequently ulcerated and rather rigid because of the underlying bone. Tumors of the deep lobe of the parotid gland usually manifest as parapharyngeal masses.

Gross Features

Most PAs are 2 cm to 6 cm and are almost invariably solitary lesions. The incidence of a primary (untreated) multifocal PAs is in the range of only 0.14% to 0.6%.[57] In the major glands they are encapsulated with a smooth, sometimes bosselated margin whereas those of the minor glands are usually devoid of a capsule. On cut surface,

Pitfalls
ADENOCARCINOMA NOT
OTHERWISE SPECIFIED

! High-grade adenocarcinomas not otherwise specified in some cases may represent the transformed component of various low-grade tumors, such as ACC, EMCa, or acinic cell carcinoma. Thus, a careful examination of the tumor for these components improves classification.

! High-grade ANOS, with a central hyalinized nodule is better classified as a CAxPA.

Key Features
PLEOMORPHIC ADENOMA

- PA is by far the most common salivary gland neoplasm.
- PAs are composed of a ductal and myoepithelial cells with broad morphologic diversity and a variety of growth patterns embedded in a chondromyxoid stroma, often with true cartilage formation.
- PAs have a low recurrence rate if completely excised.

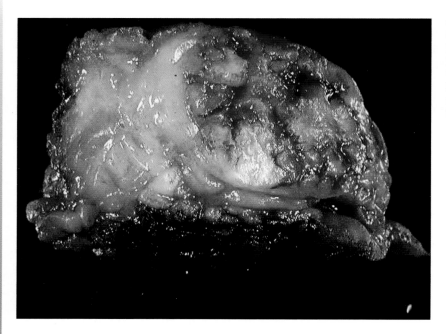

Fig. 27. Gross image of an encapsulated PA of parotid gland composed primarily of lobules of gray-white chondroid matrix. Note the central hemorrhage, secondary to prior fine-needle aspiration.

they are solid, rarely cystic, and, depending on cellular composition, vary from fleshly, tan-pink, or gray-white to opalescent blue-gray and cartilaginous (Fig. 27). In contrast, recurrences are often multinodular and multifocal mimicking a malignant process in some cases.

Microscopic Features

PAs have 4 components—capsule, epithelial cells, myoepithelial cells, and mesenchymal-stromal elements (Fig. 28). The percent composition of each of these components in any given tumor is highly variable. The term, *pleomorphic*, refers to this histologic diversity rather than to cellular pleomorphism. In general, most tumors are composed of approximately half epithelial-myoepithelial cells and half mesenchymal-stromal elements. Tumors composed of 80% or more epithelial-myoepithelial cells are sometimes referred to as cellular PAs whereas those with 80% or more mesenchymal-stromal elements are designated acellular PAs.

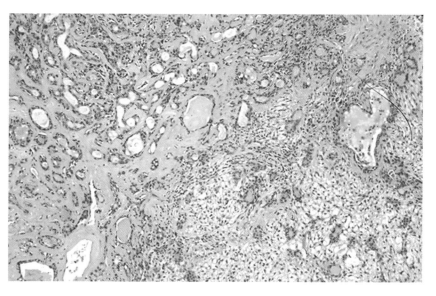

Fig. 28. Typical PA composed of approximately equal mixtures of epithelial and mesenchymal components.

Fig. 29. Hematoxylin-eosin whole mount of a PA of parotid gland. Note the variation in thickness of the capsule and scattered pseudopods.

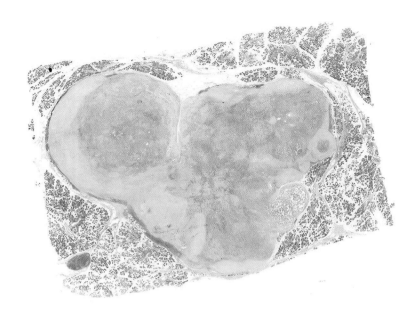

The degree of cellularity has no prognostic significance.

The capsule of a PA varies in thickness and presence, even in the same tumor (**Fig. 29**). Studies have shown that in PAs of the parotid gland that the capsule is focally absent in one-third of cases, with extrusions commonly referred to as *pseudopodia*.[58]

The epithelial cells are cuboidal to polygonal and appear as small ducts and acini surrounded by a single layer of myoepithelial cells. Tumor cells have eosinophilic to amphophilic cytoplasm and central, mildly chromatic nuclei with absent or barely discernible nucleoli. Occasionally, other cells are seen, including mucous, basaloid, squamous, sebaceous, and oncocytic. Skin adnexal differentiation is frequently observed in palate PAs.[59] Myoepithelial cells exhibit remarkable phenotypic variation and may appear spindled, plasmacytoid, epithelioid, clear, or oncocytic. The mesenchymal-stroma components range from fibrous, myxoid, chondroid, osseous, to lipomatous.

Mitoses and necroses are sparse to absent and may be related to prior fine-needle aspiration.[60] Approximately 5% to 10% of PAs focally express AR, p53 and Her-2/neu and, exceptionally, may rarely exhibit intravascular tumor deposits, yet these features do not necessarily indicate early malignant transformation, especially if seen in the vicinity of a needle tract.[61,62] DNA aneuploidy is also not uncommon, having been observed in 25% of PAs in one study.[63]

PA gene 1 (*PLAG1*) and the high-mobility group protein gene (*HMGA2*) have been implicated in the development of PAs. Alerations involving the 8p12 (*PLAG1*) locus encompass the most frequent category of genetic abnormalities in PA, with a t(3;8) the most frequent alteration, resulting in a *CTTNB1-PLAG1* fusion.[64] This 8p12 group occurs one decade younger than karyotypically normal PA and tends to be more cellular.[65] Regarding clonality, evidence suggests that all components (epithelial, myoepithelial, and mesenchymal-stromal) are derived from a common single-cell origin.[64,66–69]

Differential Diagnosis

The differential diagnosis for PA can be broad depending on cellularity and predominant cell type. Perhaps the two most common malignancies to consider, particularly for cellular PAs, are EMCa and CAxPA. The most important distinction is the

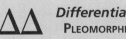

Differential Diagnosis
PLEOMORPHIC ADENOMA

- EMCa
- CAxPA
- PLGA
- Myoepithelioma
- BC

Pitfalls
PLEOMORPHIC ADENOMA

! Minor salivary gland PAs may not have a capsule.

! PAs may express p53, AR, and Her-2/neu focally; thus, these stains cannot be used alone to support malignancy.

! PAs can recur in a multinodular fashion mimicking a malignancy.

absence of true invasion in PA. Although capsular irregularities and pseudopodia may exist in PA, they are fairly myxoid and paucicellular. True invasion, even in a minimally invasive CAxPA, is typically accompanied by sclerosis. EMCa is distinguished from cellular PA by a more prominent polygonal (often clear cell) outer myoepithelial cell layer and multinodular pattern of permeation. Palate PAs can be mistaken for polymorphous low-grade adenoncarcinomas (PLGA) and both can have similar crystalloids in the stroma.[70] PLGAs are infiltrative, whereas palate PA, although not always encapsulated, is well demarcated. BCA and myoepithelioma are benign entities in the differential diagnosis. BCA may have prominent S-100 myoepithelial-derived stroma (discussed later) resembling the stroma of a PA.[71] BCA with this type of stroma has a sharp delineation between epithelial components and the adjacent stroma whereas the myoepithelial stroma of a PA blends with the ducts more readily. Additionally, BCA do not have chondrocytic differentiation. Myoepithelioma contains only one cell type whereas even myoepithelial rich PAs have a ductal component.

Treatment and Prognosis

Surgery is the treatment of choice with the extent dependent on location. For PAs of minor salivary gland origin, wide excision is used whereas those of the submandibular gland are treated by complete excision of the gland. Most PAs of the parotid gland are managed by superficial parotidectomy with facial nerve sparing.[72] The incidence of local recurrence is approximately 1% to 4% assuming negative margins.

MYOEPITHELIOMA

Myoepithelial neoplasms are tumors composed exclusively or almost exclusively of myoepithelial cells.[3,70,73–78] As a group, they are uncommon

tumors, comprising no more than 1% to 2% of all salivary neoplasms. The majority are benign (approximately 70%–90% of all cases) but some are malignant (approximately 10%–30% of all cases). The World Health Organization endorses the term, *myoepithelioma*, for benign tumors (also known as myoepithelial adenoma and benign myoepithelial tumor) and *myoepithelial carcinoma* when malignant (also known as malignant myoepithelioma).[78] This discussion pertains only to the benign variant—myoepithelioma. Myoepithelial carcinomas are discussed previously.

Overview

Approximately 75% of all cases occur in the parotid gland and palate. They are uncommon in the submandibular gland and have been described infrequently in a variety of other sites, including the sinonasal tract, oral cavity, and larynx. They involve both genders equally and occur in patients averaging age 40 to 50 years (range 9–95 years).[3]

The tumor most often presents as a slowly enlarging mass of several months to years duration. In the palate, they rarely ulcerate the mucosa.

Gross Features

The majority of myoepitheliomas are between 1 cm and 5 cm in size and are circumscribed and often encapsulated. In the parotid gland, they are almost invariably encapsulated whereas those that arise from minor salivary glands are usually not. On cut section, they are tan, gray, white, or yellow-tan.

Microscopic Features

Myoepitheliomas are composed primarily of spindle or plasmacytoid (hyaline) cells or a combination of both that grow in a solid, nodular, myxoid-mucinous, pseudoglandular, trabecular, or reticulated pattern. Epithelioid, clear cell, and oncocytic variants are less common. The spindle

Key Features
MYOEPITHELIOMA

- Myoepitheliomas are benign tumors composed solely of myoepithelial cells with a small proportion recurring if incompletely excised.

- They consist of either spindled, epithelioid, plasmacytoid, or clear cell types and can have a variety of growth patterns.

- Myoepitheliomas are immunoreactive for keratins, p63, S-100, and a variety of smooth muscle markers.

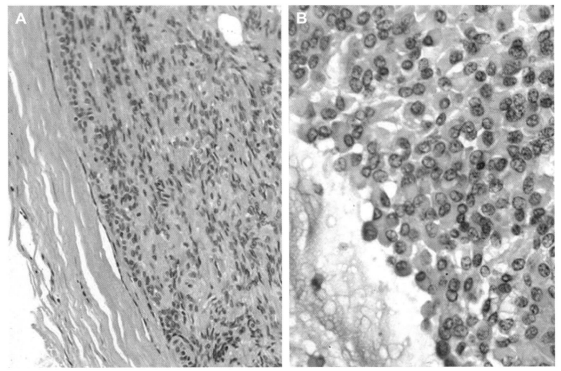

Fig. 30. Myoepithelioma. (*A*) Solid spindle cell type. Note capsule. (*B*) Plasmacytoid variant associated with mucinous stroma.

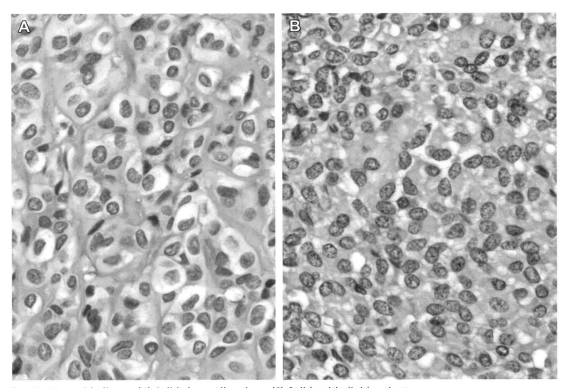

Fig. 31. Myoepithelioma. (*A*) Solid clear cell variant. (*B*) Solid epithelioid variant.

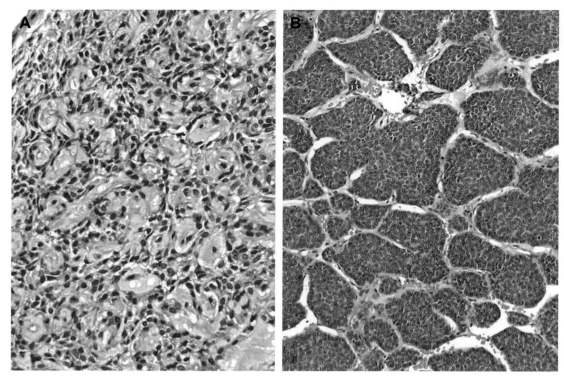

Fig. 32. Myoepithelioma. (*A*) Reticulated, spindle cell variant (*B*) Nodular pattern, epithelioid variant.

cells occur in sheets or swirls and have central oval to elongated nuclei with finely dispersed chromatin and blunt tapered ends. They cytoplasm is pink. The plasmacytoid cells have glassy, dense eosinophilic cytoplasm and eccentric, round to oval nuclei. Some may contain barely discernible nucleoli. Plasmacytoid variants are frequent in the palate. The cells of the epithelioid variant are ovoid to polygonal and contain prominent, somewhat vesicular nuclei. The clear cell type, as the name implies, contains cells with abundant glycogen, imparting a clear or empty appearance to the cytoplasm.

In the spindle cell type, as well as the epithelioid and clear cell variants, there is usually little fibrous stroma or ground substance, whereas in the plasmacytoid type, groups of plasmacytoid cells are often separated by a mucoid or myxoid stroma (**Figs. 30–32**). Mitoses, necrosis, and cartilage are typically absent. Squamous metaplasia may be focally present.

Ultrastructurally, myoepitheliomas demonstrate desmosomes, cytoplasmic filaments, and basal lamina. Myoepitheliomas are generally immunoreactive for cytokeratin, S-100 protein, p63, and vimentin and variably express glial fibrillary acidic protein, smooth muscle actin, calponin, smooth muscle myosin heavy chain, maspin, and metallothionein.[78]

Differential Diagnosis

Spindle cell myoepitheliomas are often confused with leiomyomas and neurilemomas (schwannoma). The presence of a capsule and immunoreactivity for cytokeratin and S-100 protein separate it from a leiomyoma. Neurilemomas are also

 Differential Diagnosis
MYOEPITHELIOMA

- Leiomyoma
- Schwannoma
- Extramedullary plasmacytoma
- Myoepithelial carcinoma
- EMCa
- Other clear cell tumor

> ## *Pitfalls*
> ### MYOEPITHELIOMA
>
> ! Clear cell myoepithelial tumors may have a more aggressive behavior than predicted by morphology alone.

encapsulated and S-100 protein positive, but they are negative for cytokeratin.

The plasmacytoid variant may be mistaken for an extramedullary plasmacytoma. The latter, however, is negative for cytokeratin and, unlike myoepithelioma, is positive for immunoglobulins.

Clear cell myoepithelioma can be distinguished from EMCa by the absence of ducts in the former and their presence in the latter. Other clear cell tumors that might enter the differential diagnosis include CCC and metastatic RCC. Both of the tumors, however, lack myoepithelial cells.

Treatment and Prognosis

The treatment of myoepithelioma is similar to that of a PA. In the parotid gland, a superficial lobectomy is usually indicated, whereas in other sites, a conservative excision with a margin of uninvolved tissue is indicated. Although it is commonly stated that myoepitheliomas are less prone to recur than PAs,[78,79] this has not been the authors' experience. The prognosis, in the authors' experience, parallels the PA. Both may recur if inadequately excised and both may infrequently undergo malignant transformation. Anecdotally, clear cell myoepithelial tumors may have a more aggressive course than predicted by histology alone.

BASAL CELL ADENOMA

Overview

BCA, first described by Kleinsasser and Klein in 1967,[80] is an epithelial neoplasm composed of cells with a basaloid appearance and an absence of a chondromyxoid matrix as seen in PA. It represents 1% to 3% of all salivary neoplasms and typically occurs in adults, usually in the fourth to seventh decades, and is exceptional in children.[81] The gender distribution varies according to series. Some indicate a male predominance for the membranous variant and a 1:1 to 1:2 ratio in favor of the female gender for the other subtypes.[81–83]

Most (75%–80%) occur in the parotid gland and the remainder in the submandibular and minor salivary glands, especially the upper lip and buccal mucosa. Occurrence in an intraparotid lymph node, in particular the membranous variant, is not uncommon and should not be taken as a sign of malignancy.[82]

BCA typically presents as a slowly enlarging, asymptomatic mass. The membranous BCA, also known as a dermal analog tumor, is associated in 25% to 38% of cases with the Brooke-Spiegler syndrome, an autosomal dominant syndrome characterized by numerous dermal cylindromas, trichoepitheliomas, and/or spiradenomas.[82–84] Genetic studies have show that the membranous BCA and dermal cylindroma share a similar incidence of alterations at the *CYLD1* locus in the 16q12–13 chromosome region, supporting a common origin.[85]

Gross Features

BCAs rarely exceed 3 cm and on cut surface are gray-white or tan and occasionally cystic (**Fig. 33**). In the major glands, they are solitary and encapsulated whereas in the minor glands, a capsule is usually absent. The membranous variant, in contrast, is often multifocal and may or may not be encapsulated (**Fig. 34**).

Microscopic Features

The term, *monomorphic adenomas*, historically applied to BCA is highly misleading, because they actually consist of a mixture of basal, myoepithelial, and ductal cells.[86–88] Basal cells are morphologically subdivided into small dark cells with sparse cytoplasm and round, hyperchromatic nuclei and larger pale cells that are larger and more polygonal with basophilic to slightly

> ## *Key Features*
> ### BASAL CELL ADENOMA
>
> - BCAs are predominantly located in the parotid gland.
>
> - The membranous variant of BCA is often seen in multiple cylindromatosis and trichoepithelioma syndromes typified by *CYLD1* mutations.
>
> - BCAs are triphasic tumors, consisting of peripheral, palisaded dark basal cells, pale basal cells, and central ductal cells.
>
> - The recurrence rate is low except for the membranous variant, for which tumors are often multiple and multifocal.

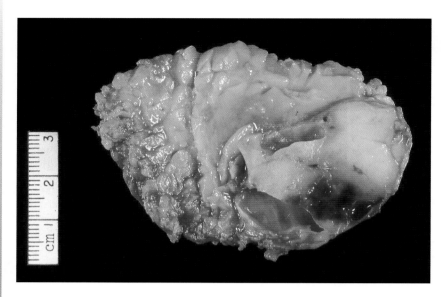

Fig. 33. Gross image of encapsulated BCA of the parotid gland with cystic changes.

eosinophilic cytoplasm and vesicular nuclei, with or without nucleoli. The small dark cells usually form the periphery of tumor nests and demonstrate peripheral palisading, whereas the larger ones rest on top of this peripheral layer. To varying degrees, within the center of tumor nests, are small ductules lined by cuboidal epithelium. The juxtaposition of peripheral dark basal cells, pale basal cells, and central ductal cells often imparts a triphasic appearance that is most prominent in the tubulotrabecular growth patterns.

Architecturally, BCAs are divided into 6 types of growth patterns: solid, trabecular, tubular, membranous, cribriform, and myoepithelial-derived stroma rich.[71] Tubular and trabecular patterns are often seen together (thus, referred to as

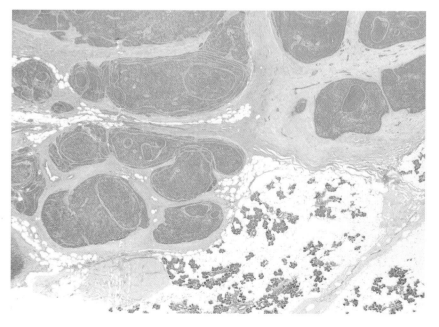

Fig. 34. BCA, membranous type of parotid gland with multifocal appearance and lack of encapsulation. This should not be mistaken for malignant change.

Fig. 35. BCA, solid type. Note predominately solid aggregates of basaloid cells with focal peripheral palisading. Capsule is at top.

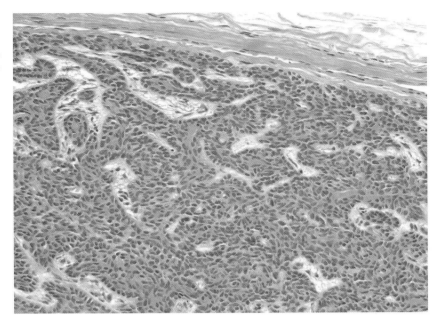

tubulotrabecular), and myoepithelial-derived stroma can be seen in any of the other patterns, although more commonly in the tubulotrabecular pattern. The more common solid type is composed of islands of varying sizes and shapes separated by strands of collagen (**Fig. 35**). The trabecular type is characterized by cords or trabeculae of cells, which often anastomose (**Fig. 36**). The presence of numerous ducts lined by cuboidal cells with slightly eosinophilic cytoplasm identifies the tubular type (**Fig. 37**). The membranous BCA is composed of islands of basaloid cells, each surrounded by

Fig. 36. BCA, trabecular variant. Note capsule at bottom and linear cords of basaloid cells.

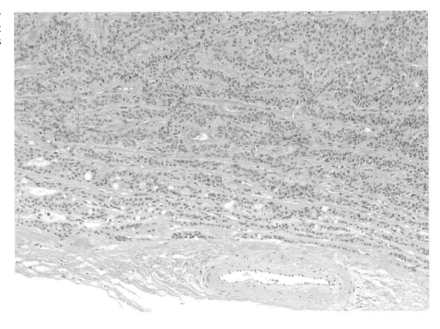

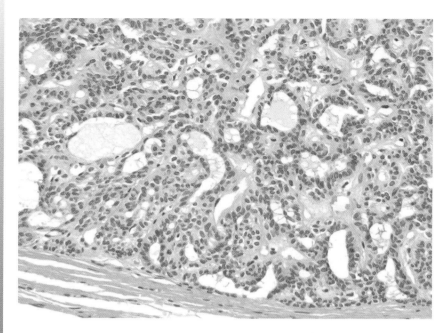

Fig. 37. BCA, tubular type. The tubules/ducts are lined by a single row of cuboidal cells. Note capsule at bottom.

a thick, eosinophilic basement membrane, which, on low magnification, appear as pieces of a jigsaw puzzle (**Fig. 38**). In the cribriform variant, the basaloid cells are arranged in a Swiss cheese pattern similar to an ACC (**Fig. 39**). Variants with myoepithelial-derived stroma contain a distinct bland, spindled, myxoid myoepithelial stroma that is distinct from the tumor nests, unlike PA, in which this stroma typically blends with the epithelial components (**Fig. 40**). Mixed patterns of BCAs

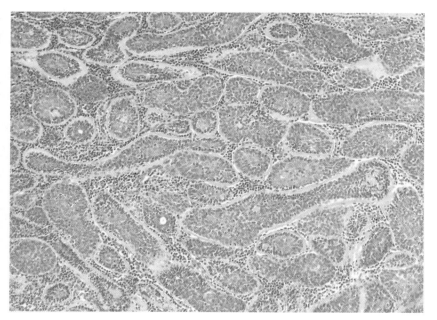

Fig. 38. BCA, membranous type. The islands of basaloid cells fit together like pieces of a jigsaw puzzle. Note the thick hyaline membrane around each and the few admixed ducts.

Fig. 39. BCA, cribriform type. It resembles ACC but is completely encapsulated.

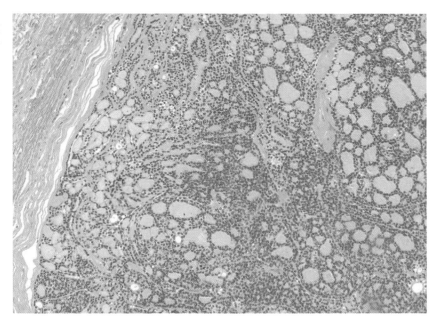

are not uncommon, although one pattern usually dominates. BCAs often show cutaneous-type elements; squamous eddies, sebaceous elements, and cystic changes can be seen in all variants.

Immunohistochemical staining varies from tumor to tumor, depending on the relative proportion of cells, with basal, luminal-ductal, and myoepithelial differentiation, but often serves to highlight the triphasic appearance of the tumor.[86–88] The dark peripheral most basal cells are typically myoepithelial in phenotype and positive for high molecular weight keratins, p63,

Fig. 40. BCA with prominent myoepithelial stroma. In this case, the basaloid cells are arranged in a mixed tubulo-trabecular pattern.

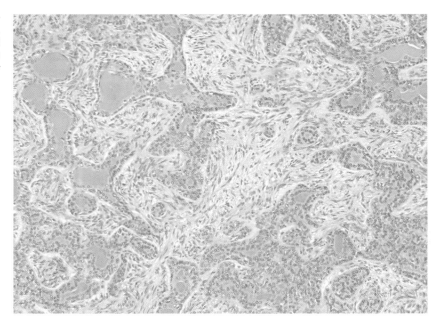

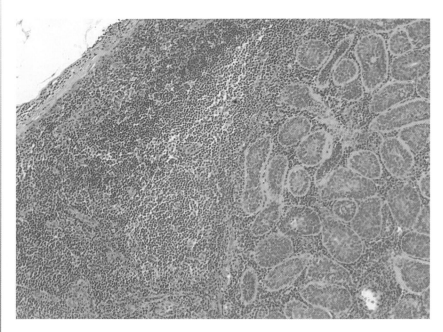

Fig. 41. BCA, membranous type arising in an intraparotid lymph node.

smooth muscle actin, calponin, and smooth muscle myosin heavy chain. The adjacent pale basal cells are purely basal in phenotype and only positive for p63 and high molecular weight keratins. Finally, the simple low molecular weight cytokeratins, carcinoembryonic antigen, and epithelial membrane antigen highlight the central luminal-ductal cells. S-100 is variably positive in the tumor. The myoepithelial-derived stroma-rich variant shows strong S-100 reactivity in the stroma. Nuclear β-catenin expression is also frequent in BCA.[89]

Differential Diagnosis

Canalicular adenoma (CA), BCAC, and ACC are of prime consideration in the differential diagnosis.

As opposed to BCA, which arises primarily in the parotid gland, CA occurs predominately in the upper lip. In addition, CA is composed of anastomosing cords of double rows of cuboidal to columnar cells lying in a well-vascularized myxoid to slightly collagenous stroma and lacks myoepithelial cells.

BCAC is invasive and either nonencapsulated or partially encapsulated at most and characteristically displays 3 or more mitoses per 10 high-power fields. It must be emphasized that the membranous BCA is often multifocal, may lack a capsule, and occasionally arises in an intraparotid lymph node and is not to be mistaken for evidence of malignancy (see **Figs. 34** and **41**).[82] In these instances, look for perineural and angiolymphatic invasion and evidence of soft tissue extension, which are unequivocal features of a malignant neoplasm.

Cribriform BCA is encapsulated and composed of cells with round to oval nuclei whereas ACC is nonencapsulated, is invasive, involves nerves, and is composed of cells with small, hyperchromatic, and angulated nuclei.

Treatment and Prognosis

Most BCAs are nonrecurrent after surgical excision. The exception is the membranous variant, which is

ΔΔ **Differential Diagnosis** BASAL CELL ADENOMA
• BCAC • ACC • CA

 Pitfalls
BASAL CELL ADENOMA

! BCAs may arise in lymph nodes from salivary gland inclusions, mimicking a metastasis.

often multifocal (50% of cases in one series) and associated with a recurrence rate of 25%.[82]

Malignant transformation of BCAs, similar to a carcinoma arising in a PA, has been described and reported as 28% for the membranous BCA and 4% for all other BCAs.[90] Most of the malignant tumors are BCACs.

CANALICULAR ADENOMA

Overview

CA is defined by the World Health Organization as a "tumor composed of columnar epithelial cells arranged in thin, anastomosing cords often with a beaded pattern. The stroma is characteristically paucicellular and highly vascular."[91] In the past, it was often referred to as a monomorphic adenoma or as a variant of BCA (BCA, canalicular type).[92–94] Differences in cell morphology, sites of occurrence, and immunohistochemical reactivity indicate that the CA is distinct from BCA.

CA typically occurs in patients over 50 years of age (range 33–87 years) and has a gender distribution of 1:1 to 1.8:1 in favor of women.[91,94] The tumor has an unexplained affinity for the upper lip (approximately 80% of all cases) but has also been described in the buccal mucosa (10%), palate (3%–10%), and exceptionally in the parotid gland (<4%).[92,94]

It presents as a painless, slowly enlarging submucosal mass covered by an intact (rarely ulcerated) mucosa that varies in color from normal to slightly bluish, often mimicking a mucocele. Although usually a solitary lesion, a few patients

> **Key Features**
> CANALICULAR ADENOMA
>
> - CA is mainly a minor salivary gland tumor with a predilection for the upper lip.
> - Tumors consist of columnar epithelial cells arranged in thin, anastomosing cords often with a beaded pattern.
> - Columnar cells are purely ductal in phenotype with keratin positivity and S-100 positivity, but no myoepithelial or basal components.
> - CAs may be multifocal.

with multiple, clinically apparent tumors have been described.[95]

Gross Features

CAs are well circumscribed and rarely exceed 2 cm. On cut section they appear pink-tan, brown, or yellow and vary from solid to cystic.

Microscopic Features

CAs may or may not be encapsulated and are composed of cuboidal to columnar cells with dark, often elongated nuclei with light eosinophilic to amphophilic cytoplasm. Nucleoli and mitoses are rare to absent. The cells are characteristically arranged in anastomosing cords of 2-cell thickness (**Fig. 42**). The 2 rows of cells alternate from

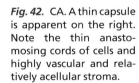

Fig. 42. CA. A thin capsule is apparent on the right. Note the thin anastomosing cords of cells and highly vascular and relatively acellular stroma.

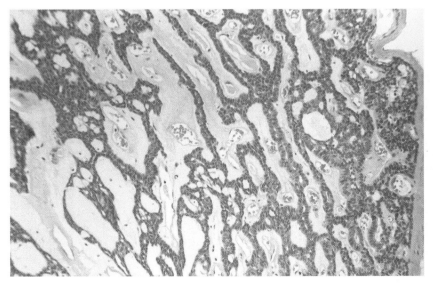

areas where they are closely apposed to those areas where they are slightly separated creating narrow channels or canaliculi. This alternating abutment and separation of the 2 rows of cells has been referred to as beading. Some CAs are more cellular than others, and if the canaliculi are seen in cross section may simulate a tubular variant of a BCA (**Fig. 43**).

The stroma is characteristic and is a useful clue to diagnosis. It is well vascularized, paucicellular, and varies from myxoid to slightly collagenous.

Although multiple clinically apparent CAs are infrequent, it is not uncommon to see multiple foci of microscopic canalicular adenomatous changes adjacent to a much larger clinically dominant tumor. The frequency of these microadenomas has been observed in up to 22% of all CAs.[95]

CAs are reactive on immunohistochemistry for cytokeratins (especially AE 1/3 and CK7) and S-100 protein and negative for carcinoembryonic antigen.[88,96] Consistent with their putative origin from excretory ducts and absence of myoepithelial cells, they are negative for smooth muscle actin, calponin, p63, and smooth muscle myosin heavy chain.[87,97,98]

Differential Diagnosis

The differential diagnosis most often includes BCA, PLGA, and ACC. Except for the fact that the CA may be multifocal (microadenomas) with a potential for developing new lesions, the

Differential Diagnosis
CANALICULAR ADENOMA

- BCA
- PLGA
- ACC

distinction between it and a BCA is largely academic. Features used to separate the 2 tumors are discussed previously.

PLGA is immunophenotypically identical to CA but is distinguished by its frankly infiltrative borders frequent perineural invasion, heterogeneity of growth patterns, and distinctive vesicular to clear nuclei. ACC distinguished from CA also by its infiltrative growth pattern and biphasic composition consisting of epithelial and myoepithelial cells characteristically arranged in a cribriform pattern. It, therefore, is positive for carcinoembryonic antigen and myoepithelial markers, both of which are negative in CA.

Treatment and Prognosis

CAs are treated by simple excision. Although local recurrences have been described, most of these are probably related to the known multifocality of this tumor (microadenomas) with the development

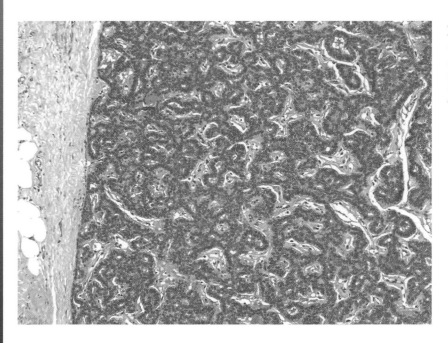

Fig. 43. CA, more cellular variant. The rows of cells have separated creating prominent canalicular channels, which, in cross section, may be mistaken for glands of tubular type of BCA.

Pitfalls
CANALICULAR ADENOMA

! Canalicular adenomas may have more cellular areas mimicking BCA.

of a new lesion rather than failure to adequately excise the original tumor.[99]

In contrast to BCA, which rarely undergoes malignant change (carcinoma ex BCA), a carcinoma arising from a CA has not been observed.

WARTHIN TUMOR

Overview

Warthin tumor was described historically as papillary cystadenoma lymphomatosum, even before the description by Warthin in 1929.[100] This is typically a tumor of the elderly, typically sixth to seventh decades, with a profound male predilection. Less than 10% occur below the age of 40. This gender predilection is in part attributable to the association with smoking.[101] In certain populations with a high prevalence of smoking, such as central Pennsylvania, it is estimated that as many as 30% of the population may have Warthin tumors.[102]

Warthin tumor is exclusively a tumor of the parotid gland and typically occurs in the tail. Reports of Warthin tumor occurring elsewhere either represent a misdiagnosis or occurrence in ectopic parotid tissue. Regarding the latter, Warthin tumors have been described in neck lymph nodes and in close apposition to submandibular gland.[103] Warthin tumor is the most common

Key Features
WARTHIN TUMOR

- Warthin tumors are exclusively of parotid tissue but may arise from ectopic salivary tissue in lymph nodes and other extraparotid sites.

- There is a strong association with smoking.

- Warthin tumor is the most common bilateral and multifocal salivary gland tumor.

- Warthin tumors have a characteristic papillary architecture and lymphoid stroma.

- Papillae are lined by a bilayer of columnar oncocytic epithelium.

multifocal and bilateral salivary gland tumor, and 12% to 19% of patients develop more than one Warthin tumor.[104]

Warthin tumors are typically slow-growing painless masses that may fluctuate periodically in size. Pain is reported in less than 10% of patients and, rarely, patients may present with earache, tinnitus, and nerve paresis. These atypical symptoms are reflective of degenerative changes, including infarction and fibrosis. Degenerative changes may result from trauma or fine-needle aspiration. Similar to other mitochondria-rich lesions, Warthin tumors are intensely sestamibi (technetium Tc 99m) avid.

Gross Features

Warthin tumors, unless infarcted, are well demarcated and fluctuant, indicative of their cystic nature. Cyst fluid is classically brown with granular tan white debris, reminiscent of motor oil. Fluid may, however, be mucoid or purulent. The parenchyma is a soft tan to brown reflective of the oncocytic nature of the epithelium. Papillary excrescences may be seen. Occasionally, Warthin tumors are more solid although they may display a soft granular cut surface (**Fig. 44**). Secondary changes include infarction and fibrosis (**Fig. 45**). Occasionally there may be separate small foci grossly.

Microscopic Features

Warthin tumors are papillary, cystic, and composed of lymphoid stroma (**Fig. 46**). Classic Warthin tumor morphology consists of papillae lined by a bilayered oncocytic columnar epithelium with lymphoid-rich stroma extending into the fibrovascular cores (**Fig. 47**). In many instances, the lymphoid stroma has true nodal architecture. Historically, Warthin tumors were subtyped based on the varying proportions of epithelium and lymphoid stroma. Warthin tumors may be fairly solid with an epithelial predominance or fairly paucicellular with a lymphoid predominance.[105] Additional elements occasionally include scattered mucocytes, sebaceous rests, and foci of squamous metaplasia (**Fig. 48**). Occasionally, there is some overlap with oncocytoma in that there may be solid foci of oncocytes within lymphoid stroma. One significant variant of Warthin tumor is the so-called infarcted or infected Warthin tumor.[104,105] This tumor is characterized by prominent secondary changes, such as stromal fibrosis, with an increased heterogeneity of inflammatory constituents ranging from neutrophils to plasma cells. Although truly infarcted papillae may be seen, the typical epithelium shows prominent

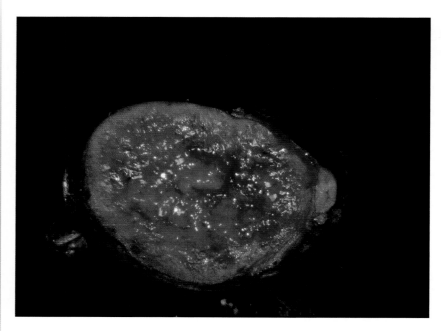

Fig. 44. Gross appearance of a Warthin tumor of the parotid tail. The cut surface demonstrates a solid red brown parenchyma similar to oncocytoma; however, centrally, there is evidence of granularity and cystic change.

squamous metaplasia and occasional mucinous metaplasia (**Fig. 49**).[104] These changes may often be seen in proximity to a fine-needle aspiration tract.

The immunophenotype and morphology of the epithelial component of Warthin tumor recapitulates that of the normal striated duct. Technically Warthin tumor is a biphasic tumor. The luminal or inner layer of oncocytic epithelium is ductal in phenotype (thus, positive for CK7, CK18, and CK19) whereas the outer layer has a basal phenotype and is positive for high molecular weight keratins (ie, CK5/6) and p63.[106,107] Similar to the abluminal cells of striated ducts, the outer layer

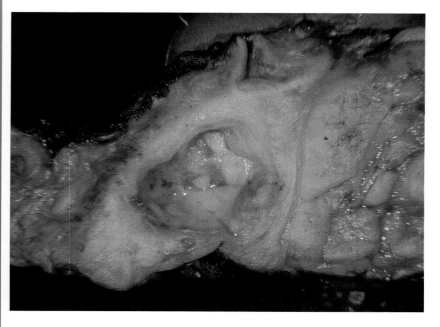

Fig. 45. Gross appearance of an infarcted Warthin tumor of the parotid gland. This lesion is cystic with a fibrous white wall and mucopurulent cyst contents.

Fig. 46. Low-power histologic features of Warthin tumor (×40). Tumors are papillary, cystic, and usually well demarcated with a lymphoid stroma reminiscent of a lymph node.

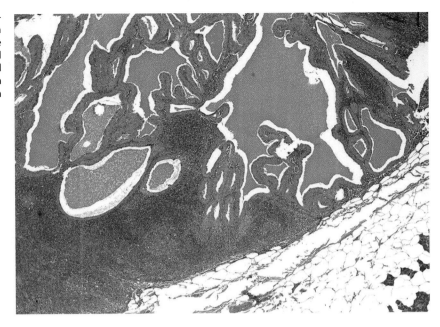

of Warthin tumor epithelium shows rare to absent myoepithelial elements that are actin and calponin negative. The inner layer of Warthin tumor is filled with mitochondria, thus is strongly positive for PTAH and antimitochondrial antibody. Unlike the intercalated duct phenotype, Warthin tumors are negative for S-100. The lymphoid stroma often recapitulates the lymphocyte distribution of a reactive lymph node. Patients with a concomitant small B-cell lymphoproliferative disorder (ie, chronic lymphocytic leukemia/small lymphocytic lymphoma), however, have been reported to have lymphomatous involvement of their Warthin tumor.[108]

Fig. 47 Characteristic epithelium of Warthin tumors (×100). The epithelial component of a Warthin tumor is typified by an oncocytic columnar bilayer.

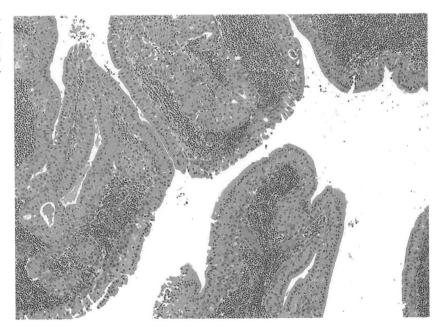

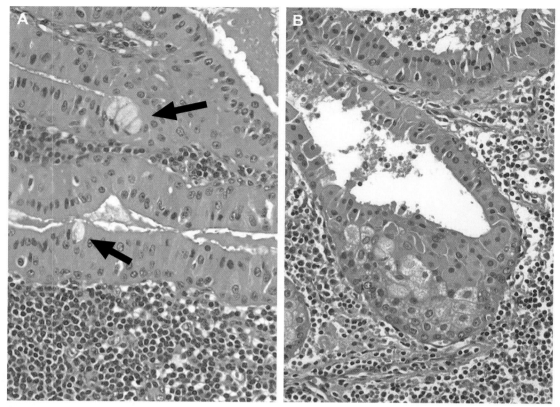

Fig. 48. Various metaplasias that may be seen in Warthin tumors. (*A*) Mucous cell metaplasia (*arrows*) (×200). (*B*) Sebaceous metaplasia (×100).

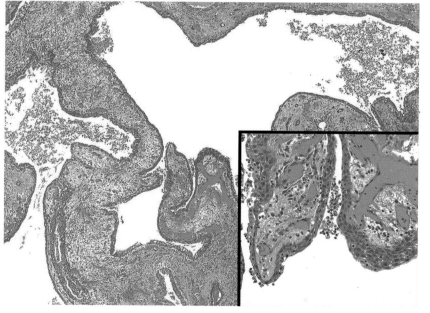

Fig. 49. Histologic appearance of an infarcted Warthin tumor (×40). These tumors, although papillary and cystic, are often composed of a more fibrous lymphoid poor stroma. Inset (×200): squamous metaplasia and neutrophilic inflammation are common in infarcted Warthin tumors.

Differential Diagnosis

Classic Warthin tumor has pathognomonic features with little diagnostic dilemma. Challenges occur with deviation from the classic bilayered morphology. Solid epithelial predominant Warthin tumors may resemble oncocytoma, and the distinction to some extent is arbitrary and of little consequence. Similarly, a Warthin tumor with prominent sebaceous elements may be designated a sebaceous lymphadenoma with oncocytic change and there is minimal clinical impact on this designation.

The more treacherous diagnostic dilemma includes the distinction of infarcted Warthin tumor from MEC or squamous cell carcinoma. An infarcted Warthin tumor should be suspected if necrotic intraluminal papillae are recognized. Additionally, unlike metastatic squamous cell carcinoma, there is only mild squamous atypia and no evidence of infiltration in a Warthin tumor with squamous metaplasia. The distinction from MEC can be more difficult particularly if the MEC is oncocytic and possesses a lymphoid stroma. Unlike Warthin tumor, on careful examination, MEC deviates from the Warthin bilayer and often contains tufts of intermediate cells and epidermoid cells underneath the surface mucous cell and columnar cell layer. Additionally, MEC shows more nuclear stratification of columnar cells. Paradoxically, true keratinization is more frequent in infarcted Warthin tumor, particularly in areas of fibrosis, reflective of a reactive metaplastic process. The conflicting features of squamous differentiation without significant cytologic atypia in a cystic lesion obviates MEC, because cystic MECs are low grade and typically mucous cell predominant. The usefulness of the MECT1/MAML2 rearrangement is controversial because some investigators think that Warthin tumors may harbor this translocation. The contention by Fehr and colleagues[109] is that so-called Warthin

tumors with the translocation are on re-review likely misdiagnosed MEC.

Minor diagnostic considerations include the distinction from lymphoepithelial cysts/HIV sialadenopathy, (nonsebaceous) lymphadenomas, and, rarely, cystic acinic cell carcinomas with prominent lymphoid stroma. Patients with lymphoepithelial cysts may have a clinical history of autoimmune disease or HIV, and the adjacent salivary tissue may show lymphoepithelial sialadenitis. Cysts are lined by a bilayer of nononcocytic cuboidal to low columnar epithelium as opposed to the tall columnar oncocytes of Warthin tumor. Lymphadenomas are often solid and more basaloid appearing. Acinic cell carcinomas that are papillary and cystic with lymphoid stroma may cause some confusion; however, these are monophasic tumors with vacuolated or granular cytoplasm and hobnail epithelium.

Treatment and Prognosis

Treatment is purely surgical. There is some debate as to the extent of surgery needed, particularly for tail of parotid lesions (ie, tail excision vs full superficial parotidectomy). With complete excision, the recurrence rate is low (<2%) and a fraction of these likely represent separate tumors because Warthin tumors are often multifocal.[104] Malignant degeneration is rare. Reported carcinoma types most commonly include squamous cell carcinoma and MEC.[110]

ONCOCYTOMA

Overview

Oncocytoma is merely one of many types of oncocytic salivary tumors. It is a designation used mainly for benign oncocytic neoplasms that are solid akin to oncocytomas of other organ sites. Similar to other oncocytic neoplasms, this is a tumor of the elderly seventh to eighth decade, although there is no gender predilection. Clear cell oncocytomas may have a female predilection.[3,111] A prior history of irradiation may be present in a subpopulation, which often presents at a younger age. Multifocal nodular oncocytic proliferations are referred to as oncocytic nodular hyperplasia, although a subset of these may be clonal neoplasms. Diffuse involvement of a salivary gland by oncocytic metaplasia is referred to as oncocytosis.

More than 80% of oncocytomas occur in the parotid gland, although they can occur in the submandibular gland and the minor salivary glands. Submandibular gland tumors may occur in slightly younger patients. Approximately 20% of oncocytoma patients have had antecedent radiation exposure.[43]

Oncocytomas tumors are typically slow growing painless masses. In general oncocytic lesions (including nodular oncocytic hyperplasia) may be bilateral in approximately 7% of patients. Similar to Warthin tumors, these may also be intensely sestamibi (technetium Tc 99m) avid and fluorodeoxyglucose 18F–positron emission tomography avid.[112,113] Oncocytomas may coexist with oncocytic cystadenomas.

Gross Features

Oncocytomas consist of uninodular, well-demarcated, encapsulated tan to mahogany brown mass with a smooth cut surface (**Fig. 50**). Occasionally, there may be central scars. Nodular oncocytic hyperplasia may have similar appearance with the exception that there are multiple nodules, and the nodules are not encapsulated. Occasionally a dominant nodule in a background of nodular oncocytic hyperplasia shows encapsulation. Some

Key Features
ONCOCYTOMA

- Oncocytoma is a benign solid oncocytic neoplasm of the elderly akin to oncocytomas seen at nonsalivary sites.

- Multonodular oncocytic nodules are referred to as oncocytic nodular hyperplasia whereas diffuse oncocytic change may be referred to as oncocytosis.

- Oncocytomas may show solid, trabecular, or compressed tubular growth and may show clear cell change if cells are heavily glycogenated.

- p63 shows a haphazard peripheral staining pattern.

designate these as oncocytomas arising on nodular oncocytic hyperplasia.

Microscopic Features

Oncocytomas are composed of polygonal oncocytes that may be arranged in solid, trabecular, and occasionally a compressed tubular growth pattern. Nuclei are round and vary from hyperchromatic to slightly vesicular with visible nucleoli (**Fig. 51**). The periphery of tumor nests contains darker cells with more scant cytoplasms. Clear

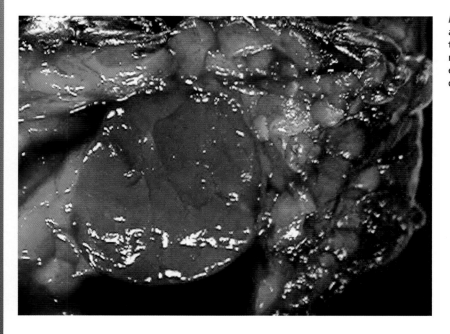

Fig. 50. Gross appearance of a parotid oncocytoma. Note the deep mahogany brown appearance of this well-demarcated nodule.

Fig. 51. Oncocytoma (×100). This parotid tumor shows an encapsulated compressed tubulotrabecular proliferation of polygonal oncocytes. Tumor nuclei are monomorphic.

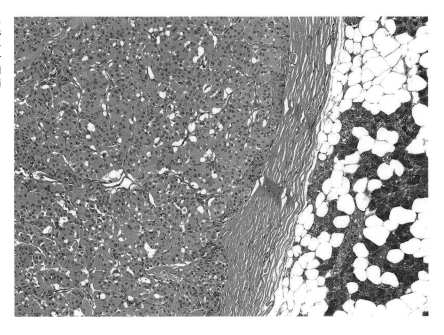

cell change may predominate in a fraction of oncocytomas and is more commonly observed in nodular oncocytic hyperplasia (**Fig. 52**). Squamous metaplasia may be seen in traumatized areas, particularly near a fine-needle tract.

Akin to many other salivary oncocytic neoplasms, oncocytomas show a striated duct phenotype. Most of the oncocytes have a ductal luminal phenotype (CK7, CK18, and CK19 positive).[114] The outermost layer in tumor nests, however, is basal in phenotype and is p63 positive (**Fig. 53**).[40] Myoepithelial cells are absent. The cytoplasm of oncocytomas consists of abundant often ultrastructurally abnormal mitochondria and are

Fig. 52. Clear cell nodular oncocytic hyperplasia (×20). Multiple well-demarcated clear cell nodules are present within the parotid parenchyma.

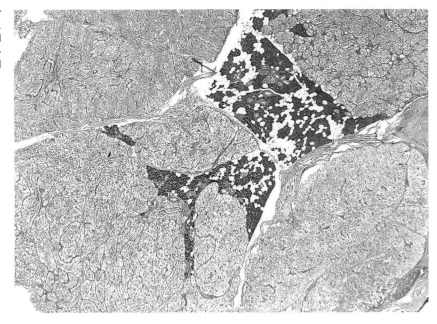

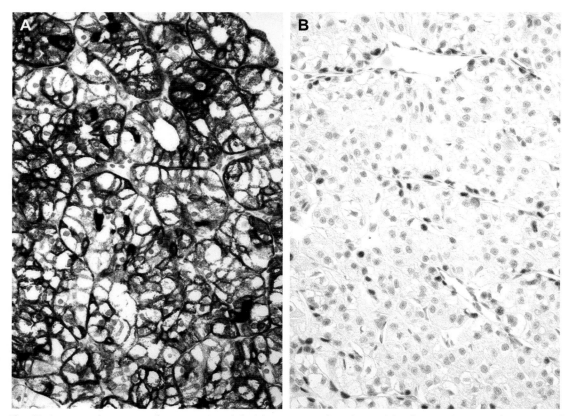

Fig. 53. Immunophenotype of oncocytoma. (*A*) This tumor tends to be positive for CK7 in a membranous and cytoplasmic fashion (×200). (*B*) Peripheral cells in tumor nests and trabeculae are p63 positive (×200), although not necessarily morphologically distinct by light microscopy.

strongly positive for PTAH and antimitochondrial antibody. Clear cell oncocytomas have a high glycogen content and may be PAS positive.[43]

Differential Diagnosis

Oncocytomas have at typical appearance for which there is minimal diagnostic dilemma. Main diagnostic considerations include oncocytic variants of other named tumor types. Oncocytic-sebaceous EMCa may have a solid appearance in areas mimicking oncocytoma. This is a more distinctly bilayered tumor, however, with the outer layer composed of myoepithelial cells compared with oncocytoma, which has only a subtle p63-positive peripheral layer.[10] Solid oncocytic MEC can be distinguished from oncocytoma by the presence of mucous cells and a more diffuse p63 reactivity.[115] Occasionally, acinic cell carcinomas may have an oncocytoid appearance but careful examination demonstrates acinar cells with basophilic zymogen granules. Oncocytic carcinoma (discussed previously) is distinguished by the

presence of infiltration, including angiolymphatic and perineural invasion. Additionally, oncocytic carcinomas have larger nuclei with more prominent nucleoli and membrane irregularities.[40]

One important diagnostic consideration in a subset of patients is metastatic RCC. The parotid gland is among the most common sites for a distant metastasis from RCC. Additionally, 37% of RCCs may not show prominent clear cell

 Differential Diagnosis
ONCOCYTOMA

- Oncocytic carcinoma
- Oncocytic-sebaceous EMCa
- Oncocytic MEC
- Acinic cell carcinoma
- Metastatic RCC

Fig. 54. Metastatic RCC (×100). This tumor resembles a clear cell oncocytoma; however, it has prominent blood lakes and more cytologic pleomorphism equating to Fuhrman nuclear grade III.

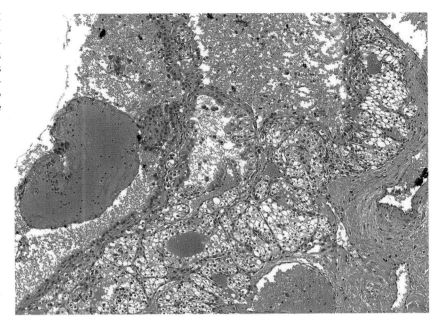

features on metastases.[40] Morphologically, they are distinguished by the presence of prominent blood lakes, and these are typically Furman nuclear grade III or IV in metastases (**Fig. 54**). Muscular arteries are more common in RCC, but may occasionally be seen in salivary oncocytic neoplasms. By immunohistochemistry, p63 is the best marker for discrimination of these 2 lesions, because RCCs are invariably p63 negative. Other markers that support a renal origin include RCC marker and CD10.[40]

Treatment and Prognosis

Treatment is surgical. Recurrences are rare and likely represent multifocality. Malignant transformation has been reported after radiotherapy in isolated cases.[116] Alternatively, based on rare reports, radioactive iodine may decrease tumor volume.[117]

LYMPHADENOMA

Overview

Lymphadenomas are rare benign tumors with prominent lymphoid stroma that do not consist of the oncocytic bilayer seen in Warthin tumor. This group of tumors usually occurs after the fifth decade with an equal gender predilection.[3,118,119]

Lymphadenomas are essentially a disease of the parotid gland, although rare cases of minor salivary glands have been reported. Lymphadenomas typically present as slow growing painless

Pitfalls
ONCOCYTOMA

! Oncocytomas may show clear cell change, and, conversely, more than a third of renal metastases to the parotid gland may not show clear cell predominant histology.

Key Features
LYMPHADENOMAS

- Lymphadenomas are benign non-Warthin epithelial lesions with prominent lymphoid stroma.
- Lymphadenomas are subcategorized as sebaceous and nonsebaceous.

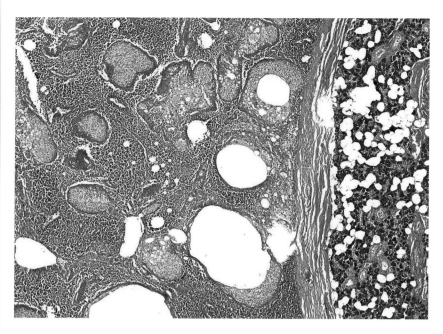

Fig. 55. Sebaceous lymphadenoma (×40). This parotid tumor shows an encapsulated proliferation of solid to cystic sebaceous nests. Lymphoid stroma is prominent.

masses. Some degree of cystic change may result in a fluctuant appearance.

Gross Features

Lymphadenomas range from solid to multicystic. They may often have a greasy yellowish sebum within the lesion. The cut surfaces are whitish or yellow. Occasionally when lymphoid stroma predominates, the cut surface is a fleshy tan resembling a lymph node. These tumors are well demarcated although the degree of encapsulation varies.

Microscopic Features

Lymphadenomas are stratified into 2 groups: sebaceous and non-sebaceous. Sebaceous lymphadenomas are more common. These consist of solid to cystic proliferations of squamoid nests with varying degrees of sebaceous differentiation

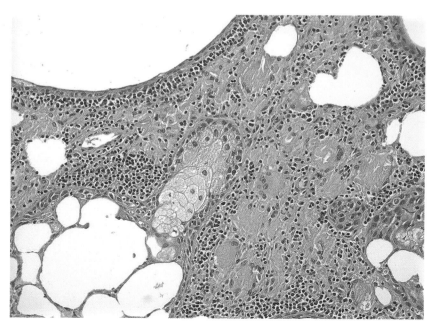

Fig. 56. Prominent lipogranulomatous reaction in sebaceous lymphadenoma (×200). The giant cells are rich in lipid from the rupture of sebaceous nests (*bottom*). Scattered cholesterol clefts are noted as well.

Fig. 57. Lymphadenoma, nonsebaceous type (×100). This tumor consists of a lymphoid rich basaloid tubulotrabecular proliferation.

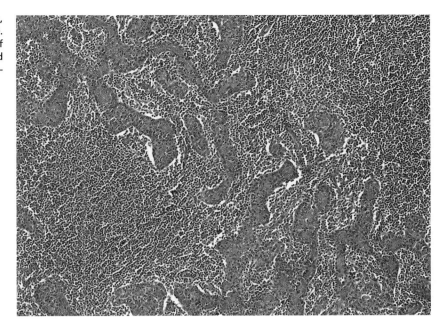

(**Fig. 55**). Similar to Warthin tumor, the lymphoid component often resembles a lymph node. Sebaceous lymphadenomas may have varying proportions of keratinization. A proportion of them may show tubular elements. Oncocytic change may be present suggesting some overlap with Warthin tumor in a subset of sebaceous lymphadenomas. One common, unique finding in sebaceous lymphadenomas is a granulomatous reaction to the keratin and sebum in the surrounding lymphoid stroma (**Fig. 56**).

The epithelial component of nonsebaceous lymphadenomas is often basaloid in appearance, ranging from solid to tubulotrabecular in growth (**Fig. 57**). Although nests are distinct, intraepithelial lymphocytes may be prominent. The epithelial

Fig. 58. Oncocytic cystadenoma (×100). This tumor resembles a Warthin tumor without lymphoid stroma and is composed of a bilayered columnar epithelium.

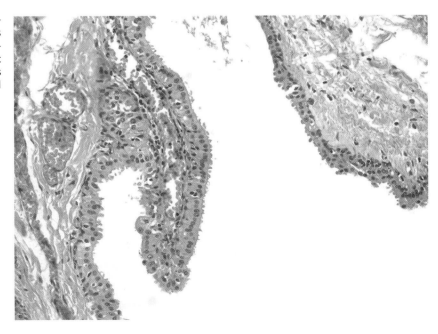

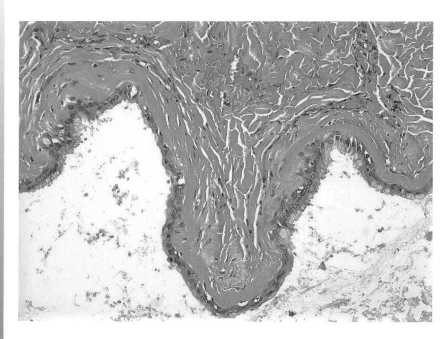

Fig. 59. Mucocytes in cystadenoma (×200). Occasionally these are prominent resembling gastric foveolar epithelium.

nests are monomorphic and bland. Similar to their sebaceous counterparts, nonsebaceous lymphadenomas may have minor oncocytic elements.

Lymphadenomas have a prominent squamoid phenotype. As such, these are positive for CK5/6 and p63 particularly at the periphery. Tubular constituents may be positive for luminal type keratins, such as CK7, CK8, CK18, and CK19. Sebaceous elements may be positive for epithelial membrane antigen and, to varying degrees, squamoid markers (CK5/6 and p63) as well as for adipophilin and perilipin but, unlike skin sebaceous lesions, they are not often positive for AR.[120]

Differential Diagnosis

Lymphadenomas do have a good deal of overlap with Warthin tumor; however, lymphadenomas, both sebaceous and nonsebaceous, have more epithelial heterogeneity whereas Warthin tumors are almost always predominantly composed of oncocytic bilayered epithelium with only minor sebaceous, squamous, or mucinous elements.

The more relevant differential diagnostic considerations for lymphadenomas are carcinomas with prominent lymphoid stroma, such as MEC and acinic cell carcinoma and metastases to intraparotid lymph nodes. Unlike acinic cell carcinomas, lymphadenomas are noninfiltrative and are composed of considerable cell type heterogeneity whereas acinic cell carcinomas are mainly of a ductoacinar phenotype with varying amounts of

zymogen granules as demonstrable by PAS after diastase treatment. MECs may have considerable overlap with sebaceous lymphadenomas, particularly low-grade to intermediate-grade MECs because the latter are also well demarcated. MECs do not typically have a prominent sebaceous component, and they should not have much keratinization. Lymphadenomas, alternatively, do not generally have mucous cells, and often have tubular elements, which are not seen in MECs. Occasionally, the solid growth pattern in nonsebaceous lymphadenomas may be mistaken for a lymphoepithelial carcinoma; unlike the syncytial growth pattern common to lymphoepithelial carcinomas, solid lymphadenomas are composed of compressed nests, tubules, and trabeculae that have distinct cell borders and tumor nest borders. Furthermore, lymphadenomas do not have the same atypia or enlarged vesicular nuclei with prominent nucleoli seen in

 Differential Diagnosis
LYMPHADENOMAS

- Warthin tumor
- MEC
- Acinic cell carcinoma
- Lymphoepithelial carcinoma

lymphoepithelial carcinoma. To date, nonsebaceous lymphadenomas have not been described to show positivity for Epstein-Barr virus early RNA, which is often seen in lymphoepithelial carcinomas.[120]

Treatment and Prognosis

Treatment is purely surgical. Recurrences are uncommon. Malignant transformation has not been convincingly described. Sebaceous lymphadenocarcinomas exist but their transition from a benign counterpart has not been described in the literature.

CYSTADENOMA

Overview

Cystadenoma is a rare category of benign cystic neoplasms that cannot be classified as cystic variants of other named neoplasms. This group of tumors occurs predominantly in the fifth decade with a female predilection of 2:1 to 3:1.[3,111] Cystadenomas typically occur in the parotid gland and submandibular gland, although they are common in the lip and oncocytic cystadenomas are common in the minor salivary tissue of the larynx.[121]

Cystadenomas usually present as fluctuant painless masses. In the oral cavity they may mimic mucoceles.

Gross Features

Cystadenomas may be unilocular or multilocular but invariably well demarcated with evidence of

a capsule in approximately one-quarter of cases. Papillary excrescences may be present, particularly in large cysts. Cyst fluid varies widely likely dependent to some extent on cell type. Minor oral salivary gland tumors are significantly smaller than parotid tumors and are seldom greater than 1 cm.

Microscopic Features

Cystadenomas may be lined by a variety of epithelial types. Most commonly the luminal epithelium is cystic to cuboidal with pale eosinophilic cytoplasm. The outer layer is lined by an indistinct layer of basal cells with scant cytoplasm and small ovoid nuclei. Oncocytic cystadenomas are a common variant, where the lining is composed of columnar oncocytic epithelium. Oncocytic cystadenomas often resemble Warthin tumors without lymphoid stroma (**Fig. 58**). Although some sources indicate that the oncocytic epithelium in cystadenomas is more haphazardly arranged, the authors' experience is that these are typically bilayered. Squamous and mucinous metaplasia may be seen (**Fig. 59**). Rarely, cystadenomas may be purely of the mucous cell type; these may be composed purely of columnar mucinous epithelium resembling gastric foveolar mucosa.[3]

The immunophenotype is nondescript and resembles that of Warthin tumor. The ductal epithelium is positive for simple low molecular weight keratins (ie, CK7 and CK18). The basal layer is positive for CK5/6, p63, and occasionally myoepithelial muscle markers, such as actin or calponin. Nononcocytic cystadenomas have more of an intercalated duct phenotype and may show an S-100–positive luminal layer.

Differential Diagnosis

The designation of cystadenoma should be made with caution. Often, there is considerable overlap between cystadenoma and reactive proliferations, such as postobstructive duct ectasia or sialocysts. The distinction to some extent is arbitrary because there is no molecular evidence that all cystadenomas are clonal neoplasms. Cystadenomas of the larynx are likely reactive. Generally, duct ectasia is distinguished by a spacing distribution more similar to the native ducts of the involved salivary gland, whereas the cysts in cystadenoma may be more densely packed and haphazardly arranged.

Oncocytic cystadenomas are separated from Warthin tumor by the absence of well-formed lymphoid stroma. Furthermore, clinically cystadenomas can occur outside the parotid gland unlike Warthin tumors.[104] Intraductal papillomas are

---

△△ *Differential Diagnosis*
CYSTADENOMA

- Sialocyst/sialectasia
- Intraductal papilloma
- Warthin tumor
- MEC
- Cystadenocarcinoma
- Acinic cell carcinoma
- Cystic EMC

Pitfalls
CYSTADENOMA

! Multiply recurrent cystadenoma may be another diagnostic entity, such as low-grade MEC and acinic cell carcinoma.

---

similar to cystadenomas. By convention, intraductal papillomas are unilocular and confined to the main duct. These entities may be related and some papillary predominant cystadenomas may be a form of intraductal papillomatosis.[2]

The malignant counterpart of cystadenoma is cystadenocarcinoma. For low-grade cystadenocarcinomas, the distinction may be subtle. Cystadenocarcinomas may show more architectural complexity, particularly more arborizing papillae. They may also show a more infiltrative growth pattern, perhaps in the form of smaller caliber cysts or tubules infiltrating from the cyst wall. Immunohistochemically, they may show loss of a delimiting basal layer around the infiltrative elements.[31] The other main carcinoma type that is in the differential is low-grade MEC, which is cystic and bland. As discussed previously, MEC shows tufts of intermediate and epidermoid cells immediately beneath overlying mucous and columnar cells. Furthermore, MECs may show more sclerosis around cysts. In difficult cases, evaluation for *MECT1/MAML2* rearrangements may delineate MEC from cystadenoma.[35] Acinic cell carcinoma, in particular the papillary cystic type, may be deceptively bland. Unlike cystadenomas, these are monophasic tumors and do not have an outer p63-positive basal layer. The cysts are line often by vacuolated cells with a hobnail epithelium, but on careful examination also show acinar cells with the characteristic basophilic zymogen granules.[122] Occasionally, EMCa may have a predominant cystic and papillary growth pattern, in particular the oncocytic variant. EMCa is delineated, however, by evidence for infiltration and increased architectural complexity. Although both cystic EMCa and cystadenoma are bilayered, the outer layer of EMCa is composed of larger polygonal cells with clear to pale cytoplasm. These are more decidedly myoepithelial with uniform co-expression of actins and basal markers, such as p63 and CK5/6, as opposed to the attenuated basal layer of cystadenomas that shows only rare myoepithelial cell constituents, if any.[8]

Treatment and Prognosis

Treatment is purely surgical. Recurrences are uncommon. The authors' experience has shown that the few recurrent cystadenomas were actually low-grade oncocytic MEC or acinic cell carcinomas. One case of malignant transformation has been reported.

REFERENCES

1. Eveson JW, Auclair PL, Gnepp DR, et al. Tumors of the salivary glands: Introduction. In: Barnes EL, Eveson JW, Reichart P, et al, editors. World health organization classification of tumours: pathology & genetics. Head and neck tumours. Lyon (France): IARC Press; 2005. p. 221–2.
2. Myers EN, Ferris RL, editors. Salivary gland disorders. Berlin: Springer; 2007.
3. Ellis G, Auclair PL. In: Tumors of the salivary glands. 4th Series. Washington, DC: Armed Forces Institute of Pathology; 2008. p. 49–140, 196–203, 269–88, 301–21, 356–63.
4. Eveson JW, Nagao T. Diseases of the salivary glands. In: Barnes L, editor. Surgical pathology of the head and neck, vol. 1. New York: Informa; 2009. p. 475–648.
5. Donath K, Seifert G, Schmitz R. Diagnosis and ultrastructure of the tubular carcinoma of salivary gland ducts. Epithelial-myoepithelial carcinoma of the intercalated ducts. Virchows Arch A Pathol Pathol Anat 1972;356(1):16–31 [in German].
6. Corridan M. Glycogen-rich clear cell adenoma of the parotid gland. J Pathol Bacteriol 1956;72:623–6.
7. Feyrter F. On glycogen-rich reticular adenoma of the salivary glands. Z Krebsforsch 1963;65: 446–54 [in German].
8. Seethala RR, Barnes EL, Hunt JL. Epithelial-myoepithelial carcinoma: a review of the clinicopathologic spectrum and immunophenotypic characteristics in 61 tumors of the salivary glands and upper aerodigestive tract. Am J Surg Pathol 2007;31(1):44–57.
9. Fonseca I, Soares J. Epithelial-myoepithelial carcinoma. In: Barnes EL, Eveson JW, Reichart P,

et al, editors. World health organization classification of tumours: pathology & genetics. Head and neck tumours. Lyon (France): IARC Press; 2005. p. 225–6.

10. Seethala RR, Richmond JA, Hoschar AP, et al. New variants of epithelial-myoepithelial carcinoma: oncocytic-sebaceous and apocrine. Arch Pathol Lab Med 2009;133(6):950–9.

11. Roy P, Bullock MJ, Perez-Ordonez B, et al. Epithelial-myoepithelial carcinoma with high grade transformation. Am J Surg Pathol 2010;34(9):1258–65.

12. Shinozaki A, Nagao T, Endo H, et al. Sebaceous epithelial-myoepithelial carcinoma of the salivary gland: clinicopathologic and immunohistochemical analysis of 6 cases of a new histologic variant. Am J Surg Pathol 2008;32(6): 913–23.

13. Dardick I, Leong I. Clear cell carcinoma: review of its histomorphogenesis and classification as a squamous cell lesion. Oral Surg Oral Med Oral Pathol Oral Radiol Endod 2009;108(3):399–405.

14. Bilodeau EA, Hoschar AP, Barnes EL, et al. Clear cell carcinoma and clear cell odontogenic carcinoma: a comparative clinicopathologic and immunohistochemical study. Head Neck Pathol 2011; 5(2):101–7.

15. Neves Cde O, Soares AB, Costa AF, et al. CD10 (Neutral Endopeptidase) Expression in myoepithelial cells of salivary neoplasms. Appl Immunohistochem Mol Morphol 2010;18(2):172–8.

16. Cho KJ, el-Naggar AK, Ordonez NG, et al. Epithelial-myoepithelial carcinoma of salivary glands. A clinicopathologic, DNA flow cytometric, and immunohistochemical study of Ki-67 and HER-2/neu oncogene. Am J Clin Pathol 1995;103(4):432–7.

17. Fonseca I, Soares J. Epithelial-myoepithelial carcinoma of the salivary glands. A study of 22 cases. Virchows Arch A Pathol Anat Histopathol 1993; 422(5):389–96.

18. Luna MA, Ordonez NG, Mackay B, et al. Salivary epithelial-myoepithelial carcinomas of intercalated ducts: a clinical, electron microscopic, and immunocytochemical study. Oral Surg Oral Med Oral Pathol 1985;59(5):482–90.

19. Ellis GL. Clear cell neoplasms in salivary glands: clearly a diagnostic challenge. Ann Diagn Pathol 1998;2(1):61–78.

20. Milchgrub S, Gnepp DR, Vuitch F, et al. Hyalinizing clear cell carcinoma of salivary gland. Am J Surg Pathol 1994;18(1):74–82.

21. Seifert G. Classification and differential diagnosis of clear and basal cell tumors of the salivary glands. Semin Diagn Pathol 1996;13(2):95–103.

22. Wang B, Brandwein M, Gordon R, et al. Primary salivary clear cell tumors—a diagnostic approach: a clinicopathologic and immunohistochemical study of 20 patients with clear cell carcinoma, clear

cell myoepithelial carcinoma, and epithelial-myoepithelial carcinoma. Arch Pathol Lab Med 2002;126(6):676–85.

23. Simpson RH, Sarsfield PT, Clarke T, et al. Clear cell carcinoma of minor salivary glands. Histopathology 1990;17(5):433–8.

24. Antonescu CR, Katabi N, Zhang L, et al. EWSR1-ATF1 fusion is a novel and consistent finding in hyalinizing clear-cell carcinoma of salivary gland. Genes Chromosomes Cancer 2011; 50(7):559–70.

25. Michal M, Skalova A, Simpson RH, et al. Clear cell malignant myoepithelioma of the salivary glands. Histopathology 1996;28(4):309–15.

26. Brandwein M, Said-Al-Naief N, Gordon R, et al. Clear cell odontogenic carcinoma: report of a case and analysis of the literature. Arch Otolaryngol Head Neck Surg 2002;128(9):1089–95.

27. Rezende RB, Drachenberg CB, Kumar D, et al. Differential diagnosis between monomorphic clear cell adenocarcinoma of salivary glands and renal (clear) cell carcinoma. Am J Surg Pathol 1999; 23(12):1532–8.

28. Fonseca I, Soares J. Basal cell adenocarcinoma of minor salivary and seromucous glands of the head and neck region. Semin Diagn Pathol 1996;13(2): 128–37.

29. Muller S, Barnes L. Basal cell adenocarcinoma of the salivary glands. Report of seven cases and review of the literature. Cancer 1996;78(12):2471–7.

30. Nagao T, Sugano I, Ishida Y, et al. Basal cell adenocarcinoma of the salivary glands: comparison with basal cell adenoma through assessment of cell proliferation, apoptosis, and expression of p53 and bcl-2. Cancer 1998; 82(3):439–47.

31. Foss RD, Ellis GL, Auclair PL. Salivary gland cystadenocarcinomas. A clinicopathologic study of 57 cases. Am J Surg Pathol 1996;20(12):1440–7.

32. Wayne S, Barnes EL, Seethala RR. Low grade intraductal carcinoma: a relative of cystadenocarcinoma, precursor to salivary duct carcinoma, or both? United States and Canadian association for pathology. Mod Pathol 2008;21(Suppl 1):242A.

33. Kapadia SB, Barnes L. Expression of androgen receptor, gross cystic disease fluid protein, and CD44 in salivary duct carcinoma. Mod Pathol 1998;11(11):1033–8.

34. Behboudi A, Enlund F, Winnes M, et al. Molecular classification of mucoepidermoid carcinomas-prognostic significance of the MECT1-MAML2 fusion oncogene. Genes Chromosomes Cancer 2006;45(5):470–81.

35. Seethala RR, Dacic S, Cieply K, et al. A reappraisal of the MECT1/MAML2 translocation in salivary mucoepidermoid carcinomas. Am J Surg Pathol 2010; 34(8):1106–21.

36. Delgado R, Klimstra D, Albores-Saavedra J. Low grade salivary duct carcinoma. A distinctive variant with a low grade histology and a predominant intraductal growth pattern. Cancer 1996; 78(5):958–67.

37. Brandwein-Gensler M, Hille J, Wang BY, et al. Low-grade salivary duct carcinoma: description of 16 cases. Am J Surg Pathol 2004;28(8):1040–4.

38. Weinreb I, Tabanda-Lichauco R, Van der Kwast T, et al. Low-grade intraductal carcinoma of salivary gland: report of 3 cases with marked apocrine differentiation. Am J Surg Pathol 2006;30(8):1014–21.

39. Cheuk W, Miliauskas JR, Chan JK. Intraductal carcinoma of the oral cavity: a case report and a reappraisal of the concept of pure ductal carcinoma in situ in salivary duct carcinoma. Am J Surg Pathol 2004;28(2):266–70.

40. McHugh JB, Hoschar AP, Dvorakova M, et al. p63 immunohistochemistry differentiates salivary gland oncocytoma and oncocytic carcinoma from metastatic renal cell carcinoma. Head Neck Pathol 2007;1(2):123–31.

41. Zhou CX, Shi DY, Ma DQ, et al. Primary oncocytic carcinoma of the salivary glands: a clinicopathologic and immunohistochemical study of 12 cases. Oral Oncol 2010;46(10):773–8.

42. Goode RK, Corio RL. Oncocytic adenocarcinoma of salivary glands. Oral Surg Oral Med Oral Pathol 1988;65(1):61–6.

43. Brandwein MS, Huvos AG. Oncocytic tumors of major salivary glands. A study of 68 cases with follow-up of 44 patients. Am J Surg Pathol 1991; 15(6):514–28.

44. Auclair PL, Van der Wal JE. Adenocarcinoma, not otherwise specified. In: Barnes L, Eveson JW, Reichart P, et al, editors. World Health Organization classification of tumours. pathology and genetics. Head and neck tumours. Lyon (France): IARC; 2005. p. 238–9.

45. Wahlberg P, Anderson H, Biorklund A, et al. Carcinoma of the parotid and submandibular glands–a study of survival in 2465 patients. Oral Oncol 2002;38(7):706–13.

46. Li J, Wang BY, Nelson M, et al. Salivary adenocarcinoma, not otherwise specified: a collection of orphans. Arch Pathol Lab Med 2004;128(12):1385–94.

47. Spiro RH, Huvos AG, Strong EW. Adenocarcinoma of salivary origin. Clinicopathologic study of 204 patients. Am J Surg 1982;144(4):423–31.

48. Seethala RR, Johnson JT, Barnes EL, et al. Polymorphous low-grade adenocarcinoma: the University of Pittsburgh experience. Arch Otolaryngol Head Neck Surg 2010;136(4):385–92.

49. Seethala RR, Hunt JL, Baloch ZW, et al. Adenoid cystic carcinoma with high-grade transformation: a report of 11 cases and a review of the literature. Am J Surg Pathol 2007;31(11):1683–94.

50. Stanley RJ, Weiland LH, Olsen KD, et al. Dedifferentiated acinic cell (acinous) carcinoma of the parotid gland. Otolaryngol Head Neck Surg 1988; 98(2):155–61.

51. Lewis JE, Olsen KD, Sebo TJ. Carcinoma ex pleomorphic adenoma: pathologic analysis of 73 cases. Hum Pathol 2001;32(6):596–604.

52. Eveson JW, Cawson RA. Salivary gland tumours. A review of 2410 cases with particular reference to histological types, site, age and sex distribution. J Pathol 1985;146(1):51–8.

53. Pinkston JA, Cole P. Incidence rates of salivary gland tumors: results from a population-based study. Otolaryngol Head Neck Surg 1999;120(6):834–40.

54. Spiro RH. Salivary neoplasms: overview of a 35-year experience with 2,807 patients. Head Neck Surg 1986;8(3):177–84.

55. Waldron CA, el-Mofty SK, Gnepp DR. Tumors of the intraoral minor salivary glands: a demographic and histologic study of 426 cases. Oral Surg Oral Med Oral Pathol 1988;66(3):323–33.

56. Ribeiro Kde C, Kowalski LP, Saba LM, et al. Epithelial salivary glands neoplasms in children and adolescents: a forty-four-year experience. Med Pediatr Oncol 2002;39(6):594–600.

57. Miliauskas JR, Hunt JL. Primary unilateral multifocal pleomorphic adenoma of the parotid gland: molecular assessment and literature review. Head Neck Pathol 2008;2(4):339–42.

58. Zbaren P, Stauffer E. Pleomorphic adenoma of the parotid gland: histopathologic analysis of the capsular characteristics of 218 tumors. Head Neck 2007;29(8):751–7.

59. Schmidt LA, Olsen SH, McHugh JB. Cutaneous adnexal differentiation and stromal metaplasia in palate pleomorphic adenomas: a potential diagnostic pitfall that may be mistaken for malignancy. Am J Surg Pathol 2010;34(8):1205–10.

60. Li S, Baloch ZW, Tomaszewski JE, et al. Worrisome histologic alterations following fine-needle aspiration of benign parotid lesions. Arch Pathol Lab Med 2000;124(1):87–91.

61. Coleman H, Altini M. Intravascular tumour in intra-oral pleomorphic adenomas: a diagnostic and therapeutic dilemma. Histopathology 1999;35(5):439–44.

62. DeRoche TC, Hoschar AP, Hunt JL. Immunohistochemical evaluation of androgen receptor, HER-2/neu, and p53 in benign pleomorphic adenomas. Arch Pathol Lab Med 2008;132(12):1907–11.

63. Martin AR, Mantravadi J, Kotylo PK, et al. Proliferative activity and aneuploidy in pleomorphic adenomas of the salivary glands. Arch Pathol Lab Med 1994;118(3):252–9.

64. Martins C, Fonseca I, Roque L, et al. PLAG1 gene alterations in salivary gland pleomorphic adenoma and carcinoma ex-pleomorphic adenoma: a combined study using chromosome banding, in

situ hybridization and immunocytochemistry. Mod Pathol 2005;18(8):1048–55.

65. Bullerdiek J, Wobst G, Meyer-Bolte K, et al. Cytogenetic subtyping of 220 salivary gland pleomorphic adenomas: correlation to occurrence, histological subtype, and in vitro cellular behavior. Cancer Genet Cytogenet 1993;65(1):27–31.

66. Debiec-Rychter M, Van Valckenborgh I, Van den Broeck C, et al. Histologic localization of PLAG1 (pleomorphic adenoma gene 1) in pleomorphic adenoma of the salivary gland: cytogenetic evidence of common origin of phenotypically diverse cells. Lab Invest 2001;81(9):1289–97.

67. Eveson JW, Kusafuka K, Stenman G, et al. Pleomorphic adenoma. In: Barnes EL, Eveson JW, Reichart P, et al, editors. World Health Organization classification of tumours: pathology & genetics. Head and neck tumours. Lyon (France): IARC Press; 2005. p. 254–8.

68. Noguchi S, Aihara T, Yoshino K, et al. Demonstration of monoclonal origin of human parotid gland pleomorphic adenoma. Cancer 1996;77(3):431–5.

69. Fowler MH, Fowler J, Ducatman B, et al. Malignant mixed tumors of the salivary gland: a study of loss of heterozygosity in tumor suppressor genes. Mod Pathol 2006;19(3):350–5.

70. Bellizzi AM, Mills SE. Collagenous crystalloids in myoepithelial carcinoma: report of a case and review of the literature. Am J Clin Pathol 2008;130(3):355–62.

71. Dardick I, Daley TD, van Nostrand AW. Basal cell adenoma with myoepithelial cell-derived "stroma": a new major salivary gland tumor entity. Head Neck Surg 1986;8(4):257–67.

72. Witt RL. The significance of the margin in parotid surgery for pleomorphic adenoma. Laryngoscope 2002;112(12):2141–54.

73. Sciubba JJ, Brannon RB. Myoepithelioma of salivary glands: report of 23 cases. Cancer 1982; 49(3):562–72.

74. Barnes L, Appel BN, Perez H, et al. Myoepithelioma of the head and neck: case report and review. J Surg Oncol 1985;28(1):21–8.

75. Alos L, Cardesa A, Bombi JA, et al. Myoepithelial tumors of salivary glands: a clinicopathologic, immunohistochemical, ultrastructural, and flow-cytometric study. Semin Diagn Pathol 1996;13(2):138–47.

76. Nagao T, Sugano I, Ishida Y, et al. Salivary gland malignant myoepithelioma: a clinicopathologic and immunohistochemical study of ten cases. Cancer 1998;83(7):1292–9.

77. Savera AT, Zarbo RJ. Defining the role of myoepithelium in salivary gland neoplasia. Adv Anat Pathol 2004;11(2):69–85.

78. Cardesa A, Alos L. Myoepithelioma. In: Barnes EL, Eveson JW, Reichart P, et al, editors. World Health Organization classification of tumours: pathology &

genetics. Head and neck tumours. Lyon (France): IARC Press; 2005. p. 259–60.

79. Peel R. Diseases of the salivary gland. In: Barnes L, editor. Surgical pathology of the head and neck, vol. 1. 2nd edition. New York: Marcel-Dekker; 2000. p. 634–90.

80. Kleinsasser O, Klein HJ. Basal cell adenoma of the salivary glands. Arch Klin Exp Ohren Nasen Kehlkopfheilkd 1967;189(3):302–16 [in German].

81. de Araujo VC. Basal cell adenoma. In: Barnes EL, Eveson JW, Reichart P, et al, editors. World Health Organization classification of tumours: pathology & genetics. Head and neck tumours. Lyon (France): IARC Press; 2005. p. 261–2.

82. Luna MA, Tortoledo ME, Allen M. Salivary dermal analogue tumors arising in lymph nodes. Cancer 1987;59(6):1165–9.

83. Zarbo RJ. Salivary gland neoplasia: a review for the practicing pathologist. Mod Pathol 2002;15(3):298–323.

84. Headington JT, Batsakis JG, Beals TF, et al. Membranous basal cell adenoma of parotid gland, dermal cylindromas, and trichoepitheliomas. Comparative histochemistry and ultrastructure. Cancer 1977;39(6):2460–9.

85. Choi HR, Batsakis JG, Callender DL, et al. Molecular analysis of chromosome 16q regions in dermal analogue tumors of salivary glands: a genetic link to dermal cylindroma? Am J Surg Pathol 2002;26(6):778–83.

86. Ferreiro JA. Immunohistochemistry of basal cell adenoma of the major salivary glands. Histopathology 1994;24(6):539–42.

87. Zarbo RJ, Prasad AR, Regezi JA, et al. Salivary gland basal cell and canalicular adenomas: immunohistochemical demonstration of myoepithelial cell participation and morphogenetic considerations. Arch Pathol Lab Med 2000;124(3):401–5.

88. Machado de Sousa SO, Soares de Araujo N, Correa L, et al. Immunohistochemical aspects of basal cell adenoma and canalicular adenoma of salivary glands. Oral Oncol 2001;37(4):365–8.

89. Kawahara A, Harada H, Abe H, et al. Nuclear beta-catenin expression in basal cell adenomas of salivary gland. J Oral Pathol Med 2011;40(6):460–6.

90. Luna MA, Batsakis JG, Tortoledo ME, et al. Carcinomas ex monomorphic adenoma of salivary glands. J Laryngol Otol 1989;103(8):756–9.

91. Ferreiro JA. Canalicular adenoma. In: Barnes EL, Eveson JW, Reichart P, et al, editors. World Health Organization classification of tumours: pathology & genetics. Head and neck tumours. Lyon (France): IARC Press; 2005. p. 267.

92. Daley TD, Gardner DG, Smout MS. Canalicular adenoma: not a basal cell adenoma. Oral Surg Oral Med Oral Pathol 1984;57(2):181–8.

93. Gardner DG, Daley TD. The use of the terms monomorphic adenoma, basal cell adenoma, and canalicular adenoma as applied to salivary gland tumors. Oral Surg Oral Med Oral Pathol 1983; 56(6):608–15.

94. Nelson JF, Jacoway JR. Monomorphic adenoma (canalicular type). Report of 29 cases. Cancer 1973;31(6):1511–3.

95. Rousseau A, Mock D, Dover DG, et al. Multiple canalicular adenomas: a case report and review of the literature. Oral Surg Oral Med Oral Pathol Oral Radiol Endod 1999;87(3):346–50.

96. Ferreiro JA. Immunohistochemical analysis of salivary gland canalicular adenoma. Oral Surg Oral Med Oral Pathol 1994;78(6):761–5.

97. McMillan MD, Smith CJ, Smillie AC. Canalicular adenoma: report of five cases with ultrastructural observations. J Oral Pathol Med 1993;22(8):368–73.

98. Edwards PC, Bhuiya T, Kelsch RD. Assessment of p63 expression in the salivary gland neoplasms adenoid cystic carcinoma, polymorphous low-grade adenocarcinoma, and basal cell and canalicular adenomas. Oral Surg Oral Med Oral Pathol Oral Radiol Endod 2004;97(5):613–9.

99. Harmse JL, Saleh HA, Odutoye T, et al. Recurrent canalicular adenoma of the minor salivary glands in the upper lip. J Laryngol Otol 1997;111(10):985–7.

100. Warthin AS. Papillary cystadenoma lymphomatosum: a rare teratoid of the parotid region. J Cancer Res 1929;13:116–25.

101. Kotwall CA. Smoking as an etiologic factor in the development of Warthin's tumor of the parotid gland. Am J Surg 1992;164(6):646–7.

102. Monk JS Jr, Church JS. Warthin's tumor. A high incidence and no sex predominance in central Pennsylvania. Arch Otolaryngol Head Neck Surg 1992; 118(5):477–8.

103. Snyderman C, Johnson JT, Barnes EL. Extraparotid Warthin's tumor. Otolaryngol Head Neck Surg 1986;94(2):169–75.

104. Simpson RH, Eveson JW. Warthin tumor. In: Barnes EL, Eveson JW, Sidransky D, editors. Pathology and classification of head and neck tumours. Lyon (France): IARC; 2005. p. 263–5.

105. Seifert G, Bull HG, Donath K. Histologic subclassification of the cystadenolymphoma of the parotid gland. Analysis of 275 cases. Virchows Arch A Pathol Anat Histol 1980;388(1):13–38.

106. Weber A, Langhanki L, Schutz A, et al. Expression profiles of p53, p63, and p73 in benign salivary gland tumors. Virchows Arch 2002;441(5):428–36.

107. Schwerer MJ, Kraft K, Baczako K, et al. Cytokeratin expression and epithelial differentiation in Warthin's tumour and its metaplastic (infarcted) variant. Histopathology 2001;39(4):347–52.

108. Saxena A, Memauri B, Hasegawa W. Initial diagnosis of small lymphocytic lymphoma in parotidectomy for Warthin tumour, a rare collision tumour. J Clin Pathol 2005;58(3):331–3.

109. Fehr A, Roser K, Belge G, et al. A closer look at Warthin tumors and the t(11;19). Cancer Genet Cytogenet 2008;180(2):135–9.

110. Williamson JD, Simmons BH, el-Naggar A. Medeiros LJ. Mucoepidermoid carcinoma involving Warthin tumor. A report of five cases and review of the literature. Am J Clin Pathol 2000;114(4): 564–70.

111. Ellis G, Auclair P, editors. Tumors of the salivary glands. 3rd Series ed. Washington, DC: Armed Forces Institute of Pathology; 1996. Atlas of tumor pathology; No. 17.

112. Miyake H, Matsumoto A, Hori Y, et al. Warthin's tumor of parotid gland on Tc-99m pertechnetate scintigraphy with lemon juice stimulation: Tc-99m uptake, size, and pathologic correlation. Eur Radiol 2001;11(12):2472–8.

113. Shah VN, Branstetter BF. Oncocytoma of the parotid gland: a potential false-positive finding on 18F-FDG PET. AJR Am J Roentgenol 2007;189(4): W212–4.

114. Zhou CX, Gao Y. Oncocytoma of the salivary glands: a clinicopathologic and immunohistochemical study. Oral Oncol 2009;45(12):e232–8.

115. Weinreb I, Seethala RR, Perez-Ordonez B, et al. Oncocytic mucoepidermoid carcinoma: clinicopathologic description in a series of 12 cases. Am J Surg Pathol 2009;33(3):409–16.

116. Coli A, Bigotti G, Bartolazzi A. Malignant oncocytoma of major salivary glands. Report of a post-irradiation case. J Exp Clin Cancer Res 1998;17(1):65–70.

117. Kosuda S, Ishikawa M, Tamura K, et al. Iodine-131 therapy for parotid oncocytoma. J Nucl Med 1988; 29(6):1126–9.

118. Gnepp DR, Brannon R. Sebaceous neoplasms of salivary gland origin. Report of 21 cases. Cancer 1984;53(10):2155–70.

119. Ma J, Chan JK, Chow CW, et al. Lymphadenoma: a report of three cases of an uncommon salivary gland neoplasm. Histopathology 2002;41(4): 342–50.

120. Seethala RR, Montone K, Kane S, et al. Salivary gland lymphadenomas: clinicopathological and immunohistochemical study. Mod Pathol 2010; 23(S1):279A.

121. Brandwein M, Huvos A. Laryngeal oncocytic cystadenomas. Eight cases and a literature review. Arch Otolaryngol Head Neck Surg 1995;121(11):1302–5.

122. Chiosea SI, Peel R, Barnes EL, et al. Salivary type tumors seen in consultation. Virchows Arch 2009; 454(4):457–66.

BONE LESIONS OF THE HEAD AND NECK

Samir K. El-Mofty, DMD, PhD*, James S. Lewis Jr, MD,
Rebecca D. Chernock, MD

KEYWORDS

- Bone lesions • Craniofacial lesions • Head and neck pathology

ABSTRACT

This article describes the clinical, radiographic, and pathologic features of tumors and tumorlike lesions affecting the bones of the head and neck region. Emphasis is placed on common bone lesions affecting the craniofacial skeleton, particularly those that occur with more frequency or those that are unique to this part of the skeleton. Several of these lesions pose a diagnostic challenge to the pathologist. To ensure that a correct diagnosis is rendered, it is of utmost importance that accurate and detailed clinical and radiographic information is available.

OVERVIEW

In this article, we describe the clinical, radiographic, and pathologic features of tumors and tumorlike lesions affecting the bones of the head and neck region. Emphasis is placed on common bone lesions affecting the craniofacial skeleton, particularly those that occur with more frequency or those that are unique to this part of the skeleton. Several of these lesions pose a diagnostic challenge to the pathologist. To ensure that a correct diagnosis is rendered, it is of utmost importance that accurate and detailed clinical and radiographic information is available. These entities are addressed within the following headings:

- Benign and Malignant Bone Tumors
- Benign and Malignant Cartilagenous Tumors
- Fibro-Osseous Lesions
- Giant Cell Lesions.

BENIGN AND MALIGNANT BONE TUMORS

BENIGN BONE TUMORS

Osteoma

Overview

Osteomas are true neoplasms composed of mature bone. They are found almost exclusively in the head and neck region and are usually diagnosed in the third and fourth decades.[1–3] Symptoms depend on location and size, with headache, visual disturbance, sinusitis, nasal obstruction, pain, and proptosis being common.[4] Frequently they are incidentally detected.[5] The most common primary site is in the paranasal sinuses.[1–4] They less often arise from the inner or outer tables of the cranial bones and in the jawbones.

Radiographic features

Osteomas appear as dense, lobulated, opaque, sharply defined masses that, if projecting into a space, are polypoid with a broad base (**Fig. 1**).[2]

Key Features
OSTEOMA

- Almost all cases arise in the head and neck.
- The most common site is the paranasal sinuses.
- They are associated with familial adenomatous polyposis/Gardner syndrome and when so, are multiple.
- Histologically, they consist of compact, lamellar bone.

Department of Pathology and Immunology, Washington University School of Medicine, 660 Euclid Avenue, Campus Box 8118, St Louis, MO 63110, USA
* Corresponding author.
E-mail address: elmofty@wustl.edu

Surgical Pathology 4 (2011) 1273–1328
doi:10.1016/j.path.2011.07.004
1875-9181/11/$ – see front matter © 2011 Elsevier Inc. All rights reserved.

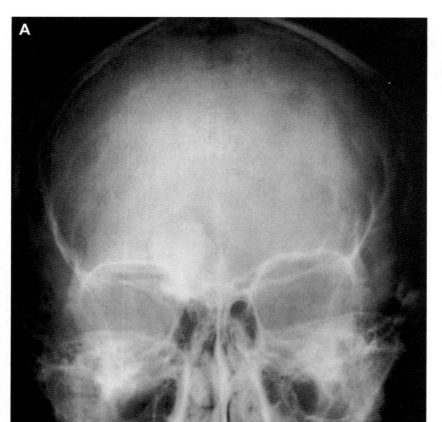

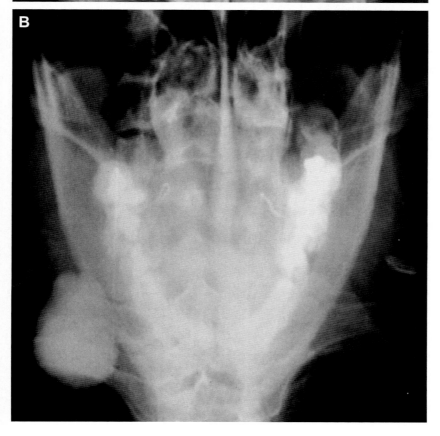

Fig. 1. (*A, B*) Radiographs of the skull showing well-circumscribed, dense, ivory osteoma of the frontal sinus. (*B*) Surface osteoma of the mandible.

Pathologic Key Features
OSTEOMA

- Well circumscribed
- Polypoid, broad-based lesions projecting into paranasal sinuses or other spaces common
- Dense, lamellar bone with varying component of fibrous tissue
- Focal "osteoblastomalike" areas occasionally present, but dense bone predominates

Differential Diagnosis
OSTEOMA

- Tori
- Osteochondroma
- Osteoid osteoma
- Osteoblastoma

Gross and microscopic features

Grossly, they are typically fragmented because they are removed in pieces and are rock hard, tan, and smooth. Most osteomas consist of dense, compact, lamellar bone with widely spaced osteocytes and little fibrous stroma (**Fig. 2**). The bone is brightly eosinophilic and looks like normal cortical bone. Dense, bony lesions are sometimes called "ivory" or "compact" type, and some lesions contain more trabecular-type bone and fibrous tissue, often termed "mature type" (**Fig. 3**). Other variants are called "osteoblastic" or "Paget-like."[4–6]

Diagnosis and differential diagnosis

Osteomas should be distinguished from exostoses, such as osteochondromas and tori (torus mandibularis or palatinus). Tori are dome-shaped, smooth, mucosal-covered, bony projections found either in the floor of the mouth or on the hard palate that are usually bilateral. They are considered developmental and not neoplastic. Tori are indistinguishable histologically from osteomas because they both consist of mature, lamellar bone so the clinical features must be taken into consideration to distinguish them.[6] Osteochondromas, unlike osteomas, have a cartilage cap with a well-defined area of endochondral ossification. Also, these almost always occur in the coronoid process or condyle of the mandible, an uncommon location for osteoma. Osteomas can also sometimes be difficult to distinguish from osteoblastoma and osteoid osteomas. Both of these latter lesions have active bone formation with osteoid lined by plump osteoblasts. Although osteomas can occasionally have these "active" areas with ongoing new bone formation ("osteoblastomalike"

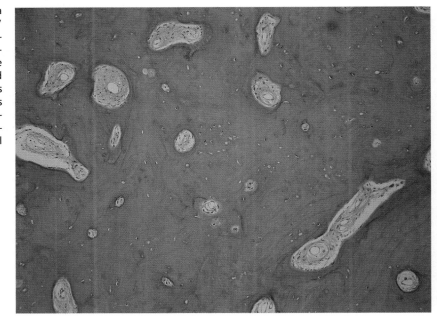

Fig. 2. Compact osteoma (sometimes termed "ivory" type) consisting predominantly of dense, eosinophilic, lamellar bone with widely spaced and inconspicuous osteocytes and only small amounts of intervening fibrovascular stroma (hematoxylin-eosin [H&E], original magnification ×100).

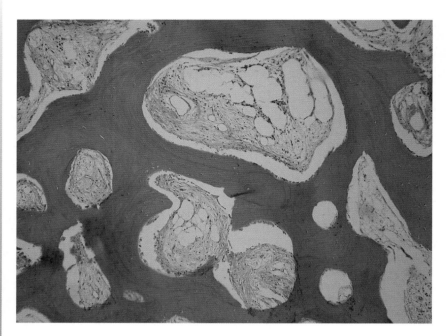

Fig. 3. Trabecular osteoma consisting of trabeculae of mature, lamellar bone with widely spaced osteocytes and a relatively prominent fibrovascular stroma with adipose tissue. Actual marrow elements can be seen (H&E, original magnification ×100).

features), these are focal and limited, with most of the lesion consisting of dense, well-formed bone. Importantly, these "active" foci in osteomas are haphazardly distributed and not just located centrally, in contrast to the niduses of osteoblastoma and osteoid osteoma, which are invariably central.[4]

Osteomas of the head and neck are capable of slow, sustained growth. They range from 1 to 8 cm.[2,5] Pathologic examination should also include review of the relevant radiographs. It is important to consider familial adenomatous polyposis (FAP)/Gardner syndrome when confronted with multiple osteomas, as they can be the first manifestation of these familial syndromes, preceding the development of other more serious manifestations by many years.[7,8]

Prognosis

If incidentally identified by imaging for other reasons, osteomas do not need to be removed. For symptomatic lesions, simple excision is curative.[1,5] There is little, if any, risk of recurrence and no risk of malignant transformation.

Osteoblastoma and Osteoid Osteoma

Overview

These histologically identical, but clinically and radiographically distinct lesions are discussed together. Both are uncommon in the head and neck, osteoblastoma being more common than osteoid osteoma. Most are located in the cervical spine followed by the skull and then jawbones.[9–15]

Radiographic features

Osteoid osteoma, in its active, proliferative phase, shows a nonaggressive-appearing, lucent, round to oval area (the "nidus") surrounded by a zone of dense, sclerotic, reactive bone (**Fig. 4**). Most are 1 cm or smaller, but some investigators have accepted sizes up to 2 cm.[16] Osteoblastoma, on the other hand, is a lucent, expansive lesion that is larger than 2 cm and may contain radiopaque areas (**Fig. 5**).[9,17] It may show cortical destruction

Pitfalls
OSTEOMA

! Tori are histologically identical, but are characteristic in location in the oral cavity (floor of mouth or hard palate).

! Osteochondroma has histologically identical mature bone at base, but has a cartilaginous cap.

! Osteomas can have focal, limited, active bone formation, which should not be confused with the florid active areas of osteoblastoma and osteoid osteoma.

Fig. 4. Osteoid osteoma of the vertebra. CT scan shows lucent area (nidus); the adjacent bone exhibits increased density.

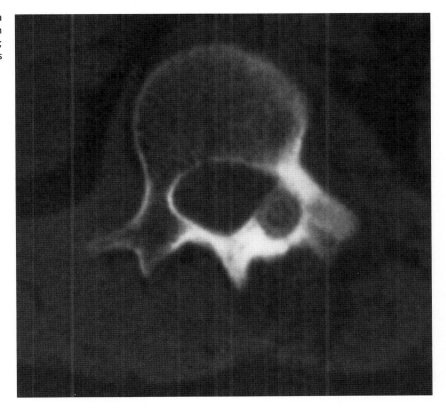

with periostitis and soft tissue extension mimicking a malignancy.[18]

Gross and microscopic features

Grossly, both lesions are well circumscribed and hemorrhagic or reddish brown. Osteoid osteoma, as it matures, can be more sclerotic and bony, blending in with the surrounding cortex in color and consistency.

The nidus of both lesions consists of active new bone in various stages of maturation, set within a loose, fibrous, and vascular stroma that resembles granulation tissue (**Fig. 6**). Streams of osteoid and woven bone are lined by plump osteoblasts with eosinophilic cytoplasm and eccentric, round nuclei (**Figs. 7** and **8**). In osteoid osteoma, they lack pleomorphism or atypia, and mitotic figures are rare. As the lesion matures, the osteoid undergoes calcification and conversion to lamellar bone.[10]

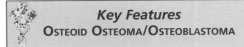

Key Features
OSTEOID OSTEOMA/OSTEOBLASTOMA

- Benign bone tumors that are rare in the head and neck, and most common in the cervical spine.

- Both are histologically indistinguishable with distinction on clinical and radiographic grounds.

- Both are clinically, radiographically, and pathologically well circumscribed.

- En bloc excision is curative; curettage yields slight recurrence risk.

Pathologic Key Features
OSTEOID OSTEOMA/OSTEOBLASTOMA

- Abundant osteoid or woven bone trabeculae lined by orderly, plump, but bland osteoblasts

- Loose, vascular "granulation tissue–like" stroma

- Well circumscribed without permeation into surrounding bone

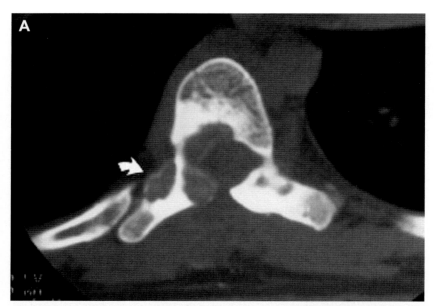

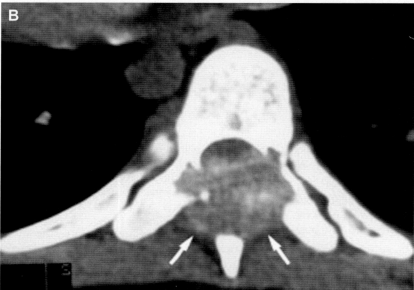

Fig. 5. Osteoblastoma of the posterior element of a vertebra. (*A*) CT scan shows an expansive lesion with an intact shell of bone. (*B*) Another view of the lesion in (*A*); arrows show bone destruction mimicking a malignancy.

Osteoblastoma, although consisting of the same basic elements, has more variation in the pattern. The trabeculae may fuse to form an anastomosing, netlike pattern. Also, osteoblastoma, unlike osteoid osteoma, usually has a significant number of osteoclasts remodeling the newly formed bone (**Fig. 9**). Although osteoblastomas are usually bland with infrequent mitotic activity, some lesions consist of larger, epithelioid osteoblasts with prominent nucleoli, occasionally in sheets, and may even have bizarre, atypical, hyperchromatic nuclei. These lesions are sometimes termed *aggressive* osteoblastoma (**Fig. 10**).[18] There are no atypical mitoses, necrosis, malignant cartilage, or infiltrative growth.[12,19]

Diagnosis and differential diagnosis
Osteoid osteoma and osteoblastoma are histologically essentially identical. As such, the distinction is made by size and clinical and radiographic

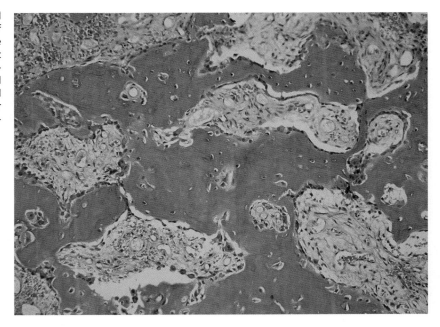

Fig. 6. Nidus of an osteoid osteoma that has cords of eosinophilic woven bone with plump, prominent osteocytes, very conspicuous rimming by round to oval osteoblasts, and set in a richly vascular stroma (H&E, original magnification ×200).

features. Osteoid osteoma is rarely ever larger than 1.5 cm, is virtually always limited to the bone, and is not "progressive." Osteoblastoma will be 2.0 cm or larger and is more "progressive" or expansive in appearance, sometimes destroying cortex. Cementoblastoma can be confused with both of these lesions in the jawbones, but the critical distinguishing feature from osteoblastoma is its intimate association with the cementum of the tooth root.[20]

Although usually straightforward, the distinction of osteoblastoma from osteosarcoma can sometimes be particularly problematic. It is distinguished

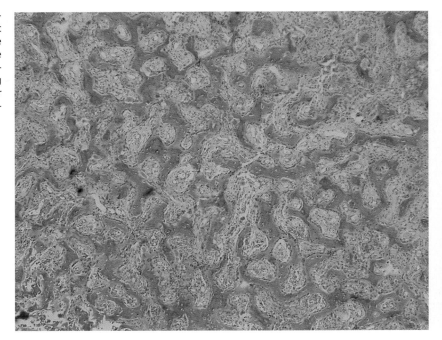

Fig. 7. Osteoblastoma demonstrating the abundant lacelike osteoid and bone formation typical of these lesions. They have abundant osteoblastic rimming and a richly vascular stroma (H&E, original magnification ×40).

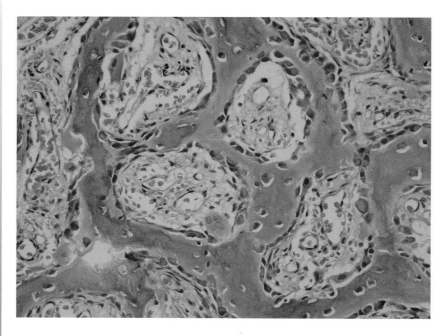

Fig. 8. High-power view of an osteoblastoma that has lacelike osteoid and woven bone formation. The prominent lining osteoblasts are "plump" with round to oval, frequently eccentric nuclei and small amounts of eosinophilic cytoplasm. There is no frank atypia (H&E, original magnification ×400).

from osteosarcoma most importantly by the orderly pattern of osteoblastic rimming of the osteoid and trabeculae with loose, vascular intervening stroma. In osteosarcoma, the intertrabecular areas are filled with disorderly collections of malignant cells (**Fig. 11**). Also, the well-circumscribed periphery of both osteoid osteoma and osteoblastoma distinguish them from the permeative pattern of osteosarcoma (**Fig. 12**). Although *aggressive* osteoblastoma can have cytologic atypia and rare mitoses, there is no atypical mitosis, necrosis, or cartilage formation.[9,20]

Given the histologic similarity, correlation with the clinical presentation and radiographic

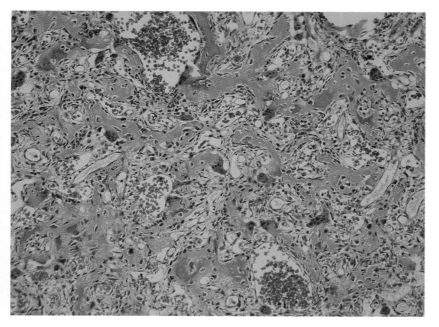

Fig. 9. Osteoblastoma, unlike osteoid osteoma, frequently has a generous amount of osteoclasts (seen as multinucleated cells with more darkly eosinophilic cytoplasm) that are actively remodeling the newly formed bone (H&E, original magnification ×200).

△△	*Differential Diagnosis*
	OSTEOID OSTEOMA/OSTEOBLASTOMA

- The 2 lesions are distinguished from each other based on size and radiographic characteristics.
- Cementoblastoma almost identical histologically but is intimately associated with tooth root.
- Osteosarcoma has overtly malignant histology and permeative/infiltrative growth.

!	*Pitfalls*
	OSTEOBLASTOMA

! Plump, epithelioid osteoblasts with prominent nucleoli and occasionally atypia and hyperchromasia (*aggressive* osteoblastoma) mimic osteosarcoma

! Aggressive radiologic features with cortical destruction and soft tissue extension can mimic osteosarcoma

appearance is critical to distinguish osteoid osteoma from osteoblastoma. Both lesions almost invariably present with pain,[13] which often goes on for long periods before imaging is performed, this being worse at night and, for osteoid osteoma, classically being dramatically relieved by aspirin.[21]

Prognosis

Both osteoid osteoma and osteoblastoma are benign lesions usually cured by en bloc resection; however, when that is not possible, curettage may be performed, but this has a 10% to 20% recurrence rate. Interestingly, osteoblastoma can spontaneously resolve after simple biopsy.[22] Unlike osteoid osteoma, malignant transformation has been rarely reported in osteoblastoma[12,23]; however, some of these cases may represent underdiagnosed osteoblastomalike osteosarcoma.[21]

MALIGNANT BONE TUMORS

Osteosarcoma

Overview

Osteosarcoma is a malignant neoplasm that is characterized by direct formation of osteoid or primitive woven bone by the malignant tumor cells. There are 4 ways by which these tumors can be classified:

1. Anatomic location: craniofacial and appendicular
2. Clinicopathologic type: conventional (intramedullary), parosteal, and periosteal

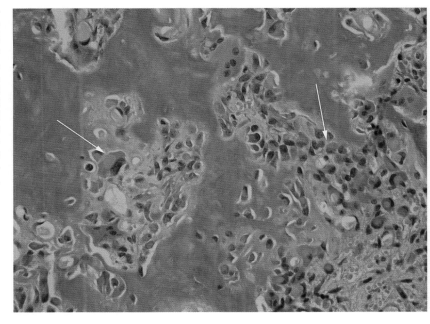

Fig. 10. So-called aggressive osteoblastoma consisting of the typical elements of osteoblastoma, but having atypical, pleomorphic osteoblasts, some with large nuclei and prominent nucleoli (*arrows*). There is minimal mitotic activity and the lesion will be well circumscribed within the native bone (H&E, original magnification ×400).

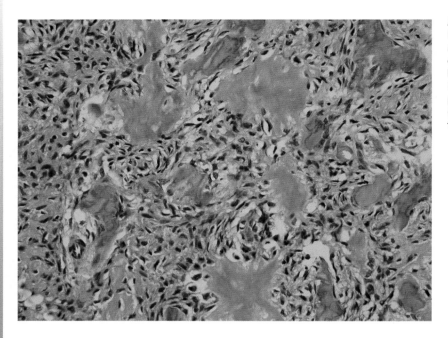

Fig. 11. Osteosarcoma showing, rather than the typical richly vascular stroma of osteoid osteoma or osteoblastoma, a filling of the intertrabecular areas by pleomorphic tumor cells (H&E, original magnification ×400).

3. Histologic type: chondroblastic, osteoblastic, fibroblastic, or other
4. Primary and secondary.

It is helpful to draw distinctions between tumors of the head and neck region and those of the non-maxillofacial skeleton, because there are several major differences. Eighty percent to 85% of osteosarcomas arise in the long bones/extragnathic sites. In large series, only 6% to 8% occurred in the head and neck.[24,25] Although extragnathic osteosarcoma is most common in the first 2 decades, head and neck cases are rare in children, being most common in the third and fourth

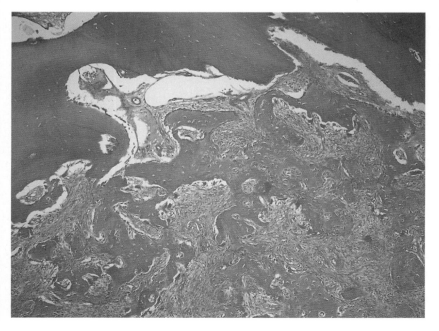

Fig. 12. Low-power view of an osteoblastoma that shows a regular and clearly circumscribed interface with the cortical bone, without permeation (H&E, original magnification ×40).

decades with an average age of approximately 36 to 38 years.[26,27] Osteosarcomas are usually primary (idiopathic) but some occur secondary to underlying conditions, most notably Paget disease,[28,29] fibrous dysplasia,[30] bone infarction,[31] and radiation.[32] In fibrous dysplasia and Paget disease, the tumors almost always occur with the polyostotic forms. A much larger percentage of head and neck osteosarcomas are secondary compared with extragnathic ones.[33–35]

The most common site in the head and neck is in the jawbones (~75%), with approximately 40% occurring in the maxilla and approximately 35% in the mandible,[24–26,34] followed by the skull bones (~20%), cervical vertebrae (fewer than 5%), and soft tissue (fewer than 5%).[21,36,37] As with extragnathic sites, any of the clinicopathologic and histologic types can occur.

Following is a more detailed discussion of each of the clinicopathologic types of osteosarcoma.

Conventional Osteosarcoma

Radiographic features

Radiographic imaging is a critical part of osteosarcoma diagnosis. Extensive bone destruction is invariably present, usually with a mixed lytic and sclerotic pattern depending on how much of the tumor is actually producing bone.[27] There is frequent extension into soft tissues (**Fig. 13**).

Gross and microscopic features

Grossly, the appearance varies greatly, depending on the relative proportions of cartilage, bone, fibrous tissue, and solid tumor (**Fig. 14**), again with most tumors consisting of a mixture of white, shiny nodules; gritty yellow tumor; and fleshy tan-white components.

Most osteosarcomas produce an abundance of osteoid and immature bone, this pattern being classified as osteoblastic (**Fig. 15**). Osteoid is the eosinophilic, collagenous precursor to bone upon

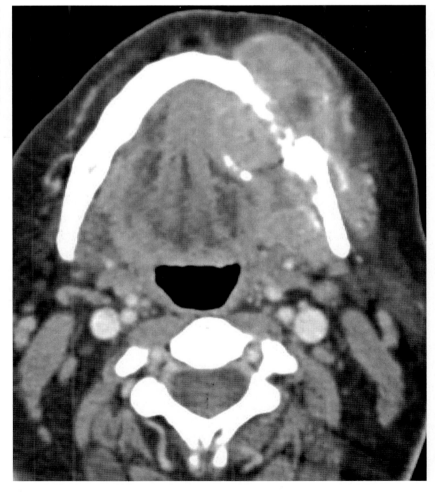

Fig. 13. Axial CT scan image of a mandibular osteosarcoma showing a mixed soft tissue and calcified, very aggressive lesion with destruction of the native cortex and extensive extension into the surrounding soft tissue.

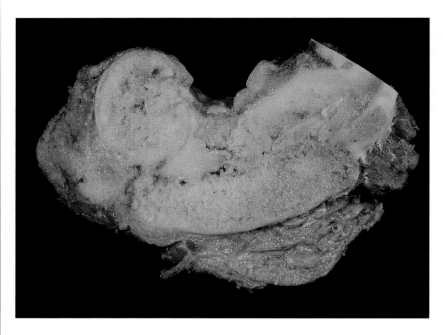

Fig. 14. Gross photograph of a surgically resected mandibular osteosarcoma showing a tan, granular, ill-defined mass permeating the bone and extending into the surrounding soft tissue.

which mineralization occurs. In benign lesions, it consists of thin, elongated, serpiginous to lacelike hyaline material distributed between, and lined by osteoblastic cells. Histologic patterns other than osteoblastic are common in head and neck osteosarcomas, including malignant cartilage-producing (chondroblastic) and spindle cell (fibroblastic). The other, rarely described, histologic types, such as telangiectatic, small cell, giant cell rich, and so forth, are exceedingly uncommon in this location.[25,26] Osteoid production is critical to the diagnosis. Unlike benign lesions, this material is not lined by an orderly proliferation of osteoblasts (**Fig. 16**).[21] The osteoid undergoes calcification so that one sees granules and lines of darker, refractile calcification in them as this

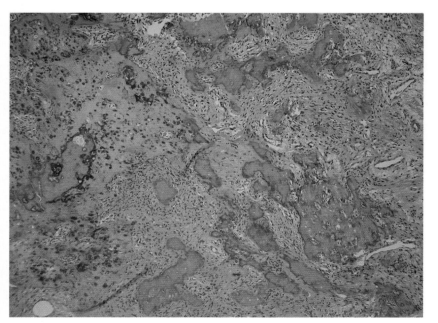

Fig. 15. Osteoblastic osteosarcoma consisting of sheets of pleomorphic tumor cells in a fibrous stroma and making abundant bone. The bone consists of irregular trabeculae of eosinophilic to partially basophilic material with no native (benign) osteoblast lining (H&E, original magnification ×100).

Fig. 16. Osteosarcoma osteoid consisting of thin strands of eosinophilic material between and around overtly malignant cells (H&E, original magnification ×400).

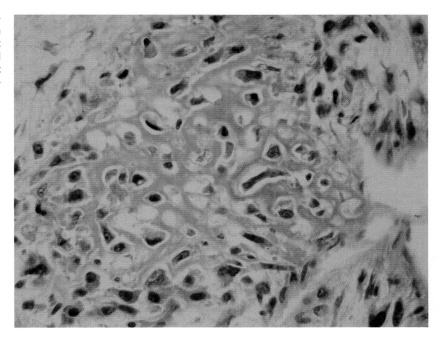

occurs. Chondroblastic osteosarcomas have a predominance of malignant cartilage arranged in lobules and with tumor cells in lacunar spaces **(Fig. 17)**. The cartilaginous stroma is refractile and basophilic. Fibroblastic osteosarcomas are composed of spindle cells that may be tightly bound and fascicular **(Fig. 18)** or more fibrohistiocytic, resembling malignant fibrous histiocytoma. Most osteosarcomas display a mixture of these different patterns, but in the head and neck, osteoblastic and chondroblastic areas predominate.[26] Postradiation and Paget disease–related osteosarcomas are typically fibroblastic.[28,32] In all forms, the tumors are infiltrative and

Fig. 17. Chondroblastic differentiation in osteosarcoma with a lobule of mixed eosinophilic and lightly basophilic cartilage with lacunae having markedly atypical and hyperchromatic tumor cells (H&E, original magnification ×200).

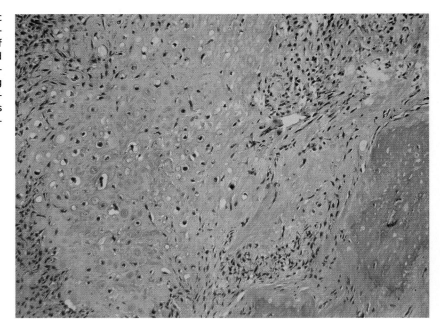

Pathologic Key Features
OSTEOSARCOMA

- Osteoid ("pre-bone") formation is the key finding. It consists of strands of brightly eosinophilic, lacelike material between malignant cells.

- Osteoblastic, chondroblastic, and fibroblastic patterns may be seen with predominance of bone-forming, cartilage-forming, or spindle cell areas dictating the type, respectively.

- Tumor infiltration of surrounding bone or soft tissue is invariably present.

Differential Diagnosis
OSTEOSARCOMA

- Chondroblastic osteosarcomas can have such extensive cartilaginous differentiation that they can mimic true chondrosarcomas: the key is finding true osteoid/bone formation by tumor cells.

- Fibroblastic or fibrohistiocytic osteosarcomas can mimic desmoplastic fibroma and malignant fibrous histiocytoma: the key is finding osteoid/bone formation by tumor cells.

- Osteoblastoma, particularly the so-called "aggressive" form, with its cellular nidus with osteoid and occasional atypia, is distinguished from osteosarcoma by lack of atypical mitoses or necrosis, but most clearly by its lack of infiltration of surrounding bone.

permeative of surrounding normal bone and soft tissue, and marked cytologic pleomorphism, mitotic activity with atypical figures (**Fig. 19**), and necrosis are common. Grading is of no prognostic value except for in the exceedingly rare well-differentiated intraosseous form where recognizing its low-grade nature is key to the diagnosis.

Diagnosis and differential diagnosis
The diagnosis of osteosarcoma is typically quite straightforward; however, there are a few situations that should be considered. For chondroblastic or fibroblastic/fibrohistiocytic osteosarcomas, the osteoid or bone formation may not be demonstrated on small biopsies. In chondroblastic cases, the distinction from chondrosarcoma may not be an easy task. Differentiation of low-grade fibroblastic osteosarcoma from desmoplastic fibroma of bone when it is bland, or from malignant fibrous histiocytoma when it is high grade, is not always

possible. Both of these scenarios require correlation with the radiographic findings and examination of the entire resection specimen to identify bone or osteoid formation. A benign entity that is sometimes difficult to distinguish from osteosarcoma is osteoblastoma, particularly in lesions of the cervical spine. These lesions can be quite cellular with osteoid production and cellular atypia. The single best discriminating histologic feature is the peripheral permeative growth of osteosarcoma, distinct from the sharp interface the nidus of osteoblastoma has with the host bone (see **Fig. 12**).

Osteosarcoma diagnosis should be coordinated with radiographic findings, particularly in cases where classic, overtly malignant cells making osteoid and/or bone are not obviously present. There are no special stains or immunostains that aid in this distinction. Some have attempted immunohistochemistry for osteonectin, osteocalcin, or osteopontin for this purpose, but they have not garnered diagnostic reliability or acceptance.[38–41] Several hereditary syndromes have been associated with an increased risk of osteosarcoma, most importantly hereditary retinoblastoma,[42] which is associated with germline mutation in the *RB1* tumor suppressor gene, and Li-Fraumeni syndrome, caused by germline mutation of the *p53* gene.[43]

Prognosis
Patients are typically treated with radical surgery followed by postoperative radiation and sometimes chemotherapy. The prognosis for conventional osteosarcoma of the head and neck is

Key Features
OSTEOSARCOMA
OF THE HEAD AND NECK

- Osteosarcoma is the most common primary head and neck sarcoma.

- Most cases arise in the jawbones, followed by the skull bones, soft tissue, and cervical vertebrae.

- Classic intramedullary is the overwhelmingly most common type.

- Although any histologic type can occur, chondroblastic is more common than osteoblastic and fibroblastic.

poor, and is strongly related to site.[21,44] Across all sites, overall 5-year survival is approximately 50% to 60%, with more recent series showing improved survival relative to older series.[21,26,34,44,45] The survival rates of jaw tumors are best, and those for cranial bones and vertebral tumors much lower. Also, osteosarcomas arising after radiation or within Paget disease have much lower survival rates.[28,32]

Parosteal Osteosarcoma

Overview

This distinctive osteosarcoma variant is rare in the head and neck,[46] with most involving the mandible and maxilla.[47–49] It is slow growing, most presenting as a painless swelling.[47]

Radiographic features

As the name parosteal (juxtacortical) suggests, it arises from the surface of the bone and forms a lobulated mass. Radiographically, the native cortex is thickened with a radiolucent cleavage plane between it and the tumor in a significant minority. The mass is well demarcated and predominantly radiodense but may have scattered areas of radiolucency.[46,50,51]

Gross and microscopic features

Grossly, the tumors are dense, tan, and firm and are limited to the bone surface.

Parosteal osteosarcoma can be diagnostically challenging. It consists predominantly of stromal and bony elements that lack obvious features of malignancy. The tumor is composed of spindle cells in a generous fibrous stroma in which there are trabeculae of woven or lamellar bone.[21] The bone is the most dense and generous in the deep aspects along the native cortex (**Fig. 20**). The fibrous stroma ranges from very hypocellular to more cellular, resembling low-grade fibrosarcoma, and the nuclei classically orient themselves parallel to the bony trabeculae. Mitotic figures are scarce. The periphery is more cellular with more irregular cells that produce osteoid.[21] Cartilaginous areas arise in more than one-half of cases, but these are not a dominant feature (see **Fig. 20**B).[46,52] Dedifferentiation occurs infrequently, usually consisting of conventional osteosarcoma.[53]

Fig. 18. Fibroblastic osteosarcoma consisting of a diffuse proliferation of pleomorphic and overtly malignant spindle cells in a collagenous stroma and admixed with thin trabeculae of woven bone (H&E, original magnification ×100).

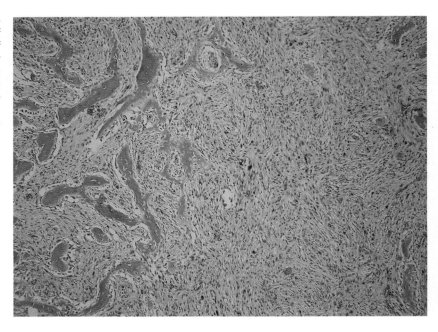

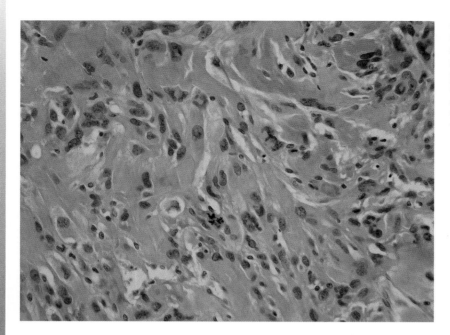

Fig. 19. High-grade osteoblastic osteosarcoma with strands of osteoid surrounding very pleomorphic tumor cells with hyperchromatic nuclei and atypical mitotic figures (H&E, original magnification ×400).

Differential diagnosis

Sessile osteochondromas can resemble parosteal osteosarcoma; however, osteochondromas are radiologically continuous with the underlying native bone. In addition, the cartilage cap of osteochondromas is completely benign appearing and, rather than having central fibrous tissue between the bony trabeculae, osteochondroma has marrow spaces.[21] Myositis ossificans rarely involves the bone but can attach itself in long-standing cases. It shows zonal distribution with the most mature bone at the periphery, whereas parosteal osteosarcoma has the most proliferative portion at the periphery where it junctions with, and infiltrates into, the soft tissue.

Prognosis

Outcomes in parosteal osteosarcoma are generally very good, although the head and neck lesions are rare enough that large studies are not available. Considering all sites, the prognosis is approximately 80% at 5 years.[46] Dedifferentiation greatly increases the risk of metastasis.[54]

Periosteal Osteosarcoma

Overview

Periosteal osteosarcoma is essentially a subperiosteal, surface-based chondroblastic osteosarcoma. These are rare in the head and neck, mostly limited to case reports.[55–57] Head and neck cases occur in individuals between 20 and 65 years old, with most occurring along the posterior mandible.[48,55–60]

Radiographic features

Although these tumors typically have a pattern of radiopaque osseous spicules radiating from the cortex, the appearance in head and neck cases is not consistent and rarely reported as such, rather being mixed sclerotic and radiolucent, but with the latter being predominant.[60]

Gross and microscopic features

Grossly, the tumor appears well circumscribed and comes off of the native cortex, which appears minimally invaded.[21,60,61] The cut surface is chondroid with glistening white lobules.[56,57]

Microscopically, the tumor consists of lobules of high-grade malignant cartilage. In between, there are spindle cells that produce fine, lacelike osteoid.[58] These latter areas can be sparse and are best seen at the periphery of the lesion (**Fig. 21**).[21,61]

Differential diagnosis

Given the surface location, parosteal osteosarcoma enters the clinical and radiographic differential more than the pathologic one, as the histology of these lesions is quite different. Parosteal osteosarcoma has large, parallel bony trabeculae and a bland fibroblastic stroma,

Fig. 20. Parosteal osteosarcoma. (*A*) Bone trabeculae show prominent reversal lines. The intertrabecular spaces are sparsely cellular. (*B*) Cartilaginous areas may be present but not as a significant component (H&E, original magnification × 100).

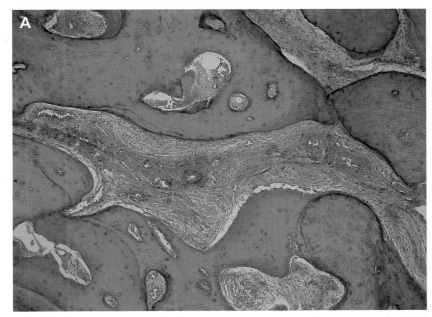

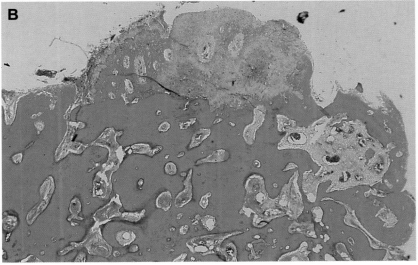

both of which are absent in periosteal osteosarcoma, which is chondroblastic and overtly malignant. Chondrosarcomas will rarely be surface or subperiosteal, but if so, will certainly lack the spindle cell component with frank osteoid production of periosteal osteosarcoma. Chondroblastic osteosarcoma with extraosseous extension is differentiated radiographically from periosteal osteosarcoma. Marrow cavity involvement by periosteal osteosarcoma is rare and has been reported only by extension along the periodontal ligament.[59] By definition,

conventional chondroblastic osteosarcoma involves marrow spaces.

Prognosis

The prognosis of non–head and neck periosteal osteosarcoma is between conventional and parosteal forms. Extremity lesions have a low but significant risk of distant metastasis.[62] In the rare head and neck cases that have been reported, the prognosis is very good after resection. Only one tumor has recurred, and this was the only lesion to develop metastases.[58,59]

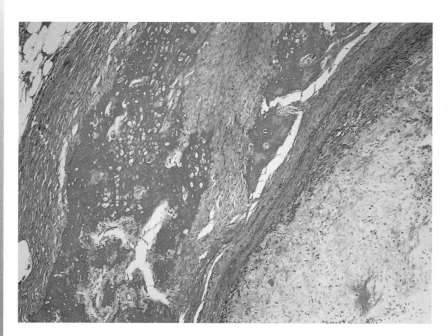

Fig. 21. Periosteal osteo-sarcoma. Lobules of cartilage are associated with lacelike osteoid at the periphery (H&E, original magnification ×200).

BENIGN AND MALIGNANT CARTILAGINOUS TUMORS

OVERVIEW

Cartilagenous lesions of the head and neck are uncommon, comprising fewer than 1% of all tumors. Of these lesions, chondrosarcoma is the most frequently encountered, particularly in the larynx where it is the most common sarcoma. Benign cartilaginous lesions of the head and neck are rare, but important to recognize, as they may be clinically and pathologically mistaken for malignant processes.

BENIGN CARTILAGENOUS TUMORS

Chondroma

Overview
Chondromas are benign cartilaginous neoplasms that rarely occur in the larynx or craniofacial bones.

Radiographic features
The imaging and gross features overlap greatly with chondrosarcoma (see discussion under chondrosarcoma). However, soft tissue invasion should not be seen in chondromas. Chondromas also tend to be smaller, measuring smaller than 2 to 3 cm.[63]

Microscopic features
Chondromas are well circumscribed and are composed of nodules of cartilage showing small uniform chondrocytes that are well separated from each other (**Fig. 22**).

Diagnosis and differential diagnosis
The main diagnostic dilemma is confusion with well-differentiated chondrosarcoma, which may be indistinguishable in biopsy material (see discussion under chondrosarcoma). The diagnosis of chondroma cannot be made without correlation of the histologic and radiographic features. Radiographic or pathologic evidence of destructive growth necessitates a diagnosis of chondrosarcoma rather than chondroma.

Prognosis
Chondromas are benign and are successfully treated with complete, conservative excision. Chondromas may recur but, unlike chondrosarcomas, they do not have metastatic potential.[64]

Chondroblastoma

Overview
Chondroblastomas are benign neoplasms that usually arise in the epiphysis of long bones. Although rare, head and neck chondroblastomas almost always involve the squamous portion of

Fig. 22. Chondroma. (*A*) A low-power image (H&E, original magnification ×100) showing a well-circumscribed hypocellular cartilaginous tumor. (*B*) On higher power (H&E, original magnification ×40), bland chondrocytes are appreciated.

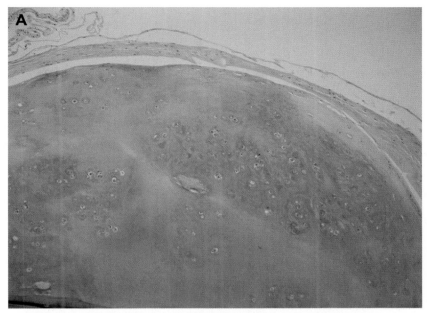

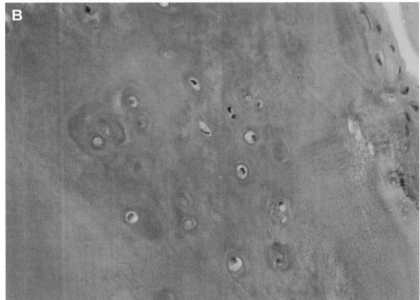

the temporal bone.[65,66] They also affect a slightly older age group (predominately 30-year-olds to 40-year-olds) than chondroblastomas at other sites and are more common in men.[65] Although chondroblastomas of the long bones often present with pain, chondroblastomas of the temporal bone are typically painless but do cause a variety of otologic complaints.[66]

Radiographic features

Radiographically, chondroblastomas appear as sharply demarcated lytic lesions with foci of calcification (**Fig. 23**).[66]

Gross and microscopic features

The gross appearance is quite variable and heterogeneous, with gray, yellow, and red to brown

Key Features
CHONDROBLASTOMA

- Predilection for the squamous portion of the temporal bone

- Affect middle-age adults (30s to 40s)

- Painless lytic lesion causing otologic symptoms

- Composed of lobules of histiocytic chondro-blasts and cartilage with "chicken-wire" calcification

- Strong and diffuse S-100 positivity

areas. Microscopically, chondroblastomas are composed of lobules of polygonal to spindled chondroblasts that have a histiocytic appearance with eccentric nuclei and abundant eosinophilic cytoplasm (**Fig. 24**). Multinucleated giant cells are often intermixed and may be numerous. Scattered chondroid areas with "chicken-wire," pericellular calcifications are characteristic. Secondary aneurysmal bone cyst change may be present as well.

Diagnosis and differential diagnosis
The main entities in the differential diagnosis are giant cell tumor—in the presence of numerous giant cells, aneurysmal bone cyst (ABC), if there is secondary ABC change, and chondromyxoid fibroma, which may contain chondroblastomalike areas.

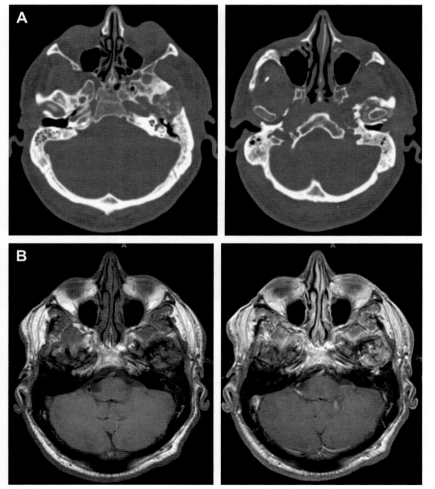

Fig. 23. Chondroblastoma of the temporal bone. (*A*) Bone window CT images demonstrate a lytic skull base mass with internal chondroid matrix arising from the left temporal bone superior to the left temporomandibular joint. Note the extension of the chondroid matrix inferiorly about the mandibular condyle, which is preserved. (*B*) Precontrast and postcontrast T1-weighted magnetic resonance images (MRIs) confirm enhancement within this mass.

Fig. 24. Chondroblastoma of the temporal bone. (*A*) A low-power image (H&E, original magnification ×200) of a chondroblastoma with sheets of chondroblasts and islands of cartilage. (*B*) On high power (H&E, original magnification ×400), the sheets of chondroblasts have a histiocytic appearance. (*C*) Pericellular "chicken-wire" calcification is also present (*arrow*) (H&E, original magnification ×600).

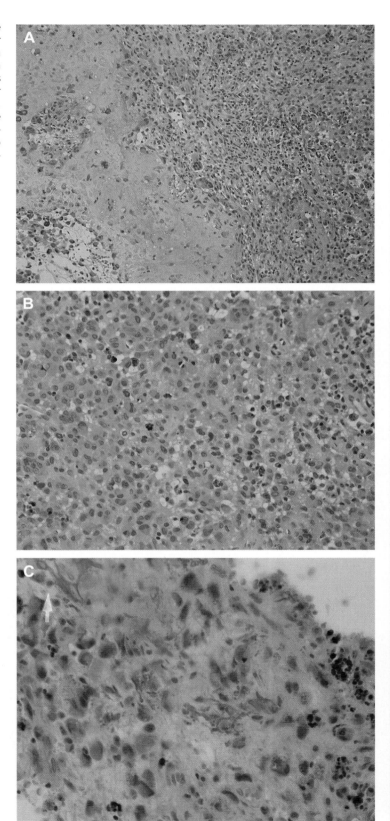

Histologic features are keys to establishing the diagnosis of chondroblastoma. Immunohistochemistry is a useful adjunct because chondroblastomas are typically strongly positive for S-100 (in 90% of cases), whereas ABC and giant cell tumor are usually negative.[67,68] S-100 is variable positive in chondromyxoid fibroma.

Prognosis
Chondroblastomas are treated with complete excision. Although benign, recurrence rates of up to 20% have been reported.[65]

Chondromyxoid Fibroma

Overview
Chondromyxoid fibroma (CMF) is a rare benign tumor representing fewer than 1% of all primary bone neoplasms. Only 2% of CMFs occur in the head and neck, most commonly involving the mandible or maxilla of young adults.

Radiographic features
On imaging, CMFs are lytic with sharply defined borders (**Fig. 25**). Calcification may be present.

Gross and microscopic features
The gross appearance is that of a well-circumscribed gray-white, lobulated lesion.

Histologically, CMFs are composed of bland chondromyxoid nodules separated by fibrous tissue (**Fig. 26**). The periphery of the nodules is more cellular than the center and often contains multinucleated giant cells. ABC change and chondroblastomalike areas may be present.

Diagnosis and differential diagnosis
The diagnosis rests on the histologic features described previously. Because these lesions may contain secondary ABC change and have chondroblastomalike areas, both of these entities need to be considered in the differential diagnosis. Chondrosarcoma, with myxoid features, may also be considered in the differential diagnosis but should have significant cytologic atypia, which is not a feature of CMF.

Prognosis
Complete excision is curative.

MALIGNANT CARTILAGINOUS TUMORS

Chondrosarcoma

Overview
Chondrosarcomas account for approximately 10% to 20% of primary malignant bone tumors, making them the second most common after osteosarcomas. Of these, fewer than 10% arise in the head and neck, where chondrosarcomas make up fewer than 0.2% of all malignancies. Chondrosarcomas of the head and neck are a heterogeneous group of tumors that can be further classified based on the

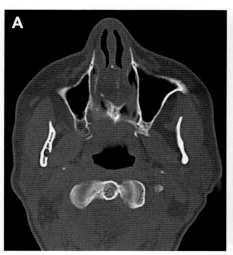
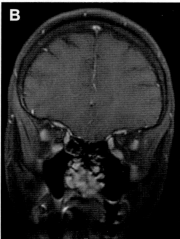

Fig. 25. CMF. (*A*) Axial CT image demonstrates a lytic expansile lesion with sharply defined borders and internal calcification arising from the hard palate and floor of the nose. (*B*) Coronal contrast-enhanced T1-weighted MRI demonstrates enhancement in this same lesion that arises from the hard palate and extending into the nasal cavity.

Fig. 26. CMF. (*A*) A low-power image (H&E, original magnification ×100) showing chondromyxoid nodule with a hypocellular center and a more cellular periphery. (*B*) Higher power (H&E, original magnification ×200) of the hypocellular center containing bland, stellate cells in a chondromyxoid stroma. (*C*) Higher power (H&E, original magnification ×200) of the more cellular periphery.

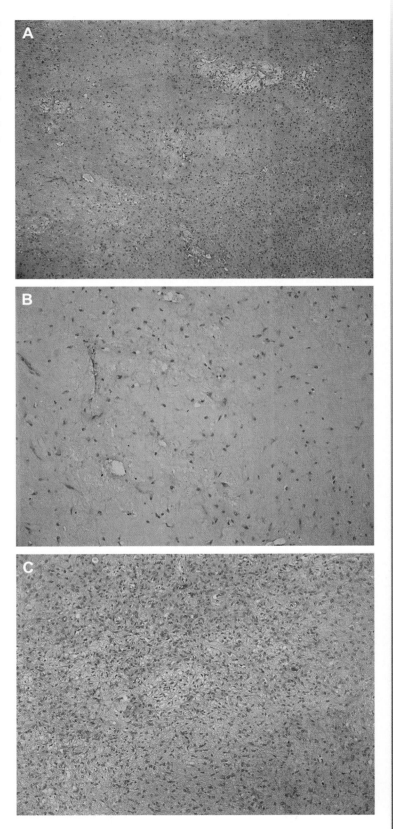

site of origin and histologic type. Almost one-half of all cases arise in the bones of the head and neck, with the maxilla being the most frequent location, followed by the mandible.[69,70] About one-fourth of cases arise in the larynx.[70] Less common sites include the sinonasal tract and soft tissues. The dominant histologic subtype is conventional chondrosarcoma, which makes up about 80% of all head and neck chondrosarcomas. Other subtypes include dedifferentiated, clear cell, extraskeletal myxoid, and mesenchymal chondrosarcoma. Dedifferentiated chondrosarcoma may develop following the local recurrence of a previous low-grade chondrosarcoma or arise de novo. Rare cases of clear cell chondrosarcoma have been reported in the head and neck.[71–75] Mesenchymal and extraskeletal chondrosarcomas are 2 uncommon but distinct clinicopathologic entities.

Conventional chondrosarcomas are typically low grade and stage. Most tumors occur in older patients (older than 50 years) and in men (approximately three-quarters of patients).[70,76] About 5% of the cases affect the head and neck. In contrast, most mesenchymal chondrosarcomas arise in the head and neck bones and sinonasal tract. Most tumors occur in younger patients (younger than 50 years), are more common in women, and are more frequently of higher grade and stage.[77,78] In addition, mesenchymal chondrosarcomas occur in African American and Latino individuals with greater frequency than in white individuals.[70] Extraskeletal myxoid chondrosarcoma is predominantly a tumor of the extremities, with the head and neck region involved in only 5% of the cases. In this anatomic site, the tumor has been reported in the tongue, nasal cavity, neck, chin, maxillary sinus, and larynx.

Radiographic features

Most chondrosarcomas of the head and neck arise in bones, including those of the craniofacial

> ## Key Features
> ### CHONDROSARCOMA OF THE HEAD AND NECK BONES
>
> - Greater numbers of mesenchymal chondrosarcomas occur at these sites than elsewhere in the head and neck
> - Higher grade and stage
> - Occur in younger patients (<50 years)
> - More common in women

region, or ossified laryngeal cartilage. Only approximately 10% to 20% arise in the soft tissue or other sites.[70] Chondrosarcomas of the craniofacial bones most often involve the maxilla or mandible, with a predilection for the alveolar portion of the maxilla and maxillary sinus.[79] In the larynx, the vast majority involve the cricoid cartilage, followed by the thyroid cartilage.[76]

Chondrosarcomas can be difficult to distinguish from benign cartilaginous entities radiographically. Imaging studies show a mass lesion with calcification in nearly all cases (**Fig. 27**).[76] Most are smaller than 10 cm. The tumors may form a well-defined or ill-defined radiolucent lesion that destroys normal cartilage and bone. Fine, punctuate to course ("popcorn") calcifications are often present. Soft tissue invasion may be seen as well, a feature that is helpful in the recognition of malignancy.

Gross and microscopic features

On gross examination, the cut surface is typically firm, bright white, and glistening, with a lobulated tumor edge (**Fig. 28**). Focal calcification may impart grittiness on sectioning. Some tumors, particularly chondrosarcomas that show myxoid features microscopically, may be more gelatinous. Dedifferentiated chondrosarcomas may have areas with a gray-tan, "fish-flesh," infiltrative appearance corresponding to areas of high-grade tumor microscopically.

Conventional chondrosarcoma

Microscopically, conventional chondrosarcomas are composed of neoplastic chondrocytes within a matrix of hyaline cartilage. By definition, malignant osteoid or bone formation is absent. Their presence in a malignant cartilaginous tumor would warrant classification as an osteosarcoma rather than a chondrosarcoma.

Chondrosarcomas have 3 grades, with emphasis on such items as nuclear morphology, mitotic activity, and degree of cellularity. Grade 1 tumors

> ## Key Features
> ### CHONDROSARCOMA OF THE LARYNX
>
> - Most common sarcoma of the larynx
> - Approximately 90% are well-differentiated conventional chondrosarcomas
> - Tend to be low stage
> - Occur in older patients (>50 years)
> - More common in men (approximately three-fourths of patients)

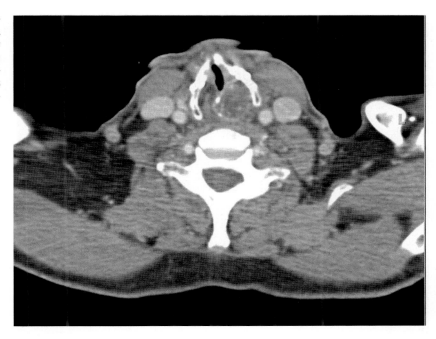

Fig. 27. CT scan of a laryngeal chondrosarcoma. A peripherally and centrally calcified mass arising from the left posterolateral aspect of the cricoids cartilage is seen. Soft tissue extension is present.

are relatively hypocellular and contain predominately small, hyperchromatic tumor cells making them difficult to recognize as malignant (**Fig. 29**). Two or more nuclei per lacuna are usually easily identified, although they can be infrequent (see **Fig. 29**). Mitotic figures are not found. Focal nuclear pleomorphism, without increased cellularity or mitotic activity, may be seen.[80] The background matrix varies from chondroid to myxoid (see **Fig. 29**). Infiltrative growth into surrounding bone is a helpful diagnostic feature in low-grade conventional chondrosarcomas. Grade 2 tumors, compared with grade 1 tumors, show increased cellularity, particularly at the periphery of tumor nodules with tumor cells beginning to form sheets.[80] The nuclei are larger in size and have more open chromatin. Mitotic figures may be present but are infrequent. The matrix tends to be more myxoid in the cellular areas. Grade 3 tumors have nuclear atypia and highly cellular areas with frequent mitoses (**Fig. 30**).[80] Chondroid differentiation may be less obvious. Tumors with higher-grade features required to warrant designation as a grade 3 are rare.[70]

Mesenchymal chondrosarcoma

Mesenchymal chondrosarcomas have an undifferentiated mesenchymal component made up of sheets or nests of small, round to spindled cells, often with a hemangiopericytomalike pattern of vasculature (**Fig. 31**). The mesenchymal component is admixed with lobules of differentiated cartilage with characteristics of conventional chondrosarcoma (see **Fig. 31**).

Extraskeletal myxoid chondrosarcoma

Histologically, extraskeletal myxoid chondrosarcomas consist of lobules of a myxoid stroma containing anastomosing strands or cords of relatively small, uniform, round to elongated cells (**Fig. 32**).

Clear cell chondrosarcoma

Clear cell chondrosarcomas are composed of chondrocytes with abundant clear cytoplasm and distinct cell borders. The histologic features are quite variable. Giant cells, osteoid, calcification, and areas of conventional chondrosarcoma may be seen (**Fig. 33**).

Dedifferentiated chondrosarcoma

Dedifferentiated chondrosarcomas are characterized by the juxtaposition of a differentiated chondrosarcoma, as described previously, with a pleomorphic sarcoma component (**Fig. 34**).

Diagnosis and Differential Diagnosis

The diagnosis of chondrosarcoma is based primarily on histologic features. Correlation with radiographic findings is important, particularly for well-differentiated conventional chondrosarcomas for which the differential diagnosis includes chondroma. If biopsy material is inconclusive,

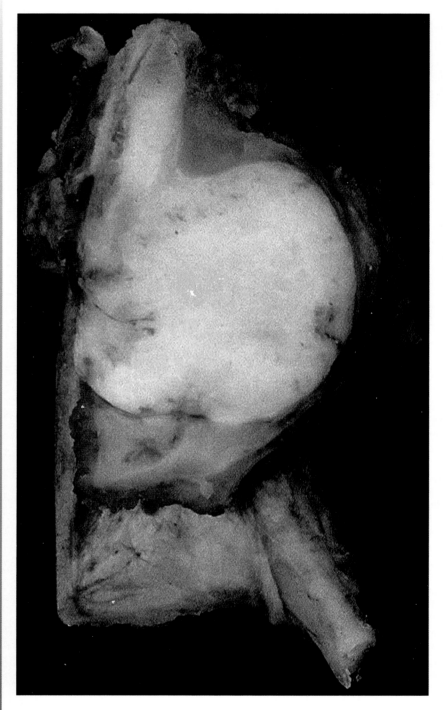

Fig. 28. Gross photograph of a well-differentiated laryngeal chondrosarcoma arising from the cricoid cartilage. The cut surface is bright white and glistening. Although the tumor is well circumscribed, soft tissue invasion is present.

radiographic evidence of malignancy (infiltrative growth) may support the diagnosis of chondrosarcoma.

Immunohistochemistry in chondrosarcomas is not specific but may be useful for excluding other entities in the differential diagnosis. Chondroid areas in chondrosarcomas are usually positive for vimentin and S-100 and negative for epithelial and muscle markers. In the case of mesenchymal chondrosarcoma, the absence of immunostaining with muscle markers excludes the diagnosis of rhabdomyosarcoma. Hematopoietic

Fig. 29. Well-differentiated chondrosarcoma arising in the larynx. (*A*) Low-power image (H&E, original magnification ×100) of a well-differentiated chondrosarcoma. The chondrocytes are bland but show increase in cellularity and bone invasion. (*B*) High-power image (H&E, original magnification ×400) of a well-differentiated chondrosarcoma showing easily identifiable lacunae containing cells with two or more nuclei. (*C*) Focal myxoid change in a well-differentiated chondrosarcoma (H&E, original magnification ×200).

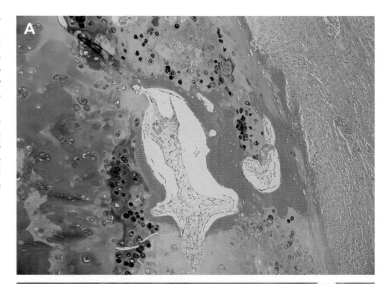

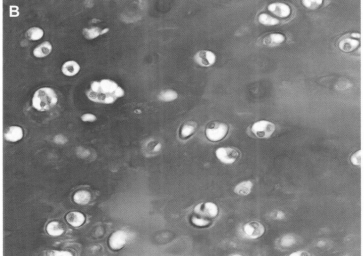

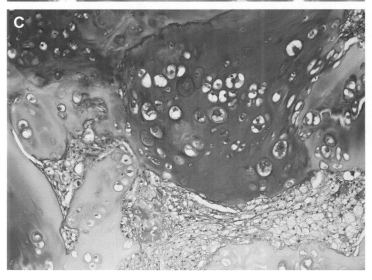

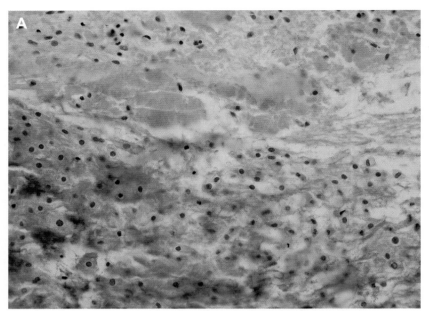

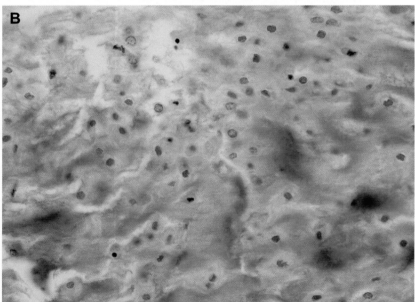

Fig. 30. High-grade chondrosarcoma with myxoid features arising in the skull base. (*A*) The tumor is cellular and has a predominately myxoid stroma (H&E, original magnification ×400). (*B*) Although the tumor cells are bland, numerous mitotic figures can be seen, warranting classification as a high-grade chondrosarcoma (H&E, original magnification ×600).

markers, such as leukocyte common antigen (CD45), would also differentiate mesenchymal chondrosarcoma from lymphoma when chondroid elements are not seen. One must use caution in relying on immunohistochemistry to distinguish mesenchymal chondrosarcoma from Ewing sarcoma/primitive neuroectodermal tumor, as the mesenchymal component may be positive for CD99 and negative for S-100.[78]

When considering the diagnosis of myxoid chondrosarcoma, absence of immunoreactivity with epithelial markers may be necessary to exclude both mucinous adenocarcinoma and chordoma.

In general, molecular studies are not particularly useful in the diagnosis of chondrosarcomas. With the exception of extraskeletal myxoid tumors, chondrosarcomas lack recurrent cytogenetic

Fig. 31. Mesenchymal chondrosarcoma of the maxilla. (*A*) A low-power image (H&E, original magnification ×100) shows a chondroid neoplasm with a vascular pattern that resembles hemangiopericytoma. (*B*) On higher power (H&E, original magnification ×400), a biphasic neoplasm composed of islands of cartilage with intervening small blue cells is seen.

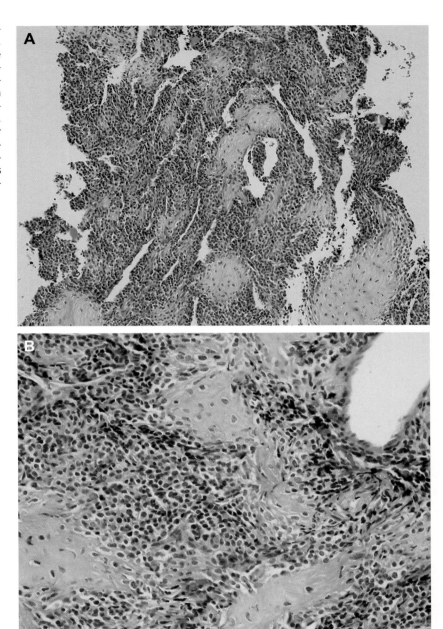

abnormalities and show complex, variable cytogenetic and molecular changes.[81,82] Extraskeletal myxoid chondrosarcoma, however, is characterized by translocations involving the *CHN* gene on chromosome 9, which may be useful in diagnostically challenging cases.[82] In addition, the lack of a translocation involving the *EWS* gene may help distinguish mesenchymal chondrosarcoma from Ewing sarcoma.

In diagnosing chondrosarcomas, it is important to report not only the histologic type and grade but also the tumor stage and margin status. Most chondrosarcomas are low grade and low stage. Margin status is important to report, as complete excision of chondrosarcomas is necessary to reduce the likelihood of local recurrence.[83]

The main considerations in the differential diagnosis of conventional chondrosarcoma are

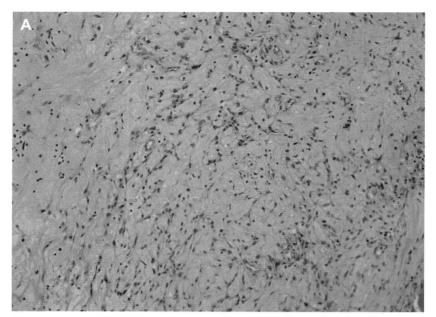

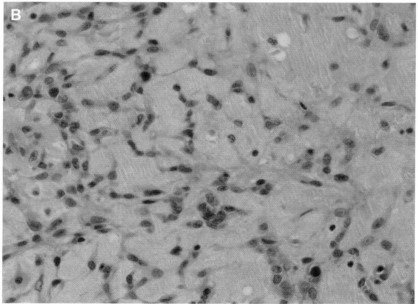

Fig. 32. Extraskeletal myxoid chondrosarcoma. Low-power (*A*, H&E, original magnification ×200) and high-power (*B*, H&E, original magnification ×600) images show myxoid stroma containing anastomosing strands or cords of relatively small, uniform, round to elongated cells.

chondroma and chondroblastic osteosarcoma. Benign chondromas consist of a well-circumscribed growth of benign cartilaginous tissue that lacks the increased cellularity and atypical chondrocytes seen in chondrosarcoma. This diagnosis should be made with caution. Benign chondromas are rare in the head and neck. In addition, chondroma and chondrosarcoma of the larynx are thought to be closely related and often occur synchronously.[63] Therefore, the finding of benign-appearing cartilaginous tissue in biopsy material does not preclude the diagnosis of chondrosarcoma, particularly in large lesions. Some have advocated the diagnosis of "low-grade cartilaginous tumor" in unclear cases. Chondroblastic osteosarcoma is also an important consideration in the differential diagnosis of chondrosarcomas occurring in the jaws, as osteosarcomas are more

Fig. 33. Clear cell chondrosarcoma. (*A*) A low-power image (H&E, original magnification ×200) showing a chondroid neoplasm with abundant clear cells. (*B*) On high-power (H&E, original magnification × 400), sheets of clear cells with scattered multinucleated giant cells are seen.

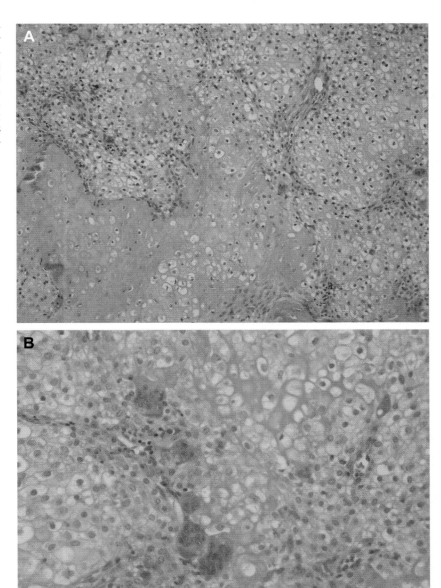

frequently encountered at this site. The finding of osteoid or bone production by tumor necessitates a diagnosis of osteosarcoma. However, chondroblastic differentiation may be extensive in osteosarcomas and careful sampling may be required to document the presence of osteoid.

Other considerations in the differential diagnosis of conventional chondrosarcoma include chondromyxoid fibroma, chondroid metaplasia, nasal chondromesenchymal hamartoma, and pleomorphic adenoma. Chondromyxoid fibroma (see previously in this article) is a benign tumor that is rare in the head and neck but may occur in the craniofacial bones. Histologically, it is composed of chondromyxoid to fibrochondroid nodules, separated by thin, fibrous bands. ABC change can occur. The nodules are centrally hypocellular and contain spindled to stellate cells. The

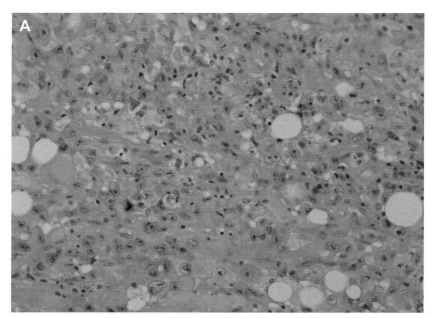

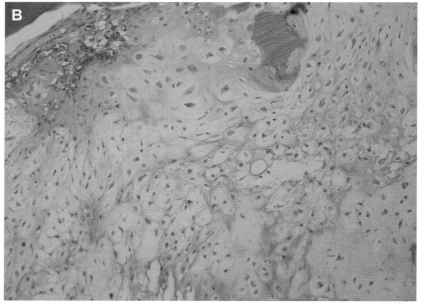

Fig. 34. Dedifferentiated chondrosarcoma. (A) A high-power image (H&E, original magnification ×400) of a high-grade sarcoma containing sheets of pleomorphic cells, some with rhabdoid features. (B) Other areas of the same tumor showed conventional chondrosarcoma (H&E, original magnification ×200).

periphery is more cellular and may mimic a high-grade chondrosarcoma. However, mitotic activity should not be seen. Nasal chondromesenchymal hamartoma is a rare, benign lesion that occurs in the nasal cavity and nasopharynx of children.[84] They are typically polypoid-containing nodules of cartilage within a variably cellular mesenchymal, myxoid to spindle-cell stroma. Giant cells and ABC change may be present. The cartilage component may be cellular and contain occasional binucleated chondrocytes, raising the differential diagnosis of chondrosarcoma. However, the absence of significant cytologic atypia, the presence of a mesenchymal component, and the pediatric age group affected help to distinguish this lesion from chondrosarcoma. Chondroid metaplasia of the larynx is a non-neoplastic, likely trauma-related condition that consists of bland

△△ *Differential Diagnosis*
WELL-DIFFERENTIATED CHONDROSARCOMA

- Benign chondroma
- Chondroblastic osteosarcoma
- Chondromyxoid fibroma
- Chondrometaplasia
- Nasal chondromesenchymal hamartoma
- Pleomorphic adenoma

△△ *Differential Diagnosis*
MESENCHYMAL CHONDROSARCOMA

- Embryonal rhabdomyosarcoma
- Ewing sarcoma
- Lymphoma
- Small cell variant of osteosarcoma

cartilaginous nodules with indistinct borders in the submucosa of the vocal cords. Most are smaller than 1 cm and, in contrast to chondrosarcomas, are not connected to the laryngeal cartilage framework. Finally, pleomorphic adenomas may have a predominant, but bland, chondromyxoid component. The identification of an epithelial component in pleomorphic adenoma easily establishes this diagnosis.

Dedifferentiated chondrosarcoma is distinguished from other high-grade sarcomas, such as fibrosarcoma or pleomorphic sarcoma, by the presence of a differentiated chondrosarcoma component, which may be only a minority of the tumor. Careful sampling of these tumors is therefore required.

The differential diagnosis for mesenchymal chondrosarcoma includes other "small blue-cell tumors" such as embryonal rhabdomyosarcoma, Ewing sarcoma, lymphoma, and the small cell variant of osteosarcoma. The presence of a chondroid component and absence of osteoid distinguishes mesenchymal chondrosarcoma from these other tumors but may not be appreciated on small biopsy material. In that case, ancillary testing, including immunohistochemistry and molecular studies, may be helpful (see previously).

Extraskeletal myxoid chondrosarcoma may share histologic similarities with chordoma and mucinous adenocarcinoma. Identification of physaliphorous cells in chordoma and epithelioid cells with cytoplasmic mucin in adenocarcinoma are distinguishing features. Immunohistochemistry and molecular studies are also useful to differentiate these tumors.

The differential diagnosis of clear cell chondrosarcoma includes other tumors that may contain clear cells, such as metastatic renal cell carcinoma.

Prognosis

Chondrosarcomas of the head and neck have a better prognosis than chondrosarcomas that arise at other sites. This may be because of anatomic constraints in the head and neck causing patients to present with symptoms at an earlier stage. A similar argument has been made for chondrosarcomas arising in the phalanges. The 5-year and 10-year disease-specific survivals reported from the National Cancer Database[70] were 87.2% and 70.6% for all head and neck chondrosarcomas. In comparison, a 10-year survival rate of 50% has been reported in the pelvis, the most frequent site of origin of all chondrosarcomas.[85] Although chondrosarcomas of the head and neck have a favorable prognosis, local recurrence is relatively common. Koch and colleagues[70] reported a local recurrence/persistence rate of 40%. On the other hand, distant metastases are relatively rare. Factors associated with decreased survival included advanced stage, higher grade, and the mesenchymal histologic subtype. Dedifferentiated chondrosarcoma has a poor prognosis; however, in comparison with their axial counterparts, dedifferentiated chondrosarcomas appear less aggressive.[72]

Pitfalls
CHONDROSARCOMA VERSUS BENIGN CHONDROMA

! Distinction between well-differentiated chondrosarcoma and benign chondroma may be difficult histologically, particularly on biopsy material

! Correlation with imaging studies may be helpful

! Benign chondromas are rare in the head and neck and should be diagnosed with caution

FIBRO-OSSEOUS LESIONS OF THE CRANIOFACIAL SKELETON

OVERVIEW

Fibro-osseous lesions are a group of benign bone lesions affecting the craniofacial skeleton and sharing similar microscopic features, characterized by fibrous stroma containing various combinations of bone and cementumlike calcified material. They include a wide variety of developmental, dysplastic, and neoplastic lesions with different clinical and radiographic features and behavior. Because of histologic similarities among these diverse disease entities, proper diagnosis requires correlation of history and clinical and radiographic findings with the microscopic features.

The more important types of fibro-osseous lesions are discussed here.

FIBROUS DYSPLASIA

Overview

Fibrous dysplasia (FD) is a skeletal anomaly in which normal bone is distorted and replaced by poorly organized and inadequately mineralized immature bone and fibrous tissue. The disease may affect multiple bones (polyostotic) or a single bone (monostotic).

Polyostotic FD is less common and a few of these cases may also be associated with skin pigmentation and endocrine abnormalities, a condition known as the McCune Albright syndrome, which is more common in female patients. The skull may be involved in either of the 2 types of FD. Monostotic FD occurs in the craniofacial skeleton, particularly the maxilla and mandible, in 25% of the cases.[86] The pathologic process in this anatomic site is not always strictly

limited to one bone, but may extend by continuity across suture lines to involve adjacent bones, thus the commonly used notation monostotic in this case is not always accurate, and the term craniofacial fibrous dysplasia is preferred.[21]

Fibrous dysplasia is a disease of growing bones. Most cases are originally identified in children and adolescents. More than 80% of craniofacial FD cases are diagnosed within the first 2 decades of life. Males and females are equally affected. Painless swelling of the facial bones with facial asymmetry is the first manifestation. Diffuse thickening of the bones with involvement of paranasal sinuses, orbits, and the foramina of the base of the skull can produce a variety of symptoms, including headache, visual loss, proptosis, nasal obstruction, anosmia, and hearing loss.[21,86,87]

Radiographic Features

Radiographic appearance of the lesions depends on the stage of the disease. Early lesions tend to be radiolucent and as it progressively calcifies it becomes more opaque. Craniofacial lesions are typically mixed radiolucent/radiopaque, producing a characteristic "ground-glass" appearance. The margins are ill defined and the lesional bone blends imperceptibly with the surrounding normal-appearing bone (**Fig. 35**).[21,87,88] The paranasal sinuses may become obliterated, and the displacement of the orbit is a common feature.

Gross and Microscopic Features

Grossly, the affected bone is rubbery, compressible, grayish white tissue that has a gritty texture when cut with a scalpel. Microscopically, normal bone is replaced with a cellular fibroblastic stroma containing variable amounts of randomly dispersed irregular, usually delicate bone trabeculae

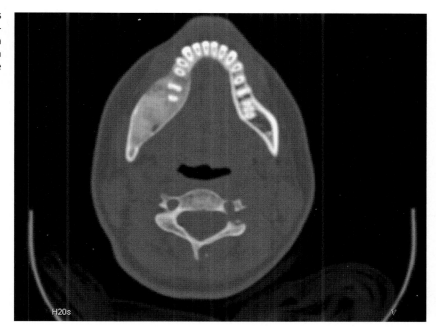

Fig. 35. CT scan of fibrous dysplasia showing expansion of the mandible by a uniformly sclerotic lesion that blends with the surrounding bone.

that evolve directly from the stroma. The bone trabeculae are described as resembling Chinese script letters. Typically, they are composed of immature woven bone that is not rimmed with osteoblasts (**Fig. 36**).[21,86,87] Rarely, FD contain nodules of hyaline cartilage that vary from microscopic foci to larger grossly evident masses.[89] It has been suggested that the bone of craniofacial FD unlike in that of long bones, may undergo a process of maturation leading to lamellar bone formation.[21,86]

Diagnosis and Differential Diagnosis

The diagnosis of FD, as in the case of other fibro-osseous lesions, could not always be established by microscopic examination alone, but is rather based, in addition, on clinical, radiographic, and intraoperative information. FD affects children and young adults, unlike cemento-ossifying fibroma,

which occurs in older adults. Radiographically, FD has ill-defined borders that blend gradually with the surrounding bone. Both cemento-ossifying fibroma and juvenile ossifying fibromas are radiographically well defined.

FD is believed to be caused by a genetic mutation effecting the activation of a G protein (Gs-alpha), which occurs early in the course of development.[90,91] The gene affected is *GNAS1*, located at 20q13.2–13.3. The gain of function mutation has been detected in McCune-Albright syndrome, isolated polyostotic FD, and monostotic FD.[90,91]

Prognosis

Many cases of craniofacial FD become quiescent after puberty; however, persistent growth in later life has been shown in multiple reports.[92,93] Simple contouring of the affected bone back to normal

---

Differential Diagnosis
FIBROUS DYSPLASIA

- Cemento-ossifying fibroma
- Juvenile ossifying fibroma
- Cemento-osseous dysplasia

Pitfalls
FIBROUS DYSPLASIA

! Because of microscopic similarity to other benign fibro-osseous lesions, accurate diagnosis may not be possible without correlation to radiographic appearance and clinical history

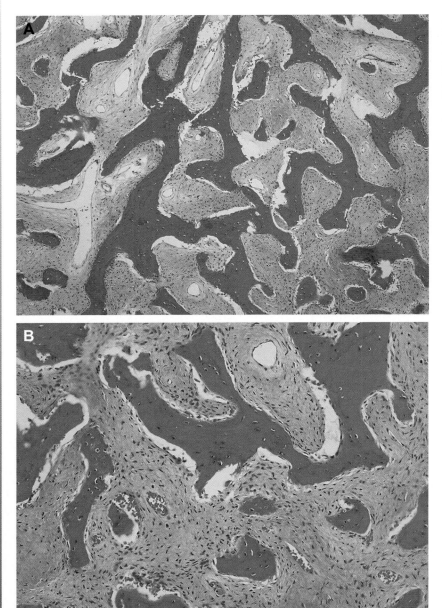

Fig. 36. Fibrous dysplasia, immature woven bone trabeculae with no osteoblastic rimming, forming irregular structures resembling Chinese letters, in a fibrous stroma. (*A*) H&E, original magnification ×200; (*B*) H&E, original magnification ×400.

dimension is usually an effective treatment. Retreatment may be required in a small percentage of patients. Partial excision followed by grafting with normal autologous bone or acrylic implants may achieve reduction in the rate of recurrence.[86,92,94]

Malignant degeneration has been reported in a few cases of FD, most of which are osteosarcomas and, less frequently, fibrosarcoma and chondrosarcoma. In most of these cases there was previous history of radiation therapy, which has been used in the past for treatment of FD.[92,95,96] Because of this risk, radiation therapy for FD is now strictly contraindicated. However, more recent reports show spontaneous sarcomatous transformation unrelated to radiation exposure in very rare cases.[21,30,97,98] It is therefore prudent to keep patients with FD under long-term follow-up. Any patient showing clinical or radiographic evidence of change should undergo an adequate biopsy to rule out sarcomatous transformation.

OSSIFYING FIBROMA

Overview

The term ossifying fibroma (OF) is used to describe benign bone-producing fibrous tumors of the craniofacial skeleton. Several lesions that differ in microscopic appearance, site of incidence, age, and gender distribution are included under the rubric *ossifying fibroma.*

In this Discussion, 2 Main Variants of Ossifying Fibroma are Addressed:

1. OF of odontogenic origin (cemento-ossifying fibroma [COF])
2. Juvenile ossifying fibroma (JOF).

The Latter is Further Subdivided into:

- Trabecular juvenile ossifying fibroma (TrJOF)
- Psammomatoid juvenile ossifying fibroma (PsJOF).

Cemento-Ossifying Fibroma

Overview

This benign odontogenic tumor has been variously called ossifying fibroma, cementifying fibroma, and cemento-ossifying fibroma. The latter is preferred because of its descriptive value and is used in the World Health Organization classification of head and neck tumors.[99] COF affects the tooth-bearing areas of the mandible and maxilla.

The neoplastic cells elaborate bone and cementum and are believed to be derived from the progenitor cells of the periodontal membrane. These cells are capable of dual differentiation into odontoblasts and cementoblasts. COF is a distinctive jaw lesion that should not be confused with other craniofacial skeleton lesions that are also termed ossifying fibroma. The tumors present as painless expansions of the jaws, particularly the mandible. They can attain a very large size with considerable deformity, if untreated. The peak age of incidence is the third and fourth decades with a definite female predilection. The female-to-male ratio is as high as 5:1.[21,99,100]

Radiographic features

The tumors are well defined and unilocular. They may be radiolucent or may show various degrees of opacification depending on the amount of calcified tissue present. In the mandible, larger lesions tend to expand inferiorly, producing a characteristic downward bowing and thinning of the inferior border (**Fig. 37**). Displacement of surrounding teeth and root resorption may be seen.[20,21,87,101]

Gross and microscopic features

An important feature of COF is that it is well defined and can be shelled out with relative ease from the surrounding tissue. Grossly, the tumor is submitted in one piece or in large fragments that are yellowish-tan, which may be hemorrhagic, and feel gritty when cut with a scalpel.

Microscopically, the tumor is well defined and may be encapsulated. It is composed of hypercellular fibroblastic stroma with sparse collagen fibers and blood vessels, containing variable amounts of calcified structures. The stromal cells show hyperchromatic nuclei. Mitosis is not easily found. The calcified structures are composed of variable amounts of osteoid or bone and lobulated

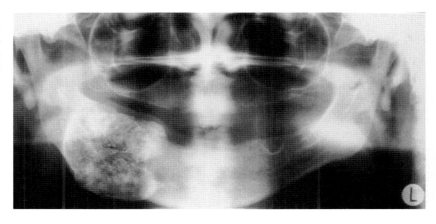

Fig. 37. Panoramic radiograph of ossifying fibroma of the mandible. The tumor is expansive with well-defined, corticated borders.

basophilic masses of cementumlike tissue resembling the cementicles that are normally found in the periodontal membrane. These structures may coalesce and form curvilinear trabeculae that may be acellular (**Fig. 38**).[20,21,87,100]

The ratio of the bone to the cementumlike tissue varies in different lesions. In some tumors, one or the other type of the calcified tissue may dominate. Osteoblastic rimming of the bone trabeculae is evident. Polarized light microscopy reveals both woven and lamellar bone. The cementumlike tissue is often woven and may show a characteristic quilted pattern.[20,21,87,101]

Diagnosis and differential diagnosis

COF is radiographically well defined. It is a lesion of the jaws affecting predominantly female patients in the third and fourth decades of life. Unlike FD, COF can be shelled out or curetted from the surrounding bone with relative ease. FD can affect any part of the craniofacial skeleton, predominantly in children and young adults. FD

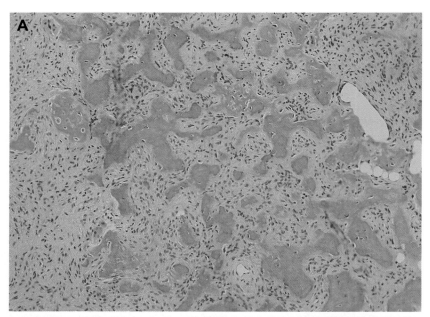

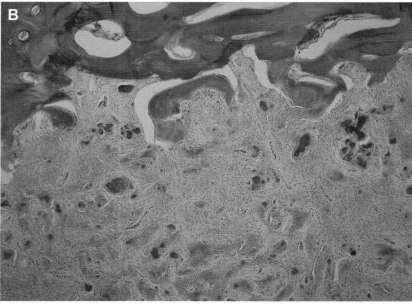

Fig. 38. Cemento-ossifying fibroma. (*A*) Bone trabeculae and cementumlike structures dispersed in hypercellular fibrous stroma (H&E, original magnification ×400). (*B*) COF showing cementumlike calcified tissue and a well-defined border with subjacent cortical bone (H&E, original magnification ×200).

has ill-defined borders that blend with the surrounding bone.

Prognosis

COF is a slow-growing benign neoplasm. It can be surgically excised conservatively by curettage, with no recurrences in most cases. Untreated tumors could attain a massive size and may require en bloc resection. Sarcomatous transformation has not been documented.[20,21,86,87]

Juvenile Ossifying Fibroma

The term JOF has been used in the literature to describe 2 distinct clinicopathologic entities:

1. TrJOF: trabecular juvenile ossifying fibroma
2. PsJOF: psammomatoid juvenile ossifying fibroma.

These tumors have been also referred to as juvenile active ossifying fibroma and juvenile aggressive ossifying fibroma.[99,100,102,103]

Trabecular juvenile ossifying fibroma

Overview TrJOF predominantly affects children and adolescents. The mean age range is 8.5 to 12.0 years.[102] Males and females are equally affected. The maxilla and mandible are the most common sites. The maxilla is more frequent than the mandible. Extragnathic occurrence is extremely rare.[99,102–104] Clinically, the lesion is characterized by progressive and sometimes rapid expansion of the affected bone. In the maxilla, obstruction of the nasal passages and epistaxis may occur.

Radiographic features The tumor is expansive and fairly well demarcated, with cortical thinning and possible perforation. The lesion shows various degrees of radiolucency or opacity depending on the amount of calcified tissue produced (**Fig. 39**). A ground-glass and multilocular appearance have been described.[20,103]

Gross and microscopic features Grossly, the tumor is described as yellowish-white and gritty. Microscopically, it is unencapsulated and shows an infiltrative growth pattern into the surrounding bone. It has a characteristic loose architecture with hypercellular stroma composed of spindle cells with little collagen production. Osteoid develops directly from the fibrous stroma and forms long, slender strands that have been likened

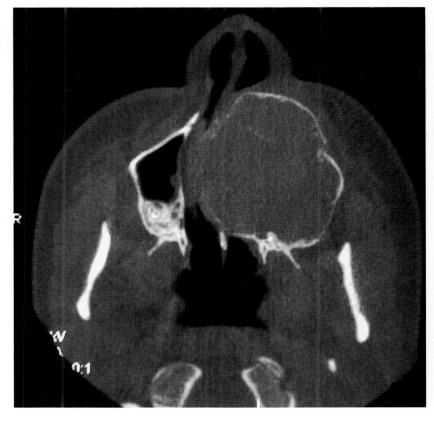

Fig. 39. CT scan of trabecular juvenile ossifying fibroma of the mandible. The lesion is expansive with ground-glass appearance and corticated border.

to paint-brush strokes. Irregular mineralization takes place at the center of the strands, resulting in the production of immature bone trabeculae that are devoid of osteoblastic rimming and do not show evidence of maturation (**Fig. 40**A). Aggregates of osteoblastic giant cells are typically found in the stroma (see **Fig. 40**B). Occasional mitosis may be observed in the stromal cells. Aneurysmal bone cyst formation has been reported in some cases.[102,103]

Prognosis Multiple recurrences have been reported following conservative excision.[102] Eventual complete cure could be achieved without resorting to radical excision. Malignant transformation has not been reported.

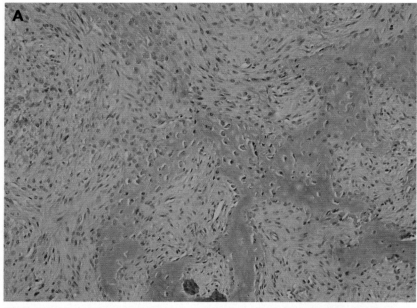

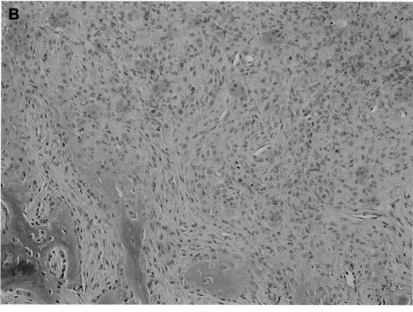

Fig. 40. (*A*) Trabecular juvenile ossifying fibroma showing cellular osteoid trabeculae in spindle cell–rich stroma (H&E, original magnification ×400). (*B*) Aggregates of osteoclast-like giant cells (H&E, original magnification ×400).

Fig. 41. Periorbital psammomatoid juvenile ossifying fibroma. CT scan shows expansive, well-defined but incompletely corticated sclerotic lesion.

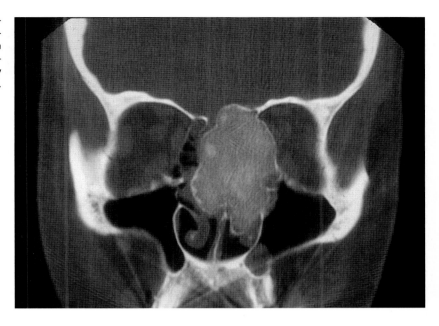

Psammomatoid juvenile ossifying fibroma

Overview PsJOF affects predominantly the extragnathic craniofacial bone. The lesions are particularly centered on periorbital frontal and ethmoid bones.[102] The average age of incidence varied in different studies from 16 to 33 years; however, the age range is wide and cases have been reported in patients as young as 3 months and as old as 72 years[21,102,104]; there is no gender predilection. Clinically, PsJOF manifests as a bony expansion that may involve the orbit or nasal bones and sinuses. Expansion of the tumor may result in proptosis, visual symptoms, and nasal obstruction.

Radiographic features Radiographically, PsJOF presents as a round well-defined osteolytic lesion. Sclerotic changes may impart it with a ground-glass appearance (**Fig. 41**).[102,105,106] The lesion may range in size from 2 to 8 cm in diameter and may appear multiloculated on computed tomography (CT) scans. Areas of low density because of cystic changes may be noted.[102,107]

Fig. 42. Psammomatoid juvenile ossifying fibroma composed of uniform, small, round ossicles (psammomatoid bodies) in a cellular stroma (H&E, original magnification ×400).

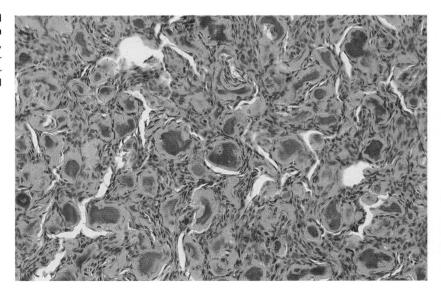

Gross and microscopic features Grossly the tumor is yellowish-white and gritty. On microscopic examination, the tumor is unencapsulated and is significant for multiple small uniform ossicles (psammomatoid bodies) imbedded in cellular stroma composed of spindle and stellate-shaped cells (**Fig. 42**).[21,99,102] The psammomatoid bodies are basophilic and bear some resemblance to dental cementum. At the periphery of the lesion, these structures may coalesce and form bone trabeculae. Cystic degeneration and ABC formation may occur. It is believed by the author (S.K.E.) that reported cases of sudden aggressive growth in both TrJOF and PsJOF may be a result of ABC formation.

Diagnosis and differential diagnosis Confusion in the literature between TrJOF and PsJOF is mainly because of the common use of the term JOF to describe these 2 clinically and pathologically distinct lesions. Microscopically, the former is characterized by trabecular bone formation, whereas in the latter the produced bone shows a characteristic psammomatoid pattern. PsJOF has a definite site predilection to the periorbital bones, whereas TrJOF affects the jaws. The latter also has a younger average age of incidence (**Table 1**).

Prognosis Recurrence, even after definitive surgery, has been reported and multiple recurrences were observed after long follow-up periods.[21,102,108]

CEMENTO-OSSEOUS DYSPLASIA

Overview
Osseous dysplasias are non-neoplastic fibroosseous lesions that affect the tooth-bearing areas of the jaws. Two types are well recognized:

1. Periapical cemento-osseous dysplasia (PCOD)
2. Florid cemento-osseous dysplasia (FCOD).

Table 1
Juvenile ossifying fibroma variants: a comparison

	TrJOF	PsJOF
Average age of incidence, y	8.5–12.0	16.0–33.0
Site predilection	Jaws	Periorbital bones
Pattern of produced bone	Trabecular	Psammomatoid

Abbreviations: PsJOF, psammomatoid juvenile ossifying fibroma; TrJOF, trabecular juvenile ossifying fibroma.

Key Features
CEMENTO-OSSEOUS DYSPLASIA

- It is a dysplastic bone condition affecting the tooth-bearing areas of the jaws.
- Two main types are recognized: periapical and florid COD.
- Middle-aged or older black women are most commonly affected.
- It is asymptomatic and usually detected on routine radiographic examination.
- Surgical intervention is contraindicated.

Ideally, these lesions should be identified clinically and radiographically without the need for a biopsy. Indeed, surgical intervention is contraindicated, because a simple biopsy, particularly in the case of FCOD, can result in persistent local infection and pain with complicated clinical course.[21,86,87]

Periapical Cemento-Osseous Dysplasia

Overview
PCOD, also known as periapical cemental dysplasia and periapical cementoma, is relatively common presumably dysplastic disorder. It typically affects the periapical area of the mandibular anterior teeth in middle-aged black female patients. The lesions are asymptomatic and are usually discovered on routine radiographic examination.

Radiographic features
The early lesions present as small periapical radiolucencies affecting the mandibular anterior teeth. Continued mineralization results in heavily calcified radiopaque areas (**Fig. 43**).[21,86,87] A similar isolated lesion affecting the posterior quadrant of

---

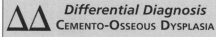

Differential Diagnosis
CEMENTO-OSSEOUS DYSPLASIA

- Inflammatory conditions
- Metastatic carcinoma
- Benign fibro-osseous neoplasms

Fig. 43. Dental radiographs showing progression of calcification in periapical cemento-osseous dysplasia over a period of several years (left to right).

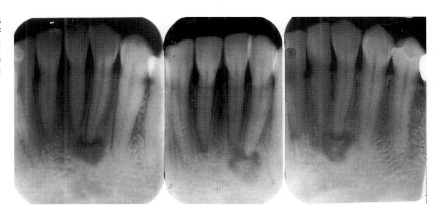

the jaws, especially the mandible, is known as focal osseous dysplasia.[21,86,87]

Microscopic features of PCOD are analogous to those of FCOD and are discussed with that entity.

Florid Cemento-Osseous Dysplasia

Overview

FCOD usually presents in middle-aged or older black women. It is asymptomatic and is typically discovered incidentally on routine radiographic examination.[21,87,109,110]

Radiographic features

A characteristic radiographic appearance is extensive sclerotic areas surrounded by a radiolucent zone and involving the posterior quadrants of both mandible and maxilla bilaterally, in a symmetric fashion (**Fig. 44**).

Microscopic features

Both periapical cemental dysplasia and FCOD have analogous microscopic features. The lesions are composed of fibrous stroma containing foci of cementum, osteoid, or bone (**Fig. 45**). More advanced lesions show increased mineralization and, in the case of FCOD, large, dense sclerotic masses that are hypocellular may form. Development of simple bone cysts in FCOD is known to occur.[111,112]

Diagnosis and Differential Diagnosis

It is of importance to know that, unlike inflammatory and neoplastic lesions, COD are asymptomatic and not associated with pain or expansion of the affected area of the jaws.

Jaw metastasis of some carcinomas, such as those of the breast and prostate, may induce osteoblastic activity and may show radiographic

Fig. 44. Florid cemento-osseous dysplasia. Panoramic radiograph showing bilateral involvement of mandible and maxilla.

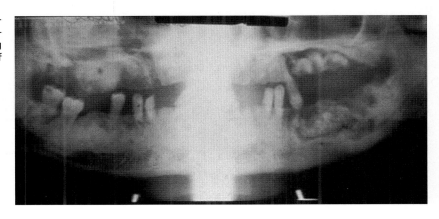

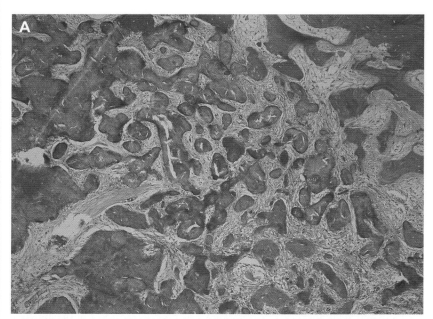

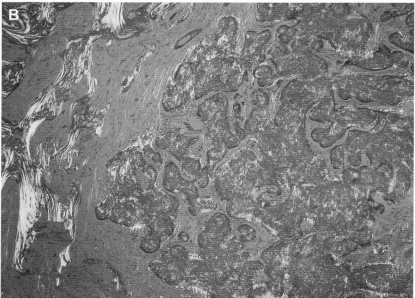

Fig. 45. Cemento-osseous dysplasia. (*A*) Hypocellular bone trabeculae and cementumlike structures coalesce and form dense sclerotic masses toward the center of the lesion (H&E, original magnification ×200). (*B*) With polarized light microscopy, the lesion appears well demarcated from the mature lamellar bone of the jaw (*upper left corner*) (original magnification ×200).

features similar to COD. However, metastatic jaw lesions are usually associated with pain, looseness of teeth, and paresthesia of the lip. A medical history of prostate or breast carcinoma should prompt a biopsy of a suspicious jaw lesion.

Prognosis

Ideally, COD should be identified clinically and radiographically, and not subjected to surgical intervention.

Pitfalls
CEMENTO-OSSEOUS
DYSPLASIA

! Surgical intervention when the lesion is not recognized by clinical and radiographic examination could result in prolonged inflammation and complicated clinical course.

GIANT CELL LESIONS

OVERVIEW

Giant cell lesions of the craniofacial skeleton are a group of clinically diverse conditions that share common microscopic features. Microscopically, they are characterized by presence of multinucleated osteoclastlike giant cells and spindle or polygonal mononuclear cells in a vascular stroma with few or no collagen fibers. These entities include the following:

- Giant cell granuloma (GCG)
- Giant cell tumor (GCT)
- Aneurysmal bone cyst (ABC)
- Cherubism.

GIANT CELL GRANULOMA

Overview

GCG, also called reparative GCG, is a common lesion. It occurs predominantly in the jaws, particularly the mandible. Cases involving the sphenoid and temporal bones have been reported.[97] They follow a benign clinical course that is unlike that of giant cell tumor of long bones. Controversy still exists concerning the relationship of GCG and GCT. Whether or not a true giant-cell tumor occurs in the jaws is a subject of debate.[21,113]

GCG can occur at any age, but most present before the age of 30 years, more commonly in female than male patients. The anterior part of the mandible crossing the midline is the favored site. The lesions usually present as a painless expansion of the affected bone.

Radiographic Features

On radiographic examination, GCG appears as a well-defined but uncorticated radiolucency, which may be either unilocular or multilocular (**Fig. 46**).

Microscopic Features

These lesions are unencapsulated and are composed of osteoclastlike multinucleated giant cells in a vascular stroma, displaying spindle, fibroblastic, and polygonal macrophagelike mononuclear cells, with little or no collagen production. Sinusoidal vascular spaces as well as endothelial-lined capillaries are present throughout the lesion

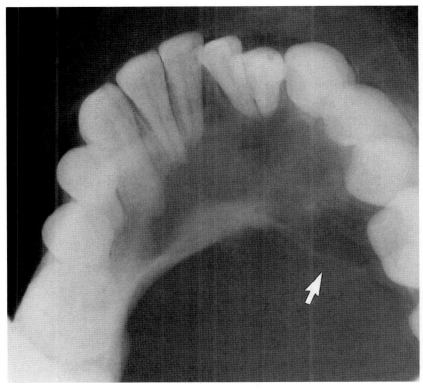

Fig. 46. Radiograph of a giant cell granuloma of the anterior mandible. The lesion caused expansion and thinning of the posterior cortex (*arrow*).

(Fig. 47).[113–115] The giant cells may be evenly dispersed or focally aggregated. They may vary in size in different cases and the number of nuclei per cell also varies from a few to several dozen. Aggregates of hemosiderin deposits and focal areas of ossification may be present.

Prognosis

GCG of the jaws is usually treated by curettage. Recurrence rates of 11% to 35% have been reported.[116,117] Recurrent lesions usually respond to further curettage. Long-term prognosis is good and malignant change or distant metastasis does not occur. It should be noted, however, that on rare occasions a giant cell lesion of the jaws, particularly in the maxilla, can behave in an aggressive fashion. These lesions are characterized by pain, rapid growth, cortical perforation, and frequent recurrences. It is suggested that these aggressive giant cell lesions may show morphologic features usually associated with giant cell tumors, particularly larger and more diffuse giant cells with more numerous nuclei.[116–119]

GIANT CELL TUMOR

Overview

Giant cell tumor is an uncommon bone neoplasm that predominantly affects the ends of long bones. It is rarely encountered in the skull, where they preferentially occur in the temporal and sphenoid bones. Patients with Paget disease of bone have an increased risk of developing GCTs of the skull.[21,97] In a review of 15 GCTs of the skull, Bertoni and colleagues[120] found that the patients tended to be generally older than those affected by GCTs of long bones. One-third of the patients were older than 50 years. The female-to-male ratio was 2:1. The most commonly affected bone was the sphenoid. The frontal, temporal, and occipital bones were other sites of involvement.

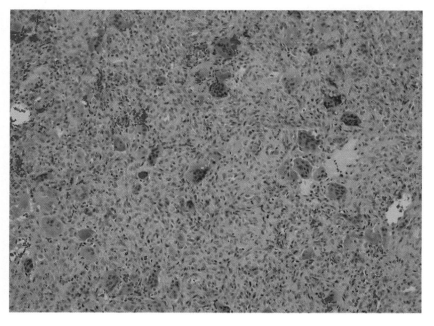

Fig. 47. Giant cell granuloma. Aggregated osteoclastlike giant cells in a stroma of spindle-shaped and polygonal mononuclear cells with little collagen deposits (H&E, original magnification ×200).

Fig. 48. (A) CT scan showing Paget disease of the skull and a giant cell tumor involving the temporal and parietal bones (arrow). (B) The tumor is translucent with well-defined borders. The bones of the skull show the characteristic cotton-wool appearance of Paget disease.

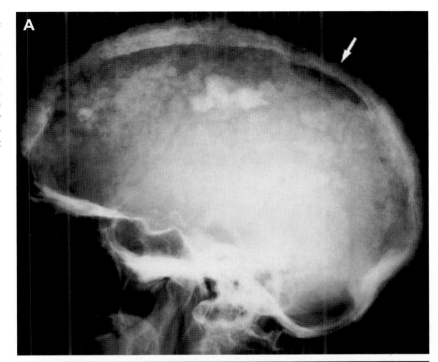

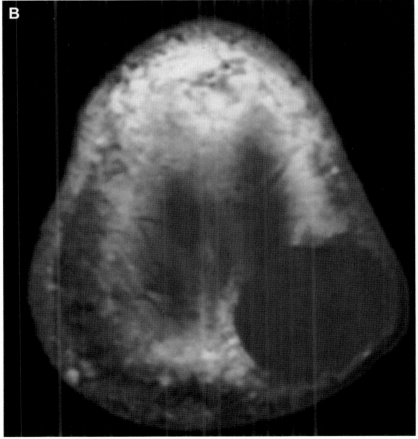

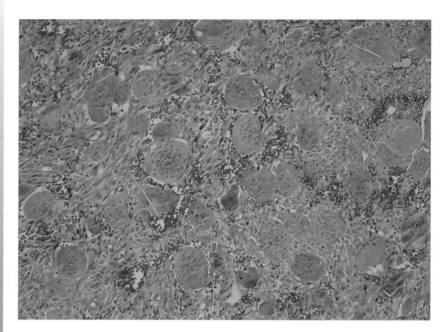

Fig. 49. Giant cell lesion with features suggestive of giant cell tumor. The giant cells are larger and with more numerous nuclei than the ones commonly seen in giant cell granuloma (H&E, original magnification ×200).

Radiographic Features

Radiographically, GCT presents as a radiolucent lesion with ill-defined borders (**Fig. 48**). There is no evidence of matrix mineralization. Bone destruction may be associated with a soft tissue mass. In the sphenoid bone, the tumor may extend into the sella tursica, the posterior nasopharynx, ethmoid sinus, and orbit.[120]

Microscopic Features

The tumors are composed of multinucleated giant cells and round and spindle-shaped mononuclear cells with little or no collagen found in the stroma. Sinusoidal vascular spaces rather than endothelial-lined capillaries are present throughout the lesion (**Fig. 49**). Mitotic activity is usually found and varies among different tumors. Atypical mitoses are not found. Permeation of surrounding marrow spaces may be present.

Diagnosis and Differential Diagnosis

True giant cell tumors in contrast to GCG are unlikely encountered in the jaws. As mentioned previously, they tend to occur in the sphenoid and temporal bones. In a comparative morphologic study, Auclair and colleagues[113] found significant differences between these two entities. GCTs are more cellular and have larger giant cells with more numerous nuclei per cell (**Fig. 50**) that GCGs. The giant cells in GCTs were

found to be more evenly dispersed in the lesions. However, a minority of cases of GCGs and GCTs are morphologically similar.

Prognosis

GCT of the skull bones can be aggressive, and because of their location, adequate excision is not always possible. Postoperative radiation is used with some success in achieving local control. Malignant transformation has been reported de novo as well as after radiation therapy.[121]

Differential Diagnosis
CELL GRANULOMA AND GIANT CELL TUMOR

- Morphologic differences include distribution of the giant cells, their size, and number of nuclei per cell. GCTs show larger giant cells that have more nuclei and show diffuse distribution.

- GCGs are histologically identical to brown tumors of hyperparathyroidism. The latter are associated with clinical and radiographic manifestations of hyperparathyroidism and resolves after managing the parathyroid disease.

Pitfalls
GIANT CELL GRANULOMA AND GIANT CELL TUMOR

! A minority of cases of GCG and GCT are microscopically identical but with marked differences in clinical aggressiveness.

! GCGs may morphologically resemble Brown tumors of hyperparathyroidism.

Key Features
ANEURYSMAL BONE CYST

- ABC may present as a primary lesion or secondary with a bone tumor.
- It characteristically affects growing bones.
- Sudden expansion of the involved bone is a typical feature.

ANEURYSMAL BONE CYST

Overview

ABC is a benign bone cyst of probable neoplastic potential.[122,123] It is a lesion of growing bones. The greatest majority occur in patients who are younger than 20 years. Male and female patients are equally affected.[124,125] ABC can affect any bone, but, judging from reported cases, the craniofacial bones, the vertebrae, and the flat bones of the pelvis are the most common sites. In the long bones, the femur and tibia are more likely to be affected. In the skull, the jaws are more frequently involved than other bones, with somewhat more predilection for the mandible.[126]

ABC may develop either as a primary lesion or secondary, in association with a variety of bone tumors including chondroblastoma, osteoblastoma, GCT, COF, and JOF.[127–129] A secondary ABC shows a sudden expansion of a preexisting bone lesion. ABC may present clinically as painless expansion of bone or may be associated with pain. The symptoms may last from days to months. On palpation, the deformity is found to be firm and boney. In the mandible, numbness of the lower lip, trismus, and displacement of teeth may be evident.[125,130,131]

Radiographic Features

Radiographically ABCs present as a rapidly expanding benign cystic lesion (see **Fig. 50**). The rate of expansion can be illustrated in serial radiographs. More frequently, it is unilocular but less frequently may be multilocular, even with a "soap bubble" appearance.[127,131,132] The rapid expansion may result in loss of cortication and even loss of marginal definition in plain film radiographs; however, a thin cortical shell is usually identifiable in CT scans.[132] Fluid levels may also be seen in the scans.

Gross and Microscopic Features

When the lesion is exposed at surgery, welling of nonclotted blood without spurting is noticed.[106,133] Grossly, the cut surface of the lesion appears spongy and resembles honeycomb.[106] On microscopic examination, ABC may be either primary, if the characteristic microscopic features are represented throughout the specimen, or secondary, when ABC is associated with another bone tumor. Approximately 30% of ABCs are secondary.[128]

On microscopic examination, ABC is typically composed of sinusoidal spaces of variable sizes that are not lined with endothelial cells. The

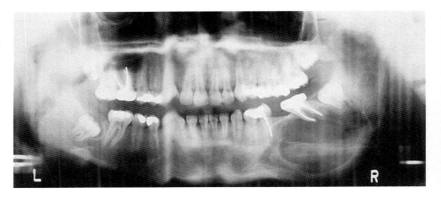

Fig. 50. Panoramic radiograph showing aneurysmal bone cyst of the right mandible. The lesion is expansive, well-defined, and unilocular.

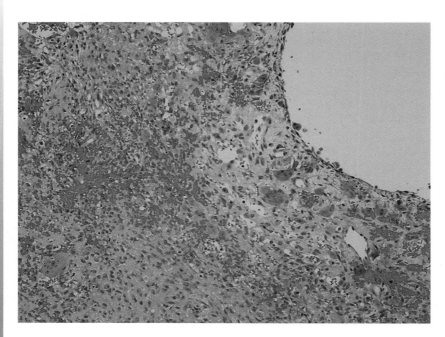

Fig. 51. Aneurysmal bone cyst of the mandible. Wide sinusoidal spaces surrounded by a stroma that resembles giant cell granuloma (H&E, original magnification ×200).

surrounding stroma, forming the intersinusoidal septa, bears some resemblance to GCG, and is composed of both spindle and epithelioid mononuclear cells, in addition to osteoclastic giant cells, interspersed with small vascular spaces (**Fig. 51**). Hemosiderin deposits in addition to reactive bone are commonly present. Amorphous calcification with chondroid appearance may be present.[125]

Prognosis

Curettage is the most common treatment modality of ABC of any site. A recurrence rate of 19% is reported for the jaw lesions.[126] Factors associated with increased risk of recurrence include the patient's age, size of lesion, and increased mitotic activity[134–136]; however, incomplete surgical excision is probably the most important single factor. Recurrences have occurred 4 months to 3 years after treatment.[124] Malignant transformation of ABCs has rarely been reported.[122]

CHERUBISM

Overview

Cherubism is a hereditary disease transmitted as an autosomal dominant trait with variable expressivity in different patients. The disease is characterized by bilateral expansion of the jaws caused by giant cell lesions. The jaw deformity starts to

be obvious during the first years of life, becomes progressively larger until puberty, and abates by middle age. The boney expansion may start unilaterally, but eventually it affects both sides of the jaws. In the mandible, the molar coronoid area is particularly involved. In the maxilla, the tuberosity is initially affected, but anterior and orbital bones may follow.[137,138] The boney expansion is painless and hard. Involvement of other bones in the skeleton has rarely been reported.[139]

 Differential Diagnosis
ANEURYSMAL BONE CYST

- Wide sinusoidal spaces distinguish ABCs from solid giant cell lesions, such as GCG and GCT.

- On radiographic examination, telangiectatic osteosarcoma has ill-defined borders with extensive cortical destruction and microscopically shows atypical pleomorphic cells with excessive mitosis.

Fig. 52. Cherubism. Panoramic radiograph showing expansive multilocular radiolucent lesions affecting the mandible and maxilla bilaterally.

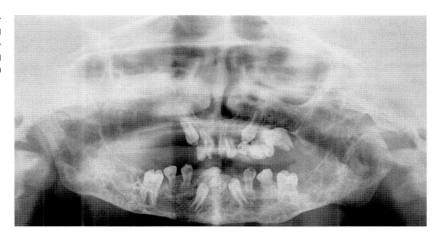

Key Features
CHERUBISM

- It is a hereditary disease inherited as an autosomal dominant trait.

- Childhood onset, which is characterized by gradual expansion of the jaws, bilaterally.

- Radiographic examination reveals expansive, well-defined, multilocular radiolucency.

- Microscopic examination shows giant cell lesion that resembles GCG.

Radiographic Features

The lesions are expansive and radiolucent with well-demarcated outline. They may be unilocular but are usually multilocular (**Fig. 52**).[97,137,140] Many of the developing teeth may be affected by the growing lesions, including misplacement, uneruption, and root resorption.[137,140]

Microscopic Features

The microscopic findings of the lesions of cherubism are essentially similar to those of GCG described previously. However, the vascular stroma in cherubism seem to be more loosely arranged with

Fig. 53. Cherubism. Sparse giant cells in a background of spindle-shaped and macrophagelike mononuclear cells. Note the perivascular eosinophilic deposits (H&E, original magnification ×200).

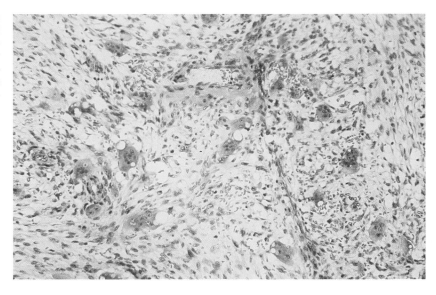

fewer and smaller giant cells that tend to be focally aggregated (**Fig. 53**). Eosinophilic, perivascular, cufflike deposits are characteristic features of cherubism but they are not always present.[140–142] Hemosiderin deposits and metaplastic bone may be found.

Prognosis

Cherubism is a self-limiting process and may even be reversed by age. Treatment is usually limited to curettage and cosmetic contouring of the affected bone. Some cases of cherubism show active disease persistence in adult life, and cases showing rapid regrowth after surgery have been reported.[141,143] An association between Noonan syndrome and cherubism has been shown.[144–146]

REFERENCES

1. Boysen M. Osteomas of the paranasal sinuses. J Otolaryngol 1978;7(4):366–70.
2. Earwaker J. Paranasal sinus osteomas: a review of 46 cases. Skeletal Radiol 1993;22(6):417–23.
3. Samy LL, Mostafa H. Osteomata of the nose and paranasal sinuses with a report of twenty one cases. J Laryngol Otol 1971;85(5):449–69.
4. McHugh JB, Mukherji SK, Lucas DR. Sino-orbital osteoma: a clinicopathologic study of 45 surgically treated cases with emphasis on tumors with osteoblastoma-like features. Arch Pathol Lab Med 2009;133(10):1587–93.
5. Fu YS, Perzin KH. Non-epithelial tumors of the nasal cavity, paranasal sinuses, and nasopharynx. A clinicopathologic study. II. Osseous and fibro-osseous lesions, including osteoma, fibrous dysplasia, ossifying fibroma, osteoblastoma, giant cell tumor, and osteosarcoma. Cancer 1974;33(5):1289–305.
6. Bouquot JE, Müller S, Nikai H. Lesions of the oral cavity. In: Gnepp DR, editor. Diagnostic surgical pathology of the head and neck. Philadelphia: Saunders Elsevier; 2009. p. 210–1.
7. Chang CH, Piatt ED, Thomas KE, et al. Bone abnormalities in Gardner's syndrome. Am J Roentgenol Radium Ther Nucl Med 1968;103(3):645–52.
8. Takeuchi T, Takenoshita Y, Kubo K, et al. Natural course of jaw lesions in patients with familial adenomatosis coli (Gardner's syndrome). Int J Oral Maxillofac Surg 1993;22(4):226–30.
9. Della Rocca C, Huvos AG. Osteoblastoma: varied histological presentations with a benign clinical course. An analysis of 55 cases. Am J Surg Pathol 1996;20(7):841–50.
10. Jackson RP, Reckling FW, Mants FA. Osteoid osteoma and osteoblastoma. Similar histologic lesions with different natural histories. Clin Orthop Relat Res 1977;128:303–13.
11. Jones AC, Prihoda TJ, Kacher JE, et al. Osteoblastoma of the maxilla and mandible: a report of 24 cases, review of the literature, and discussion of its relationship to osteoid osteoma of the jaws. Oral Surg Oral Med Oral Pathol Oral Radiol Endod 2006;102(5):639–50.
12. Lucas DR, Unni KK, McLeod RA, et al. Osteoblastoma: clinicopathologic study of 306 cases. Hum Pathol 1994;25(2):117–34.
13. Pettine KA, Klassen RA. Osteoid-osteoma and osteoblastoma of the spine. J Bone Joint Surg Am 1986;68(3):354–61.
14. Prabhakar B, Reddy DR, Dayananda B, et al. Osteoid osteoma of the skull. J Bone Joint Surg Br 1972;54(1):146–8.
15. Yang C, Qiu WL. Osteoid osteoma of the eminence of the temporomandibular joint. Br J Oral Maxillofac Surg 2001;39(5):404–6.
16. Swee RG, McLeod RA, Beabout JW. Osteoid osteoma. Detection, diagnosis, and localization. Radiology 1979;130(1):117–23.
17. Kroon HM, Schurmans J. Osteoblastoma: clinical and radiologic findings in 98 new cases. Radiology 1990;175(3):783–90.
18. Dorfman HD, Weiss SW. Borderline osteoblastic tumors: problems in the differential diagnosis of aggressive osteoblastoma and low-grade osteosarcoma. Semin Diagn Pathol 1984;1(3):215–34.
19. Lypka MA, Goos RR, Yamashita DD, et al. Aggressive osteoblastoma of the mandible. Int J Oral Maxillofac Surg 2008;37(7):675–8.
20. El-Mofty SK. Cemento-ossifying fibroma and benign cementoblastoma. Semin Diagn Pathol 1999;16(4):302–7.
21. El-Mofty S. Bone lesions. In: Gnepp DR, editor. Diagnostic surgical pathology of the head and neck. 2nd edition. Philadelphia: Saunders Elsevier; 2009. p. 729–84.
22. Eisenbud L, Kahn LB, Friedman E. Benign osteoblastoma of the mandible: fifteen year follow-up showing spontaneous regression after biopsy. J Oral Maxillofac Surg 1987;45(1):53–7.
23. Merryweather R, Middlemiss JH, Sanerkin NG. Malignant transformation of osteoblastoma. J Bone Joint Surg Br 1980;62(3):381–4.
24. Harvei S, Solheim O. The prognosis in osteosarcoma: Norwegian National Data. Cancer 1981;48(8):1719–23.
25. Uribe-Botero G, Russell WO, Sutow WW, et al. Primary osteosarcoma of bone. Clinicopathologic investigation of 243 cases, with necropsy studies in 54. Am J Clin Pathol 1977;67(5):427–35.
26. Smith RB, Apostolakis LW, Karnell LH, et al. National cancer data base report on osteosarcoma of the head and neck. Cancer 2003;98(8):1670–80.
27. Unni K. General aspects and data on 11,087 cases. In: Unni KK, editor. Dahlin's bone tumors. 5th edition. Philadelphia: Lippincott-Raven; 1996. p. 143–84.

28. Huvos AG, Butler A, Bretsky SS. Osteogenic sarcoma associated with Paget's disease of bone. A clinicopathologic study of 65 patients. Cancer 1983;52(8):1489–95.

29. Schajowicz F, Santini Araujo E, Berenstein M. Sarcoma complicating Paget's disease of bone. A clinicopathological study of 62 cases. J Bone Joint Surg Br 1983;65(3):299–307.

30. Taconis WK. Osteosarcoma in fibrous dysplasia. Skeletal Radiol 1988;17(3):163–70.

31. Torres FX, Kyriakos M. Bone infarct-associated osteosarcoma. Cancer 1992;70(10):2418–30.

32. Huvos AG, Woodard HQ, Cahan WG, et al. Postradiation osteogenic sarcoma of bone and soft tissues. A clinicopathologic study of 66 patients. Cancer 1985;55(6):1244–55.

33. Bennett JH, Thomas G, Evans AW, et al. Osteosarcoma of the jaws: a 30-year retrospective review. Oral Surg Oral Med Oral Pathol Oral Radiol Endod 2000;90(3):323–32.

34. Guadagnolo BA, Zagars GK, Raymond AK, et al. Osteosarcoma of the jaw/craniofacial region: outcomes after multimodality treatment. Cancer 2009;115(14):3262–70.

35. Huvos AG. Osteogenic sarcoma of bones and soft tissues in older persons. A clinicopathologic analysis of 117 patients older than 60 years. Cancer 1986;57(7):1442–9.

36. Allan CJ, Soule EH. Osteogenic sarcoma of the somatic soft tissues. Clinicopathologic study of 26 cases and review of literature. Cancer 1971;27(5):1121–33.

37. Rao U, Cheng A, Didolkar MS. Extraosseous osteogenic sarcoma: clinicopathological study of eight cases and review of literature. Cancer 1978;41(4):1488–96.

38. Fanburg JC, Rosenberg AE, Weaver DL, et al. Osteocalcin and osteonectin immunoreactivity in the diagnosis of osteosarcoma. Am J Clin Pathol 1997;108(4):464–73.

39. Park YK, Yang MH, Kim YW, et al. Osteocalcin expression in primary bone tumors—in situ hybridization and immunohistochemical study. J Korean Med Sci 1995;10(4):263–8.

40. Park YK, Yang MH, Park HR. The impact of osteonectin for differential diagnosis of osteogenic bone tumors: an immunohistochemical and in situ hybridization approach. Skeletal Radiol 1996;25(1):13–7.

41. Serra M, Morini MC, Scotlandi K, et al. Evaluation of osteonectin as a diagnostic marker of osteogenic bone tumors. Hum Pathol 1992;23(12):1326–31.

42. Issing WJ, Wustrow TP, Oeckler R, et al. An association of the RB gene with osteosarcoma: molecular genetic evaluation of a case of hereditary retinoblastoma. Eur Arch Otorhinolaryngol 1993;250(5):277–80.

43. Porter DE, Holden ST, Steel CM, et al. A significant proportion of patients with osteosarcoma may belong to Li-Fraumeni cancer families. J Bone Joint Surg Br 1992;74(6):883–6.

44. Kassir RR, Rassekh CH, Kinsella JB, et al. Osteosarcoma of the head and neck: meta-analysis of nonrandomized studies. Laryngoscope 1997;107(1):56–61.

45. Ha PK, Eisele DW, Frassica FJ, et al. Osteosarcoma of the head and neck: a review of the Johns Hopkins experience. Laryngoscope 1999;109(6):964–9.

46. Okada K, Frassica FJ, Sim FH, et al. Parosteal osteosarcoma. A clinicopathological study. J Bone Joint Surg Am 1994;76(3):366–78.

47. Banerjee SC. Juxtacortical osteosarcoma of mandible: review of literature and report of case. J Oral Surg 1981;39(7):535–8.

48. Millar BG, Browne RM, Flood TR. Juxtacortical osteosarcoma of the jaws. Br J Oral Maxillofac Surg 1990;28(2):73–9.

49. Roca AN, Smith JL Jr, Jing BS. Osteosarcoma and parosteal osteogenic sarcoma of the maxilla and mandible: study of 20 cases. Am J Clin Pathol 1970;54(6):625–36.

50. Kumar R, Moser RP Jr, Madewell JE, et al. Parosteal osteogenic sarcoma arising in cranial bones: clinical and radiologic features in eight patients. AJR Am J Roentgenol 1990;155(1):113–7.

51. Smith J, Ahuja SC, Huvos AG, et al. Parosteal (juxtacortical) osteogenic sarcoma. A roentgenological study of 30 patients. J Can Assoc Radiol 1978;29(3):167–74.

52. van der Heul RO, von Ronnen JR. Juxtacortical osteosarcoma. Diagnosis, differential diagnosis, treatment, and an analysis of eighty cases. J Bone Joint Surg Am 1967;49(3):415–39.

53. Bertoni F, Bacchini P, Staals EL, et al. Dedifferentiated parosteal osteosarcoma: the experience of the Rizzoli Institute. Cancer 2005;103(11):2373–82.

54. Sheth DS, Yasko AW, Raymond AK, et al. Conventional and dedifferentiated parosteal osteosarcoma. Diagnosis, treatment, and outcome. Cancer 1996;78(10):2136–45.

55. Bras JM, Donner R, van der Kwast WA, et al. Juxtacortical osteogenic sarcoma of the jaws. Review of the literature and report of a case. Oral Surg Oral Med Oral Pathol 1980;50(6):535–44.

56. Minic AJ. Periosteal osteosarcoma of the mandible. Int J Oral Maxillofac Surg 1995;24(3):226–8.

57. Patterson A, Greer RO Jr, Howard D. Periosteal osteosarcoma of the maxilla: a case report and review of literature. J Oral Maxillofac Surg 1990;48(5):522–6.

58. Piattelli A, Favia GF. Periosteal osteosarcoma of the jaws: report of 2 cases. J Periodontol 2000;71(2):325–9.

59. Yoon JH, Yook JI, Kim HJ, et al. Periosteal osteosar-coma of the mandible. J Oral Maxillofac Surg 2005; 63(5):699–703.

60. Zarbo RJ, Regezi JA, Baker SR. Periosteal osteo-genic sarcoma of the mandible. Oral Surg Oral Med Oral Pathol 1984;57(6):643–7.

61. Schajowicz F, McGuire MH, Santini Araujo E, et al. Osteosarcomas arising on the surfaces of long bones. J Bone Joint Surg Am 1988;70(4):555–64.

62. Unni KK, Dahlin DC, Beabout JW, et al. Parosteal osteogenic sarcoma. Cancer 1976;37(5):2466–75.

63. Baatenburg de Jong RJ, van Lent S, Hogendoorn CW. Chondroma and chondrosar-coma of the larynx. Curr Opin Otolaryngol Head Neck Surg 2004;12:98–105.

64. Casiraghi O, Martinez-Madrigal F, Pineda-Daboin K, et al. Chondroid tumors of the larynx: a clinicopathologic study of 19 cases, including two dedifferentiated chondrosarcomas. Ann Diagn Pathol 2004;8(4):189–97.

65. Bian LG, Sun QF, Zhao WG, et al. Temporal bone chondroblastoma: a review. Neuropathology 2005; 25:159–64.

66. Watanabe N, Yoshida K, Shigemi H, et al. Temporal bone chondroblastoma. Otolaryngol Head Neck Surg 1999;121(3):327–30.

67. Monda L, Wick MR. S-100 protein immunostaining in the differential diagnosis of chondroblastoma. Hum Pathol 1985;16:287–93.

68. Oliveira AM, Dei Tos AP, Fletcher CD, et al. Primary giant cell tumor of soft tissues: a study of 22 cases. Am J Surg Pathol 2000;24(2):248–56.

69. Gadwal SR, Fanburg-Smith JC, Gannon FH, et al. Primary chondrosarcoma of the head and neck in pediatric patients. Cancer 2000;88(9):2181–8.

70. Koch BB, Karnell LH, Hoffman HT, et al. National cancer database report on chondrosarcoma of the head and neck. Head Neck 2000;22:408–25.

71. Ceylan K, Kizilkaya Z, Yavanoglu A. Extraskeletal myxoid chondrosarcoma of the nasal cavity. Eur Arch Otorhinolaryngol 2006;263:1044–7.

72. Garcia RE, Gannon FH, Thompson LD. Dedifferen-tiated chondrosarcomas of the larynx: a report of two cases and review of the literature. Laryngo-scope 2002;112:1015–8.

73. Kleist B, Poetsch M, Lang C, et al. Clear cell chon-drosarcoma of the larynx: a case report of a rare histologic variant in an uncommon localization. Am J Surg Pathol 2002;26(3):386–92.

74. Rinaggio J, Duffey D, McGuff S. Dedifferentiated chondrosarcoma of the larynx. Oral Surg Oral Med Oral Pathol Oral Radiol Endod 2004;97:369–75.

75. Said S, Civantos F, Whiteman M, et al. Clear cell chondrosarcoma of the larynx. Otolaryngol Head Neck Surg 2001;125:107–8.

76. Thompson LD, Gannon FH. Chondrosarcoma of the larynx: a clinicopathologic study of 111 cases with a review of the literature. Am J Surg Pathol 2002;26(7):836–51.

77. Knott PD, Gannon FH, Thompson LD. Mesen-chymal chondrosarcoma of the sinonasal tract: a clinicopathological study of 13 cases with review of the literature. Laryngoscope 2003;113: 783–90.

78. Pellitteri PK, Ferlito A, Fagan JJ, et al. Mesen-chymal chondrosarcoma of the head and neck. Oral Oncol 2007;43:970–5.

79. Atkins KA, Mills SE, editors. Diseases of bones and joints. 3rd edition. New York: Informa Healthcare USA; 2009.

80. Evans HL, Ayala AG, Romsdahl MM. Prognostic factors in chondrosarcoma of bone: a clinicopatho-logic analysis with emphasis on histologic grading. Cancer 1977;40:818–31.

81. Sandberg A, Bridge JA. Updates on the cytogenetics and molecular genetics of bone and soft tissue tumors: chondrosarcoma and other cartilaginous neoplasms. Cancer Genet Cytogenet 2003;143:1–31.

82. Sandberg A. Genetics of chondrosarcoma and related tumors. Curr Opin Oncol 2004;16:342–54.

83. Ruark DS, Schlehaider UK, Shah JP. Chondrosar-comas of the head and neck. World J Surg 1992; 16(5):1010–5.

84. McDermott MB, Ponder TB, Dehner LP. Nasal chondromesenchymal hamartoma: an upper respi-ratory tract analogue of the chest wall mesen-chymal hamartoma. Am J Surg Pathol 1998;22(4): 425–33.

85. Ozaki T, Hillmann A, Lindner N, et al. Chondrosar-coma of the pelvis. Clin Orthop Relat Res 1997; 337:226–39.

86. Waldron CA. Fibro-osseous lesions of the jaws. J Oral Maxillofac Surg 1993;51(8):828–35.

87. Eversole R, Su L, El-Mofty S. Benign fibro-osseous lesions of the craniofacial complex: a review. Head Neck Pathol 2008;2:177–202.

88. Kransdorf MJ, Moser RP Jr, Gilkey FW. Fibrous dysplasia. Radiographics 1990;10(3):519–37.

89. Ishida T, Dorfman HD. Massive chondroid differen-tiation in fibrous dysplasia of bone (fibrocartilagi-nous dysplasia). Am J Surg Pathol 1993;17(9): 924–30.

90. Marie PJ. Cellular and molecular basis of fibrous dysplasia. Histol Histopathol 2001;16(3):981–8.

91. Lietman SA, Ding C, Levine MA. A highly sensitive polymerase chain reaction method detects acti-vating mutations of the GNAS gene in peripheral blood cells in McCune-Albright syndrome or iso-lated fibrous dysplasia. J Bone Joint Surg Am 2005;87(11):2489–94.

92. Stompro BE, Wolf P, Haghighi P. Fibrous dysplasia of bone. Am Fam Physician 1989;39(3):179–84.

93. Ricalde P, Horswell BB. Craniofacial fibrous dysplasia of the fronto-orbital region: a case series

and literature review. J Oral Maxillofac Surg 2001; 59(2):157–67 [discussion: 167–8].

94. Moore AT, Buncic JR, Munro IR. Fibrous dysplasia of the orbit in childhood. Clinical features and management. Ophthalmology 1985;92(1):12–20.

95. Barat M, Rybak LP, Mann JL. Fibrous dysplasia masquerading as chronic maxillary sinusitis. Ear Nose Throat J 1989;68(1):42, 4–6.

96. Yabut SM Jr, Kenan S, Sissons HA, et al. Malignant transformation of fibrous dysplasia. A case report and review of the literature. Clin Orthop Relat Res 1988;228:281–9.

97. Huvos A. Bone tumors: diagnosis, treatment, and prognosis. 2nd edition. Philadelphia: W B Saunders; 1991.

98. Ruggieri P, Sim FH, Bond JR, et al. Malignancies in fibrous dysplasia. Cancer 1994;73(5):1411–24.

99. Slootweg P, El-Mofty S. Ossifying fibroma. In: Barnes L, Eveson J, Reichart P, et al, editors. Pathology and genetics of head and neck tumors. Lyon: IARC Press; 2005. p. 319–20.

100. Eversole LR, Leider AS, Nelson K. Ossifying fibroma: a clinicopathologic study of sixty-four cases. Oral Surg Oral Med Oral Pathol 1985; 60(5):505–11.

101. Eversole LR, Merrell PW, Strub D. Radiographic characteristics of central ossifying fibroma. Oral Surg Oral Med Oral Pathol 1985;59(5):522–7.

102. El-Mofty S. Psammomatoid and trabecular juvenile ossifying fibroma of the craniofacial skeleton: two distinct clinicopathologic entities. Oral Surg Oral Med Oral Pathol Oral Radiol Endod 2002;93(3): 296–304.

103. Slootweg PJ, Muller H. Juvenile ossifying fibroma. Report of four cases. J Craniomaxillofac Surg 1990;18(3):125–9.

104. Slootweg PJ, Panders AK, Koopmans R, et al. Juvenile ossifying fibroma. An analysis of 33 cases with emphasis on histopathological aspects. J Oral Pathol Med 1994;23(9):385–8.

105. Margo CE, Weiss A, Habal MB. Psammomatoid ossifying fibroma. Arch Ophthalmol 1986;104(9): 1347–51.

106. Margo CE, Ragsdale BD, Perman KI, et al. Psammomatoid (juvenile) ossifying fibroma of the orbit. Ophthalmology 1985;92(1):150–9.

107. Khoury NJ, Naffaa LN, Shabb NS, et al. Juvenile ossifying fibroma: CT and MR findings. Eur Radiol 2002;12(Suppl 3):S109–13.

108. Marvel JB, Marsh MA, Catlin Fl. Ossifying fibroma of the mid-face and paranasal sinuses: diagnostic and therapeutic considerations. Otolaryngol Head Neck Surg 1991;104(6):803–8.

109. Melrose RJ, Abrams AM, Mills BG. Florid osseous dysplasia. A clinical-pathologic study of thirty-four cases. Oral Surg Oral Med Oral Pathol 1976; 41(1):62–82.

110. El-Mofty SK. Lesions of the head and neck. In: Wick M, Humphrey P, Ritter J, editors. Pathology of pseudoneoplastic lesions. Philadelphia: Lippincott - Raven; 1997. p. 69–96.

111. Mupparapu M, Singer SR, Milles M, et al. Simultaneous presentation of focal cemento-osseous dysplasia and simple bone cyst of the mandible masquerading as a multilocular radiolucency. Dentomaxillofac Radiol 2005;34(1):39–43.

112. Wakasa T, Kawai N, Aiga H, et al. Management of florid cemento-osseous dysplasia of the mandible producing solitary bone cyst: report of a case. J Oral Maxillofac Surg 2002;60(7):832–5.

113. Auclair PL, Cuenin P, Kratochvil FJ, et al. A clinical and histomorphologic comparison of the central giant cell granuloma and the giant cell tumor. Oral Surg Oral Med Oral Pathol 1988;66(2): 197–208.

114. El-Mofty SK, Osdoby P. Growth behavior and lineage of isolated and cultured cells derived from giant cell granuloma of the mandible. J Oral Pathol 1985;14(7):539–52.

115. Waldron CA, Shafer WG. The central giant cell reparative granuloma of the jaws. An analysis of 38 cases. Am J Clin Pathol 1966;45(4):437–47.

116. Ficarra G, Kaban LB, Hansen LS. Central giant cell lesions of the mandible and maxilla: a clinicopathologic and cytometric study. Oral Surg Oral Med Oral Pathol 1987;64(1):44–9.

117. Whitaker SB, Waldron CA. Central giant cell lesions of the jaws. A clinical, radiologic, and histopathologic study. Oral Surg Oral Med Oral Pathol 1993; 75(2):199–208.

118. Chuong R, Kaban LB, Kozakewich H, et al. Central giant cell lesions of the jaws: a clinicopathologic study. J Oral Maxillofac Surg 1986;44(9): 708–13.

119. Stolovitzky JP, Waldron CA, McConnel FM. Giant cell lesions of the maxilla and paranasal sinuses. Head Neck 1994;16(2):143–8.

120. Bertoni F, Unni KK, Beabout JW, et al. Giant cell tumor of the skull. Cancer 1992;70(5):1124–32.

121. Leonard J, Gokden M, Kyriakos M, et al. Malignant giant-cell tumor of the parietal bone: case report and review of the literature. Neurosurgery 2001; 48(2):424–9.

122. Kyriakos M, Hardy D. Malignant transformation of aneurysmal bone cyst, with an analysis of the literature. Cancer 1991;68(8):1770–80.

123. Morton KS. Aneurysmal bone cyst: a review of 26 cases. Can J Surg 1986;29(2):110–5.

124. Mankin HJ, Hornicek FJ, Ortiz-Cruz E, et al. Aneurysmal bone cyst: a review of 150 patients. J Clin Oncol 2005;23(27):6756–62.

125. Vergel De Dios AM, Bond JR, Shives TC, et al. Aneurysmal bone cyst. A clinicopathologic study of 238 cases. Cancer 1992;69(12):2921–31.

126. Gingell JC, Levy BA, Beckerman T, et al. Aneurysmal bone cyst. J Oral Maxillofac Surg 1984;42(8):527–34.

127. Kershisnik M, Batsakis JG. Aneurysmal bone cysts of the jaws. Ann Otol Rhinol Laryngol 1994;103(2):164–5.

128. Martinez V, Sissons HA. Aneurysmal bone cyst. A review of 123 cases including primary lesions and those secondary to other bone pathology. Cancer 1988;61(11):2291–304.

129. Svensson B, Isacsson G. Benign osteoblastoma associated with an aneurysmal bone cyst of the mandibular ramus and condyle. Oral Surg Oral Med Oral Pathol 1993;76(4):433–6.

130. Citardi MJ, Janjua T, Abrahams JJ, et al. Orbitoethmoid aneurysmal bone cyst. Otolaryngol Head Neck Surg 1996;114(3):466–70.

131. Toljanic JA, Lechewski E, Huvos AG, et al. Aneurysmal bone cysts of the jaws: a case study and review of the literature. Oral Surg Oral Med Oral Pathol 1987;64(1):72–7.

132. Trent C, Byl FM. Aneurysmal bone cyst of the mandible. Ann Otol Rhinol Laryngol 1993;102(12):917–24.

133. Dahlin D, Unni KK. Bone tumors, general aspects and data on 8,542 cases. 4th edition. Springfield (IL): Charles C. Thomas; 1986.

134. Biesecker JL, Marcove RC, Huvos AG, et al. Aneurysmal bone cysts. A clinicopathologic study of 66 cases. Cancer 1970;26(3):615–25.

135. Ruiter DJ, van Rijssel TG, van der Velde EA. Aneurysmal bone cysts: a clinicopathological study of 105 cases. Cancer 1977;39(5):2231–9.

136. Tillman BP, Dahlin DC, Lipscomb PR, et al. Aneurysmal bone cyst: an analysis of ninety-five cases. Mayo Clin Proc 1968;43(7):478–95.

137. Arnott DG. Cherubism—an initial unilateral presentation. Br J Oral Surg 1978;16(1):38–46.

138. Ayoub AF, el-Mofty SS. Cherubism: report of an aggressive case and review of the literature. J Oral Maxillofac Surg 1993;51(6):702–5.

139. Wayman JB. Cherubism: a report on three cases. Br J Oral Surg 1978;16(1):47–56.

140. Kaugars GE, Niamtu J 3rd, Svirsky JA. Cherubism: diagnosis, treatment, and comparison with central giant cell granulomas and giant cell tumors. Oral Surg Oral Med Oral Pathol 1992;73(3):369–74.

141. Koury ME, Stella JP, Epker BN. Vascular transformation in cherubism. Oral Surg Oral Med Oral Pathol 1993;76(1):20–7.

142. Peters WJ. Cherubism: a study of twenty cases from one family. Oral Surg Oral Med Oral Pathol 1979;47(4):307–11.

143. Hamner JE 3rd, Ketcham AS. Cherubism: an analysis of treatment. Cancer 1969;23(5):1133–43.

144. Addante RR, Breen GH. Cherubism in a patient with Noonan's syndrome. J Oral Maxillofac Surg 1996;54(2):210–3.

145. Betts NJ, Stewart JC, Fonseca RJ, et al. Multiple central giant cell lesions with a Noonan-like phenotype. Oral Surg Oral Med Oral Pathol 1993;76(5):601–7.

146. Dunlap C, Neville B, Vickers RA, et al. The Noonan syndrome/cherubism association. Oral Surg Oral Med Oral Pathol 1989;67(6):698–705.

Index

Note: Page numbers of article titles are in **boldface** type.

Surgical Pathology 4 (2011) 1329–1336
doi:10.1016/S1875-9181(11)00256-X
1875-9181/11/$ – see front matter © 2011 Elsevier Inc. All rights reserved.

United States Postal Service

Statement of Ownership, Management, and Circulation
(All Periodicals Publications Except Requestor Publications)

1. Publication Title	2. Publication Number									3. Filing Date
Surgical Pathology Clinics	0	2	5	-	4	7	8			9/16/11

4. Issue Frequency	5. Number of Issues Published Annually	6. Annual Subscription Price
Mar, Jun, Sep, Dec	4	$170.00

7. Complete Mailing Address of Known Office of Publication (Not printer) (Street, city, county, state, and ZIP+4®)

Elsevier Inc.
360 Park Avenue South
New York, NY 10010-1710

Contact Person
Amy S. Beacham

Telephone (Include area code)
215-239-3687

8. Complete Mailing Address of Headquarters or General Business Office of Publisher (Not printer)

Elsevier Inc., 360 Park Avenue South, New York, NY 10010-1710

9. Full Names and Complete Mailing Addresses of Publisher, Editor, and Managing Editor (Do not leave blank)

Publisher (Name and complete mailing address)

Kim Murphy, Elsevier, Inc., 1600 John F. Kennedy Blvd. Suite 1800, Philadelphia, PA 19103-2899

Editor (Name and complete mailing address)

Joanne Husovski, Elsevier, Inc., 1600 John F. Kennedy Blvd. Suite 1800, Philadelphia, PA 19103-2899

Managing Editor (Name and complete mailing address)

Barton Dudlick, Elsevier, Inc., 1600 John F. Kennedy Blvd. Suite 1800, Philadelphia, PA 19103-2899

10. Owner (Do not leave blank. If the publication is owned by a corporation, give the name and address of the corporation immediately followed by the names and addresses of all stockholders owning or holding 1 percent or more of the total amount of stock. If not owned by a corporation, give the names and addresses of the individual owners. If owned by a partnership or other unincorporated firm, give its name and address as well as those of each individual owner. If the publication is published by a nonprofit organization, give its name and address.)

Full Name	Complete Mailing Address
Wholly owned subsidiary of	4520 East-West Highway
Reed/Elsevier, US holdings	Bethesda, MD 20814

11. Known Bondholders, Mortgagees, and Other Security Holders Owning or Holding 1 Percent or More of Total Amount of Bonds, Mortgages, or Other Securities. If none, check box ☑ None

Full Name	Complete Mailing Address
N/A	

12. Tax Status (For completion by nonprofit organizations authorized to mail at nonprofit rates) (Check one)
The purpose, function, and nonprofit status of this organization and the exempt status for federal income tax purposes:
☐ Has Not Changed During Preceding 12 Months
☐ Has Changed During Preceding 12 Months (Publisher must submit explanation of change with this statement)

PS Form 3526, September 2007 (Page 1 of 3 (Instructions Page 3)) PSN 7530-01-000-9931 PRIVACY NOTICE: See our Privacy policy in www.usps.com

---

13. Publication Title				14. Issue Date for Circulation Data Below
Surgical Pathology Clinics				June 2011

15. Extent and Nature of Circulation			Average No. Copies Each Issue During Preceding 12 Months	No. Copies of Single Issue Published Nearest to Filing Date
a. Total Number of Copies (Net press run)			1270	1216
b. Paid Circulation (By Mail and Outside the Mail)	(1)	Mailed Outside-County Paid Subscriptions Stated on PS Form 3541. (Include paid distribution above nominal rate, advertiser's proof copies, and exchange copies)	538	519
	(2)	Mailed In-County Paid Subscriptions Stated on PS Form 3541 (Include paid distribution above nominal rate, advertiser's proof copies, and exchange copies)		
	(3)	Paid Distribution Outside the Mails Including Sales Through Dealers and Carriers, Street Vendors, Counter Sales, and Other Paid Distribution Outside USPS®	41	33
	(4)	Paid Distribution by Other Classes Mailed Through the USPS (e.g. First-Class Mail®)		
c. Total Paid Distribution (Sum of 15b (1), (2), (3), and (4))		▶	579	552
d. Free or Nominal Rate Distribution (By Mail and Outside the Mail)	(1)	Free or Nominal Rate Outside-County Copies Included on PS Form 3541	48	42
	(2)	Free or Nominal Rate In-County Copies Included on PS Form 3541		
	(3)	Free or Nominal Rate Copies Mailed at Other Classes Through the USPS (e.g. First-Class Mail)		
	(4)	Free or Nominal Rate Distribution Outside the Mail (Carriers or other means)		
e. Total Free or Nominal Rate Distribution (Sum of 15d (1), (2), (3) and (4))		▶	48	42
f. Total Distribution (Sum of 15c and 15e)		▶	627	594
g. Copies not Distributed (See instructions to publishers #4 (page #3))		▶	643	622
h. Total (Sum of 15f and g)		▶	1270	1216
i. Percent Paid (15c divided by 15f times 100)			92.34%	92.93%

16. Publication of Statement of Ownership
☐ If the publication is a general publication, publication of this statement is required. Will be printed in the December 2011 issue of this publication.   ☐ Publication not required

17. Signature and Title of Editor, Publisher, Business Manager, or Owner

Amy S. Beacham — Senior Inventory Distribution Coordinator   Date: September 16, 2011

I certify that all information furnished on this form is true and complete. I understand that anyone who furnishes false or misleading information on this form or who omits material or information requested on the form may be subject to criminal sanctions (including fines and imprisonment) and/or civil sanctions (including civil penalties).

PS Form 3526, September 2007 (Page 2 of 3)

Moving?

Make sure your subscription moves with you!

To notify us of your new address, find your **Clinics Account Number** (located on your mailing label above your name), and contact customer service at:

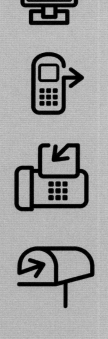

Email: journalscustomerservice-usa@elsevier.com

800-654-2452 (subscribers in the U.S. & Canada)
314-447-8871 (subscribers outside of the U.S. & Canada)

Fax number: 314-447-8029

Elsevier Health Sciences Division
Subscription Customer Service
3251 Riverport Lane
Maryland Heights, MO 63043

*To ensure uninterrupted delivery of your subscription, please notify us at least 4 weeks in advance of move.

ELSEVIER